Zinc:
Clinical and Biochemical Significance

Author

Stephen C. Cunnane, Ph.D.
Assistant Professor
Department of Nutritional Sciences
Faculty of Medicine
University of Toronto
Toronto, Canada

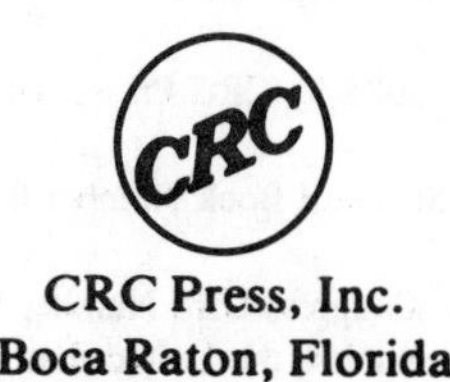

CRC Press, Inc.
Boca Raton, Florida

Library of Congress Cataloging-in-Publication Data

Cunnane, Stephen C.
Zinc: clinical and biochemical significance.

Bibliography: p.
Includes index.
1. Zinc in the body. 2. Zinc — Metabolism.
3. Zinc deficiency diseases. I. Title. [DNLM: 1. Zinc
— deficiency. 2. Zinc — metabolism. QV 298 C973z]
QP535.Z6C86 1988 616.3'96 87-35523
ISBN 0-8493-6735-2

This book represents information obtained from authentic and highly regarded sources. Reprinted material is quoted with permission, and sources are indicated. A wide variety of references are listed. Every reasonable effort has been made to give reliable data and information, but the author and the publisher cannot assume responsibility for the validity of all materials or for the consequences of their use.

Direct all inquiries to CRC Press, Inc., 2000 Corporate Blvd., N.W., Boca Raton, Florida, 33431.

International Standard Book Number 0-8493-6735-2

Library of Congress Card Number 87-35523
Printed in the United States

FOREWORD

Several trace elements such as iron, copper, zinc, chromium, selenium, manganese, cobalt, iodine, and fluorine are known to be essential for human health; but only a few have clinical relevance. Deficiency of manganese in human subjects has not been established. Flourine, although important for dental health, is not essential for life.

The essentiality of iron for heme synthesis and iodine for thyroid metabolism has been recognized for over a century. Clinical deficiencies of chromium and selenium are not well established thus far, although their potentially useful role in clinical medicine has been realized. Deficiencies of zinc and copper in human subjects have been recognized only during the past two decades. Copper deficiency in human subjects appears to be uncommon.

As recently as 20 years ago, deficiency of zinc in human subjects was considered improbable. Today it is being recognized with greater frequency under a variety of clinical circumstances. During the past two decades, considerable progress has been made in the field of zinc metabolism. Three events led to these advances.

The first was the recognition of the many biochemical roles of zinc that were reported in the 1960s. The second was the development of accurate and simple methodology with the use of atomic absorption spectrophotometry in the early 1960s, which made it simple to assess the status of zinc in human subjects. The third, and most important, event was the documentation that zinc deficiency in human subjects could occur under the most practical dietary conditions. Indeed, nutritional deficiency of zinc has been reported today in many developing countries; and, perhaps, it may turn out to be a world health problem second only to iron deficiency.

Zinc is known to regulate the activity of almost 200 enzymes. It is needed for DNA synthesis and is required at each step of the cell cycle. Zinc is involved in the gene amplification of at least one small molecular weight protein, metallothionein. The zinc-dependent nature of certain hormones, such as thymulin, testosterone, prolactin, and possibly somatomedin, is a truly fascinating area for further research.

Perhaps the most impressive and promising development in the zinc field in recent years has been the recognition that zinc may have an important role in immune functions. The influence of zinc on thymic-dependent lymphocytes (T cells) is now well documented. The implications of this finding extend to other areas as well, such as the development of malignancies in the elderly, inasmuch as T-natural killer cells appear to be zinc dependent.

Recently, the use of zinc as a therapeutic agent has emerged. Zinc may act as an antisickling agent and play a role in the prevention of pain crisis in sickle-cell disease. Zinc has been utilized to decrease the copper burden of patients with Wilson's disease. It is, therefore, very obvious that investigations of many aspects of zinc metabolism in humans will continue for a period of time in the foreseeable future.

Dr. Stephen Cunnane has undertaken the formidable task of putting the current knowledge about zinc together in this book. In my opinion, he has done an admirable job. This book should prove very valuable to everyone interested in the field of zinc metabolism.

Ananda S. Prasad, M.D., Ph.D.
Wayne State University
School of Medicine
Detroit, Michigan

PREFACE

When first approached about writing this book in 1984, my first reaction was to do it because I felt that in spite of many excellent reviews, the secondary zinc literature was very patchy, with much of the primary literature never reviewed. My second reaction, which followed rapidly on the first, was not to try to do it because it was going to be almost impossible. Evidently, the first reaction prevailed, but the reality of the situation made it quite a challenge.

I have been involved with research on zinc since 1977 and have always felt the need for a more comprehensive reference source. This book is an attempt to provide such a source. My priorities were that the book be comprehensive and up-to-date, features which are almost contradictory in a book about a heavily researched topic such as zinc. I also felt that approaching the clinical aspects of the subject from an etiological standpoint — zinc deficiency, depletion, therapy, and toxicity — would be more refreshing and perhaps more revealing than the standard organ-by-organ or disease-by-disease method. Both systems have their advantages and disadvantages. The idea of discussing secondary zinc depletion as an entity is to be able to describe together conditions that have this abnormality in common. Thus, it is intended to emphasize the *common* aspects of diseases as they relate to zinc, rather than their differences. This will hopefully influence therapeutic strategy.

In keeping with the etiology theme, it also became apparent that the clinical aspects needed to be strictly separated from the animal aspects of zinc metabolism, a separation that has never previously been attempted. Although this division, like the separation of primary from secondary zinc depletion, may be somewhat arbitrary, it is my impression that current knowledge of the truly clinical aspects of zinc metabolism is too often confused with its effects in animals. The two will frequently be similar, but not always. In this book, therefore, animal studies are considered in Part II (Biochemistry). Only a handful of references to animal studies has been included in Part I (Clinical). The purpose of this separation is to clearly distinguish animal from human, experimental from clinical. Too many of the animal studies have involved severe and prolonged zinc deficiency or other exaggerated nutritional conditions that cannot be realistically applied in the clinical setting. Furthermore, animal studies are mainly of primary (dietary) zinc depletion, whereas in humans, secondary zinc depletion is more prevalent and has a more diverse etiology.

Another unique feature is that the book contains a comprehensive summary of the interaction of zinc with lipids, essential fatty acids, and prostaglandins and membranes, something that has been conspicuously lacking previously. Clinical aspects of this interaction, including its usefulness in assessing zinc status and descriptions of clinical conditions in which the interaction is well founded are included. A list of general reading (short bibliography) follows the list of referenced citations at the end of the book.

Stephen Cunnane
July 1, 1987
Toronto

THE AUTHOR

Stephen C. Cunnane, Ph.D., is Assistant Professor of Nutritional Sciences in the Faculty of Medicine at the University of Toronto, Toronto, Canada.

Dr. Cunnane received his B.S. from Bishop's University, Lennoxville, Quebec in 1975. After completing a Ph.D. in Physiology at McGill University, Montréal, Québec in 1980, he was awarded a postdoctoral fellowship by the Lalor Foundation (Wilmington, Del.), which was spent at the Rowett Research Institute (Aberdeen, Scotland) and at the Institute of Zoology (London, England) during 1980 to 1982. After spending four years as an Industrial Fellow of the National Science and Engineering Research Council at the Efamol Research Institute in Kentville, Nova Scotia, he was appointed to his current position at the University of Toronto.

He is a Fellow of the American College of Nutrition and a member of the Nutrition Society (U.K.), Canadian Society for Nutritional Sciences, American Institute of Nutrition, Society for Experimental Biology and Medicine, and the International Society for Trace Element Research in Humans.

Dr. Cunnane has published over 70 research papers and his major research interest is in establishing the implications for human nutrition of the role of essential trace metals in lipid metabolism.

ACKNOWLEDGMENTS

I would like to acknowledge the encouragement of David Horrobin, who persuaded me to write this book. It has been a rewarding, challenging, and hopefully fruitful experience. Drs. Noel Solomons (Instituto de Nutricion de Centro América y Panamá [INCAP], Guatemala), Stephen Davies (East Grinstead, U.K.), Jim Smith, Jr. (Human Nutrition Research Center, Bethesda, Md.), Janet King and Leslie Wada (University of California, Department of Biochemistry, Berkeley), Joe Prohaska (University of Minnesota, Department of Biochemistry, Duluth), and Stan Zlotkin (Hospital for Sick Children, Toronto) have reviewed the manuscript at various stages as I wrote it. I owe them a great deal for their editing, suggestions, and considerable help. My colleagues, past and present, including Drs. Michel Bégin, Ronnie Hancock, Vic Huang, Trevor Kent, and Mehar Manku, have all shown considerable tolerance and encouragement, which has been very much appreciated. Christina Toplack completed the citations for numerous references and accessed many others, for which I am most grateful. Finally, I wish to thank my wife, Karen Stanworth, who made writing this book both possible and worthwhile.

TABLE OF CONTENTS

PART I — CLINICAL

PART II — BIOCHEMISTRY

INTRODUCTION

It has been 118 years since zinc was recognized as an element essential to the growth of the bread mold, *Aspergillis niger,*[1338] 73 years since it was demonstrated to be essential to plant growth,[1075] and 53 years since its essentiality for animals was proven.[1614] Comparatively recently, the essentiality of zinc for normal human growth and development was established.[1308,1309] In both plants and animals, zinc intake can be artificially manipulated to unequivocally establish its essentiality. In young animals, growth retardation and skin lesions occur shortly after the omission of zinc from the diet and are readily corrected by the addition of zinc. In humans, experiments in which adult volunteers have subsisted on zinc-deficient diets have only recently been conducted.[89,207,737,1316] Unequivocal evidence of the role of zinc in spermatogenesis was thereby established.[1316]

Prior to the realization that zinc was essential to humans, parenteral i.v. solutions were frequently used that contained no added zinc. Accidental zinc deficiency resulted, characterized principally by growth retardation and dermal lesions, thereby confirming the essentiality of zinc from a different angle.[536,537,1602] Acrodermatitis enteropathica, (AE), a rare genetic disease in which zinc absorption is impaired, is completely corrected by zinc supplementation.[103] Thus, evidence from conditions of specific zinc depletion has corroborated the earlier studies in which zinc depletion, albeit complicated by protein-energy malnutrition, was demonstrated in the Middle East.[1308]

However, recognizing conditions in which an ''induced'' or secondary zinc depletion exists, as opposed to dietary deficiency, is a greater problem. The more obvious causes of zinc depletion are currently well-understood, e.g., zinc malabsorption in AE, increased zinc excretion caused by certain drugs and alcohol, and increased zinc requirement in chronic infection or burn patients. Whether pregnant women, slow-growing children, or the aged constitute populations at risk of zinc depletion is much more difficult to determine.

Two main hurdles exist that have made it difficult to appreciate the extent to which zinc depletion may exist in apparently well-nourished populations: (1) inadequate means of assessment of zinc status and (2) insufficient understanding of the diversity of the metabolic role of zinc, especially in relation to other nutrients. Progress on the assessment of zinc status was initially impeded by inaccurate zinc measurement, which allowed spurious and conflicting results to be published. Having largely solved the problem of standardizing the methodology of zinc measurement, the problem that has emerged is one of knowing in which tissues to measure zinc and how best to recognize differences in zinc levels that are indicative of altered zinc status.

Of the readily biopsied tissues/cells (hair, skin, erythrocytes, leukocytes, and platelets) and fluids (blood plasma/serum or urine), blood plasma has been most widely used to measure zinc status. It is now appreciated that plasma proteins that transport zinc, especially albumin, also fluctuate in disease. Thus, without measurement of the plasma transport proteins, zinc analysis of plasma is of limited value, except in the severest (and rarest) causes of zinc depletion. Assessment of zinc status by other methods, including its measurement in nucleated cells, e.g., leukocytes, and use of short-lived radionuclides and functional tests, including the zinc-tolerance test, dark adaptation, and taste-smell tests, offer considerable promise. These tests are restricted by confounding influences, e.g., drug treatments and excesses or deficiencies of other nutrients. Their usefulness is as a secondary test done in conjunction with direct measurement of zinc in appropriate tissues. The ultimate indicator of zinc nutriture is still the clinical evaluation of an individual's response to zinc supplementation. In spite of a diagnosis based on biochemical assessment, the clinical response to zinc is the only realistic indicator of preexisting zinc deficiency or depletion. In view of the negligible toxicity of zinc when used in moderate amounts, clinical response to zinc supplementation is a safe and effective test.

Assessment of zinc status is also impeded by lack of understanding of the relationship of zinc to other nutrients, in other words, lack of understanding of the function of zinc beyond its biochemical function in enzymes and protein synthesis. It is well recognized that zinc is a component of many enzymes. Research on the function of zinc has centered around this role. In most cases, the activity of zinc metalloenzymes is retained, even in conditions of severe zinc depletion. Death through inanition or infection usually occurs before the activity of the enzyme is reduced. Thus, activity of enzymes such as alkaline phosphatase and carbonic anhydrase infrequently mirrors zinc status. Exploitation of other indexes of zinc status, including functional tests, and appreciation of the role of zinc in relation to other nutrients may be more fruitful in eventually defining truer indexes of zinc status, as well as understanding the important metabolic functions of zinc.

The function of zinc in relation to other nutrients has been alluded to since the essentiality of zinc in animals was established in 1934. Aside from its role in protein and nucleic acid synthesis, an interaction of zinc has been established experimentally with vitamins A, E, B_6, folic acid, with other metals, including copper, cadmium, iron, calcium, and selenium, and with the essential fatty acids (EFAs). Interactions with lipoproteins, phospholipids, cholesterol, insulin, and steroids have yielded provocative results concerning the effect of zinc not directly related to protein synthesis or specific metalloenzymes. Ionic zinc also influences membrane function and membrane receptors. In the future, diagnosis of zinc depletion may be made by measurement of a nutrient or metabolite of a nutrient not currently known to be affected by changes in zinc status.

Part I — Clinical

Chapter 1

HISTORICAL

I. CLINICAL

The first definitive demonstration of clinical zinc deficiency was in the early 1960s in Iranian adolescent dwarfs.[1308,1309] The dwarfism was a consequence of protein-energy malnutrition, anemia, and zinc deficiency. Although increased growth and sexual maturation was observed in dwarfs fed a nutritionally adequate diet without zinc supplementation, zinc supplementation consistently shortened the period of time required to develop sexual maturity and improve growth.[672] It was these studies of the effects of zinc supplementation which finally demonstrated that zinc deficiency could and did exist in humans.

For the purpose of providing a background to clinical zinc studies, the period prior to 1961 will be considered as historical. The rest of the chapter is an outline of studies on zinc, both animal and human, which were carried out prior to 1961. By separating the period prior to 1961, one can see that the wide range of the biochemical importance of zinc was largely established during that period. Since 1961, we have refined, but not significantly extended, our understanding of zinc biochemistry. What certainly has been achieved is the establishment of zinc as a nutrient of critical clinical importance whose homeostasis is very finely regulated.

The use of zinc in such preparations as calamine (contains zinc oxide) and zinc ointment for skin irritations, abrasions, and burns, has been documented since pre-Christian times, e.g., in the Ebers papyrus.[439] Oral zinc salts (zinc oxide and sulfate) have been given since the 18th century for the treatment of epilepsy[765] and convulsive disorders.[1355] One of the earliest reports of the clinical use of zinc as a medication was by Graham.[629] who described the use of zinc sulfate pills prepared with turpentine. These pills were fed orally to cure gleet and leukorrhea, conditions of vaginal infection. The biochemical effects of zinc oxide against staphylococci and streptococci were reported by Haxthausen[702] who also observed that the acid conditions produced by the bacteria enhanced the bactericidal effects of zinc oxide. Eggleton[451] noted that zinc levels in hair, skin, and nails of Chinese patients with beriberi were 50% of those of healthy controls and suggested that coexisting zinc deficiency might exacerbate beriberi.

Zinc was also shown to complex with uroporphyrin, the excretion of which is increased in idiopathic porphyria.[1684] The etiology of porphyria was later hypothesized to be zinc-related. Zinc chelating agents, e.g., 2,3-dimercaptopropanol and ethylenediaminetetraacetic acid (EDTA), were successfully used to treat porphyria.[1270,1271]

Vallee and Gibson[1637] studied zinc levels in various anemias. With the exception of pernicious anemia in which erythrocyte zinc was found to be increased, anemia was not associated with a change in blood zinc. Treatment of pernicious anemia with liver extracts caused a decline in erythrocyte zinc, an effect suggested to be due to an increase in the rate of erythrocyte death.

A paper frequently quoted is that by Vikbladh[1657] on the analysis of zinc in human blood plasma, erythrocytes, and leukocytes. Vikbladh showed that about a third of plasma zinc transport proteins bound zinc tightly and two thirds bound it loosely. Transferrin was suggested as a possible zinc transport protein. Diurnal rhythms in plasma zinc were observed, as was the decrease in plasma zinc during pregnancy and increase in the newborn. Plasma zinc was also shown to decrease during acute infection, an effect that correlated well with the increase in body temperature. Vikbladh made the comment that zinc was "indispensable" for mammals, but its lack, however, causes no specific pathological syndrome (in humans).[1657]

Vallee and Altschule[1636] published an excellent and detailed review on zinc. They made particular reference to effects of zinc toxicity, e.g., leukocytosis and anemia. The elevation of blood zinc in pernicious anemia was also noted. Vallee has published further reviews on zinc,[1634,1635] with extensive discussion of enzymes and zinc deficiency effects on plants.

The sharp decrease in serum levels of zinc concomitant with increased levels of malic and lactic dehydrogenase were suggested by Wacker et al.[1665] to be a reliable indicator of the occurrence of a myocardial infarction. Shortly after, Vallee's group also demonstrated that serum zinc was decreased and urinary zinc excretion was increased in alcoholic cirrhosis.[1640] In this context, zinc was noted to be required for ethanol metabolism to acetaldehyde.

Zinc was implicated in the epidemiology of cancer by Stocks and Davies.[1561] They found that both zinc and cobalt in the soil were positively correlated with the incidence of stomach cancer. Two tumor cell types, spindle cell sarcoma and mammary adenocarcinoma, when transplanted into mice, were shown to more rapidly take up zinc-65 than the normal surrounding tissue.[703]

II. ZINC MEASUREMENT

Prior to the application of atomic absorption spectrophotometry to trace element analysis in 1955, zinc analysis was done mainly by colorimetric methods using agents such as dithizone (diphenylthiocarbazone) or its analogs. Most of the methods used in the studies described below will have used the colorimetric method.

Birckner[145] demonstrated that human milk and cow's milk contained zinc. Zinc was reported by Bertrand and Vladesco[134] to be present in the prostate of men, bulls, and pigs. The zinc content of the human body was calculated by Lutz[1030] to be about 2 g, a figure still quoted today. In human semen the majority of zinc was shown to be of prostatic origin.[1072]

Incorporation of zinc-65 into tissues of the mouse and dog was studied by Sheline et al.[1460] They demonstrated that, after an oral dose, zinc-65 disappeared from the plasma within 10 hr. Uptake was continuous into the erythrocyte and liver with significant amounts also appearing in the pancreatic acinar cell.[1143] Excretion was mainly via the feces. Similar studies by McCance and Widdowson[1080] using unlabeled zinc, corroborated these results. From zinc analysis of average diets, they suggested that a normal intake of zinc would be in the region of 10 to 15 mg/day. Spray and Widdowson[1542] reported on the effect of maturation on tissue zinc levels in mammals. They observed that total body zinc (per gram of body weight) did not change significantly from birth to 300 days.

Feaster et al.[501] reported on the placental transfer of zinc-65 in the rat. They noted that ^{65}Zn was readily transferred across the placenta with peak amounts being transferred at 20 days gestation (near term). Similar results were reported for the rabbit intravenously infused with zinc-65.[1606] Maternal milk was also shown to be a major route of zinc transfer to the neonate.[1606] Zinc was also found in the *Tapetum lucidum* in the eye of the dog and fox.[1703] The zinc in acetone-dried extracts of *T. lucidum* amounted to 10 to 20% by weight and was found in a 1:1 ratio with cysteine.

III. ZINC DEFICIENCY IN ANIMALS

Todd et al.[1614] were the first to clearly demonstrate that the rat could be fed a diet deficient only in zinc. Growth retardation and alopecia were observed and both were corrected by zinc supplementation.[1560] Hart's group also demonstrated that zinc deficiency in the rat affected the glucose and alanine tolerance tests and enhanced fecal excretion of nitrogen.[783] At the same time, Bertrand and Bhattacherjee[133] established the essentiality of zinc to the mouse. Both groups recognized that inanition was a consequence of prolonged severe zinc deficiency.

Elcoate et al.[454] reported that the submaxillary gland was significantly increased in size and that it contained no secretory granules in rats fed a diet containing zinc at 0.5 mg/kg (virtually zinc free). These data suggested that impaired salivation may have contributed to reduced food intake in zinc deficiency.

Hove et al.,[784] postulated that since zinc deficiency did not result in lower zinc levels in soft tissues of zinc-deficient rats than in controls, a critical minimum zinc concentration was maintained by each organ at the expense of growth and proliferation of new tissue. The features of zinc-deficient rats were extended by Follis et al.[546] to include esophageal parakeratosis, hyperpigmentation of the skin, rapid loss of subcutaneous fat, and leukocyte infiltration of the cornea.

Zinc deficiency in the pig was first demonstrated in 1955 and was shown to be one of the main factors contributing to parakeratosis.[1623] O'Dell and Savage[1212] first proposed the essentiality of zinc to the chick. Their observations were confirmed by Lease et al.[980] who reported zinc deficiency in chicks fed 52 mg/kg zinc in a diet based on sesame meal. The deficiency symptoms were reversible with zinc supplementation or with addition of EDTA to the diet. Subsequently, it was reported that eggs of zinc-deficient hens had lower hatchability and gross embryonic abnormalities and that chicks hatched from zinc-deficient hens were weaker than controls.[150]

IV. ZINC TOXICITY

Excess dietary zinc was demonstrated to adversely affect the outcome of pregnancy in the rat.[1586] At 5 to 10 g/kg in the diet, zinc caused stillbirths, fetal growth retardation, and decreased maternal hematocrit. Sadasivan[1384-1386] conducted in-depth studies of zinc toxicity. It was noted that zinc excess and deficiency had similar characteristics in the rat, e.g., less body fat, growth retardation, and increased fecal nitrogen excretion. The effects of zinc excess were also dependent on the level of fat in the diet. With 30% fat in the diet, effects of 5 g/kg dietary zinc were similar to those of 10 g/kg zinc and 10% fat in the diet, suggesting a possible exacerbation of the effects of zinc toxicity by higher dietary fat.

V. METALLOENZYMES

The long and illustrious history of zinc as a metalloenzyme began with the reports by Keilin and Mann[889] that zinc was a structural component of erythrocyte carbonic anhydrase. The zinc was later shown to be bound in a 1:1 ratio with the cysteine residues of carbonic anhydrase.[1358] As has been subsequently shown for most zinc metalloenzymes, carbonic anhydrase in erythrocytes did not take up ^{65}Zn, even though the erythrocyte rapidly incorporated zinc-65.[1625] In view of the increased excretion of nitrogen and increased plasma levels of uric acid in zinc deficiency, liver uricase levels were analyzed but no differences with controls were observed.[1634,1663] NAD-dependent oxidative phosphorylation was shown to be inhibited by zinc.[807] Pyridoxal kinase was reported to be activated by zinc at a lower concentration than by magnesium.[1090,1091] The effect of zinc was biphasic; $<0.1\ M$ was stimulatory, but $> 0.1\ M$ was inhibitory.[1090]

VI. REPRODUCTION

An early indication of the interaction of zinc with steroids was the study by Bischoff[146] in which copper was shown to augment the in vitro growth-promoting effect of pituitary gonadotrophic extracts on the ovary in incubations at acid pH, whereas at alkaline pH, zinc was stimulatory. In the horse, zinc was shown to reduce the stimulatory effect of gonadotrophin on the ovary, but to have no effect on the testes.[981] The relationship between zinc and taste acuity was reported by Allara[39] who showed that in rats the decrease in taste acuity caused by castration was preventable by zinc.

Both corticotrophin[920] and adrenocorticotrophic hormone (ACTH) extracts were reported to contain about 200 μg/g zinc. Sperm were reported by Mawson and Fisher[1072] to contain very high amounts of zinc. Zinc has been shown to prolong the activity of ACTH in hypophysectomized rats.[762] In the presence of testosterone, gonadotrophin caused zinc accumulation in the prostate.[1124] Castration decreased the prostatic uptake of zinc, an effect prevented by treatment with testosterone.

Fujii et al.[575] observed that the rapid increase in motility of sea urchin sperm occurred on contact with seawater. This occurred only in the presence of histidine, an effect related to a decrease in the zinc concentration of the sperm. It was concluded that zinc probably inhibited the respiration and motility of the sperm, an effect blocked after chelation of the zinc by histidine.

VII. MUSCLE CONTRACTION

Zinc has been shown to influence the contraction of striated muscle fiber bundles; at 1 μ*M*, contraction was increased, whereas at 10 μ*M*, zinc caused relaxation.[448] The inhibition of contraction was suggested to be due to sulfhydryl groups binding to the zinc, thereby inhibiting its contractile effect.[449,450] Issacson and Sandow[832] noted that stimulation of the twitch of the sartorious muscle of the frog by acridine orange was potentiated by 1 m*M* zinc chloride. However, zinc delayed the onset of tetanus.

VIII. SUBCELLULAR LOCALIZATION

The initial observation by Harrison[696] that zinc was located in the cytoplasm of the liver cell was further investigated by Thiers and Vallee.[1607a] They reported that the percentage distribution of zinc in the liver cell was: 43% supernatent (cytoplasm), 37% nucleus, 13% microsomes, 5% mitochondria, and 2% connective tissue. Carbon tetrachloride was shown to increase the microsomal and mitochondrial content of zinc. In sea urchin eggs, zinc distribution was altered in association with mitosis; at the onset of mitosis, the zinc shifted from the nucleolus to the chromosomes.[574]

IX. INTERACTION WITH OTHER DIETARY COMPONENTS

Zinc has been shown to interact with several other elements, including calcium, copper, and cadmium. In the young rapidly growing pig, zinc deficiency results in parakeratosis, a disorder characterized by scaly skin, dermatitis, and growth retardation. Excess dietary calcium[551,1027,1722] and cadmium[999] have been shown to contribute to parakeratosis by inhibition of zinc absorption. Cadmium was also shown to compete with zinc for clearance from the blood.[313] High zinc intake (0.5% by weight in the diet of rats) was shown to decrease the copper content of the liver, kidney, and blood in the rat by decreasing copper absorption.[663,1037] The decrease in erythrocyte hemoglobin and cytochrome c oxidase activity caused by zinc were shown to be reversible by copper.[421,1494]

Essential fatty acid deficiency has also been shown to cause parakeratosis. Essential fatty acids, in combination with zinc, are an effective treatment for parakeratosis.[691] O'Dell and Savage[1213] published one of the earliest reports demonstrating an inhibitory effect of phytate on zinc absorption. This was shown in a comparison of casein-based (phytate-free) compared to soybean-based (contains phytate) diets; the soybean diet caused a more rapid onset of the symptoms of zinc deficiency, an effect shown to be due to its content of phytate.

X. SUMMARY

The three decades preceding the definitive establishment of human zinc deficiency[1308,1309] were a very exciting period of zinc research. During that period, although methods of zinc analysis probably left something to be desired, most of the currently interesting areas of zinc research were opened up; both whole body and subcellular zinc levels were established, zinc-65 was in use, zinc metalloenzymes were identified, effects of zinc deficiency and toxicity in animals were documented, and some wide-ranging physiological effects of zinc were reported. Only an understanding of the clinical importance of zinc was lacking and information on that subject, as this book will attest, is accumulating rapidly.

Chapter 2

ASSESSMENT OF ZINC NUTRITURE

I. INTRODUCTION

Assessment of zinc nutriture or status is at a crossroads. Difficulties which plagued early studies were primarily of a technical nature. Measurements were compared between laboratories that used the dithizone colorimetric method and those that used atomic absorption spectrophotometry.[1123] In addition, some labs recognized and prevented sources of contamination, e.g., hemolysis and inadequately washed glassware and syringe plungers, and others did not.[688] Variations between results were not nearly as great for blood samples as for tissue samples. The latter require wet digestion or dry-ashing, whereas the former, being aqueous already, do not. Different methods of wet (acid) or dry (furnace) ashing can yield different results. Now, standard reference materials are available from the National Bureau of Standards, Washingon, D.C., for which zinc values are assigned by lot. These values are set after independent analyses by reputable laboratories using different methodologies. Thus, standardization of the methodology of sample preparation and analysis can largely eliminate the difficulty of two laboratories arriving at the same value for two aliquots of the same sample.

The problem has become one of establishing what to measure, under what conditions to measure it, and from this information, how to recognize altered zinc status (reviewed by Solomons[1499]). Zinc status is a measure of total *available* body zinc. Unexchangeable zinc, e.g., in metalloenzymes and most intracellular zinc, is not included in the measurement of total available zinc. Of the zinc which is measurable in extracellular sites, there is generally a poor correlation between zinc levels and clinical diagnosis.[1299]

II. ZINC ANALYSIS

Current tests of zinc nutriture involving direct zinc analysis are listed in Table 1.

A. Zinc in Body Fluids

The available body fluids, plasma or serum, milk, urine, saliva, and semen are of limited usefulness in the assessment of zinc status. Their zinc concentration is subject to changes induced by physiological variability — time of day, season, and degree of fasting.[383,740] Therefore, a change in the level of zinc in plasma may reflect a clinically significant change in zinc status, but it may also reflect a physiological change, e.g., during pregnancy or acute infection. Normal values for zinc in body fluids or humans and tissues of humans, rats, and pigs are given in Tables 17 and 18, Chapter 9.

1. Plasma

Serum zinc levels were originally suggested to be about 15% higher than plasma levels due to contamination from platelets and invisible hemolysis.[545] More recently, it has been demonstrated that this need not be the case.[935,1045] Over 95% of zinc in plasma is carried by either albumin of α_2-macroglobulin. The remainder is bound primarily to microligands including free cysteine, histidine, and histamine.[132,602,1310] Changes in the levels of the transport proteins cause changes in plasma zinc levels.[548,1238,1417] Albumin carries >65% of the protein-bound zinc[600] and its levels are more variable in response to disease than those of α_2-macroglobulin. The amount of zinc carried by α_2-macroglobulin has recently been reported to be only 5 to 6% of the total in plasma[902] compared to the 20 to 30% previously thought.[601]

Table 1
TESTS OF ZINC NUTRITURE UTILIZING DIRECT ZINC ANALYSIS

- Zinc in body fluids
  - Plasma
  - Urine
  - Semen
  - Saliva
  - Sweat
  - Ascites
  - Amniotic fluid
  - Milk
  - Cerebrospinal fluid
- Zinc in blood cells
  - Erythrocyte
  - Leukocyte
  - Platelet
- Hair
- Zinc tolerance test
- Zinc balance
- Zinc radionuclides

In healthy individuals, albumin-bound zinc is correlated with total serum zinc ($r = 0.91$), whereas α_2-macroglobulin-bound zinc does not correlate with total serum zinc or total α_2-macroglobulin.[601,1078] Thus, variations in total plasma zinc may be due to a number of factors, excluding any influence of altered zinc intake, utilization, or disease.

Zinc-free total parenteral nutrition is an example of a condition in which plasma albumin is significantly decreased and in which zinc deficiency readily occurs. Zinc supplementation reverses both the symptoms of the induced zinc deficiency and restores the plasma albumin to normal.[106] The question therefore arises as to whether the decreased plasma albumin is the cause of the low plasma zinc level or the effect of low zinc intake.

Since >65% of plasma zinc is transported by albumin and the albumin-bound zinc appears to accurately reflect total plasma zinc,[549] it is essential that serum or plasma albumin be measured at the time of plasma zinc measurement. This has recently been done and will probably lead to a better evaluation of the usefulness of plasma zinc measurements: in alcoholic cirrhosis[1418] and in hemodialysis[550] a decrease in the affinity of albumin for zinc has been reported. Measurement of albumin-bound as well as total plasma zinc therefore yields more meaningful information than plasma zinc alone.

It is also important that the interpretation of the analysis of serum zinc levels takes into account the circadian and seasonal rhythms which, in healthy individuals, can account for differences of as much as 40%.[334,1002,1055] Thus, if a diagnosis is to be based solely on plasma or serum zinc levels, multiple sampling is required at a standard time of day (preferably morning and while fasting).

2. *Urine*

Feces, rather than urine, are the primary route of zinc excretion. Only 400 to 600 μg/day of an average total zinc excretion of about 10 mg/day is via the urine.[1502] Whether this amount represents "overflow" or is metabolically excreted is not known.

In humans, urinary zinc levels have been shown to decrease rapidly and consistently in experimental[89] and clinical[1299] zinc depletion. The urinary excretion of zinc-65 in the first 24 hr period following its oral administration has been shown to be directly proportional to zinc absorption,[714] suggesting that the measurement of urinary zinc immediately after an oral dose of zinc might be a useful index of zinc status. However, this may only be applicable in conditions of zinc depletion in which intake or absorption are decreased.

In alcoholic liver disease, a condition of induced zinc deficiency, urinary zinc excretion is markedly elevated.[886] Catabolic states including starvation and anorexia also greatly increase zinc excretion, without necessarily influencing plasma zinc.[1537] In such a situation, zinc depletion may exist, but neither the plasma nor urine zinc levels necessarily reflect the altered zinc status. Hence, the cause of zinc depletion is critical to the evaluation of the usefulness of measuring changes in urinary zinc excretion.

3. Semen

The zinc content of human ejaculate is predominantly in semen.[567] Semen zinc levels may be diagnostic of infertility in men.[1446,1477,1546a] Low semen zinc has been shown to correlate with low sperm motility and a reduced percentage of active sperm, both of which are responsive to zinc supplementation.[1283] More recently, however, infertile men with low sperm counts have been shown to have low *serum* zinc but normal semen zinc.[1035] Sperm count also varied as did semen zinc in fertile but not infertile men. Whether semen zinc levels are indicative of zinc status is therefore still unknown.

4. Saliva

Salivary zinc levels reflect whole-body zinc status in zinc-deficient animals (sheep, monkeys, rats, and pigs) but in humans does not seem to correlate well with other parameters of zinc status. In patients with idiopathic hypogeusia, parotid zinc levels were shown to be only 20% of those in people with normal taste acuity.[718] In a metabolic study in which zinc intakes of 11.4 and 14.7 mg/day were compared, the lower zinc intake reduced zinc in saliva supernatant (free of cells) but not in whole saliva.[640] Zinc in whole saliva does not appear to correlate with hair or serum zinc. This appears largely due to wide diurnal variations in salivary zinc concentration.[1766]

5. Sweat

Sweat zinc levels vary with dietary zinc intake and may represent as much as 10% of total zinc losses.[1133] In malnourished zinc-deficient adolescents in the Middle East, zinc concentration in sweat was not different from controls.[1321] Sweat zinc levels do, however, increase after zinc supplementation.[388] The potential usefulness of this parameter would appear to be mainly as a research tool because of the cumbersome nature of measuring sweat zinc levels.

6. Ascites

Zinc levels have been measured in ascites and have been shown to correlate positively with the total protein levels of ascites.[210,373] The exchangeability of zinc from ascites is unknown. If it is unexchangeable, accumulation of ascites would be a potential source of zinc depletion.

7. Amniotic Fluid

Amniotic fluid zinc levels have been shown to rise gradually from values of 0.01 to 0.02 μg/mℓ to 0.05 to 0.25 μg/mℓ at 13 to 19 weeks and higher again after 34 weeks.[271,1391] Nonprotein-bound zinc is considerably higher in amniotic fluid than in plasma, but its diagnostic value has not been established.[154]

Less of an increase in amniotic fluid zinc levels at 34 weeks has been reported in pregnancies of high fetal risk.[426,500,964] Rosick et al.,[1374] in a study of 227 pregnancies, did not find that amniotic fluid zinc was indicative of pregnancy outcome. Laitinen et al.,[968,969] have distinguished between pregnancies involving normal fetal development (no correlation with amniotic fluid zinc) and those involving fetal malformations; in the latter, zinc and α-fetoprotein were directly correlated. In 80% of the abnormal cases, zinc was 2.5 times higher than the normal value. Evidently, further research is necessary to clear up these opposing findings and to determine the possible *prospective* value of zinc measurements in amniotic fluid.

8. Milk

Zinc levels in milk have been frequently measured but, to my knowledge, this information has not been used to assess zinc status in neonates or mothers. The content of zinc in the milk has been shown to be unresponsive to zinc supplementation of the mother.[503,943]

9. Cerebrospinal Fluid

Cerebrospinal fluid is not a readily accessible fluid for routine zinc measurements and has not been reported as reflecting zinc status.

B. Zinc In Blood Cells

1. Erythrocyte

The erythrocyte contains 10 to 14 μg of zinc per mℓ of packed cells.[1299] This represents 75 to 90% of total blood zinc. Zinc in the erythrocyte is primarily located in the cytosol as a component of the enzyme, carbonic anhydrase,[578,1220] and is not in equilibrium with extracellular zinc.[1637] Only very long-term zinc depletion is therefore likely to change erythrocyte zinc levels.

Erythrocyte zinc is generally rated as being of minimal value in assessing zinc nutriture. One limitation to the usefulness of erythrocyte zinc is its relatively slow response to changes in zinc status measured by other techniques.[1301] In some liver diseases, for example, plasma and leukocyte zinc levels have been shown to decrease, but the zinc of erythrocytes may remain unchanged.[886]

Another limitation is the lack of standardization of analytical techniques, which has contributed to irreproducibility of results.[1299,1559] Thus, results may be expressed as milligrams per gram, milligrams per milliliter, milligrams per 10^{10} cells, milligrams per gram of protein, and milligrams per gram of hemoglobin. Some of these methods of expressing zinc values may be more physiologically relevant than others. Until this is established, erythrocyte zinc should not be dismissed as a marker of zinc status.

Furthermore, in diseases such as chronic renal failure, in which zinc depletion is presumed to exist,[20] changes in erythrocyte zinc may be similar or opposite to those of plasma. This suggests that the mechanism controlling erythrocyte zinc levels is not necessarily linked to that affecting plasma zinc levels. In fact, there are genetic and age-related influences on the regulation of erythrocyte zinc; monozygotic twins have a higher positive correlation of erythrocyte zinc levels than do dizygotic twins, and parent-offspring erythrocyte zinc levels often have a good positive correlation.[378] From 1 month up to 10 to 12 years of age, erythrocyte zinc steadily increases, at which point adult values are usually observed.[829]

The observation that increased zinc levels in erythrocytes of patients with multiple sclerosis[410] are confined to the membrane and, within the membrane, to the lipid component[753,754] suggests that greater attention needs to be paid to the possible changes in zinc in membrane components of the erythrocyte rather than to zinc levels in the whole cell. In view of the increase in erythrocyte zinc in other conditions including bone metastases,[628] uremia,[116,1543] and Duchenne muscular dystrophy,[1454] the etiology of raised erythrocyte zinc is worth assessing. Conversely, zinc deficiency in rats is associated with decreased zinc in erythrocyte *membranes* but the difference is not detectable in whole erythrocytes.[135,143] Hence, the erythrocyte membrane may be of considerable value in diagnosing altered zinc homeostasis due to pathological changes; its use for the nutritional assessment of zinc is as yet unproven.

2. Leukocyte

Measurement of zinc levels in peripheral blood leukocytes was first described by Vallee and Gibson.[1637] Recently, the assessment of zinc status by measurement of zinc in total mixed leukocytes or in separated neutrophils has been widely applied[550,749,750,1721] and reviewed by Patrick and Dervish.[1246] The leukocyte may be a more reliable indicator of whole-body intracellular zinc than plasma, urinary, or erythrocyte zinc because leukocyte zinc is thought to be in equilibrium with plasma zinc.[866]

Leukocyte zinc has been measured in various clinical conditions and in human experimental zinc deficiency.[1305] A good correlation has been demonstrated between leukocyte zinc and skeletal muscle zinc in both healthy controls and patients with various liver diseases.[867] No correlation was observed between leukocyte zinc and liver zinc or plasma zinc.[867]

In primary biliary cirrhosis, alcoholic cirrhosis, and chronic active hepatitis, leukocyte zinc has been shown to be significantly decreased.[886,1633] In these liver diseases, leukocyte zinc values decreased in parallel with zinc in plasma but not in erythrocytes. Nevertheless, the clinical state of the patients and their leukocyte zinc levels were not in agreement. This suggests that although leukocyte zinc is representative of muscle zinc (the largest single zinc pool in the body), it may not be truly representative of whole-body zinc status in liver disease. Other clinical conditions in which leukocyte zinc has been measured include diabetes, arthritis and scleroderma,[1588] and uremia.[300]

Leukocyte zinc has also been measured during pregnancy. In comparison with women delivering normal term or appropriate-for-gestational-age preterm babies in which leukocyte zinc was normal, lower zinc was found in leukocytes of women delivering small-for-gestational-age babies.[1101,1471] The leukocyte zinc values correlated with muscle zinc values, but not plasma zinc. Zinc depletion in the cord-blood leukocytes has been observed in babies with intrauterine growth retardation.[1100] Again, there was no correlation with fetal or maternal plasma zinc.

A potential therefore exists for leukocyte zinc to be a useful measure of zinc nutriture. In the majority of studies, however, the total peripheral blood leukocyte population has been used. Some of the poor correlations with clinical state and with other measures of zinc status may have resulted from changes in the size of leukocyte subpopulations, e.g., the monocytosis of Crohn's disease. Separated lymphocytes or neutrophils may yield more accurate information. Zinc measurement based on DNA as a reference unit might also be useful in view of the possible changes in leukocyte water content due to changes in sodium transport which occur, for instance, in malnourished children.[1247]

3. Platelet

The platelet is largely unassessed as a marker for changes in zinc status. One study of plasma and blood cell zinc levels in arthritis and scleroderma found that platelets had the most significant decrease in zinc content of any blood cells. Blood cell zinc, however, did not correlate with disease duration.[1588]

4. Lymphocyte

Lymphocyte zinc levels in leukemic children have been reported to contain less zinc and higher copper and iron than those of age-matched controls.[228]

C. Hair

Evidence concerning the validity of hair zinc analysis has occasionally shown a good correlation between hair zinc levels and other measures of zinc status but, in general, there are too many variables influencing hair zinc values to make them of real usefulness.[409]

Like erythrocyte zinc, lower zinc levels in hair only reflect zinc depletion over long periods and tend to be less accurate in adults than in children.[1299] Hambidge and Walravens[684] have shown that, in comparison with adults, hair zinc levels are lower in infants, particularly those that are formula-fed. They also noted that lower plasma and hair zinc levels did not necessarily correlate with clinically detectable zinc depletion, although those infants with the lowest hair zinc (< 70 μg/g) also had the poorest growth. Similar results have been reported in Chinese[1748] and Canadian children.[1481]

Nor do hair and plasma zinc necessarily correlate with each other.[650,1077,1349,1662] Gentile et al.[587] have shown that hair zinc did not correlate with age, weight, or height in adults, but these variables all positively correlated with hair zinc in infants and adolescents (<20 years). Therefore, age is a determinant of the reliability of hair zinc analysis. Water hardness is also a factor; higher hair zinc values have been observed in areas of hard drinking water.[594] Gibson and deWolfe[595] did not find any correlation between birthweight, which is normally correlated with plasma zinc[1161] and hair zinc in neonates. Hair zinc has been reported to be lower in parents of children with achondroplasia, a condition characterized by hydrocephalus.[298]

In protein-energy malnutrition, hair growth is decreased. Bradfield and Hambidge[166] have therefore noted that it is possible to maintain normal hair zinc levels even though zinc deficiency may be evident clinically or by other means of assessment. Hence, in conditions of severe zinc depletion, Hambidge feels that zinc analysis of hair may also be of little value.[675] As with plasma zinc levels, hair zinc levels are variable according to the time of year,[539,1566] thus making it imperative that multiple sampling be carried out to verify initial results.

D. Nails

Toenail zinc concentration has been reported to bear no relation to hair, serum, or urinary zinc.[1092]

E. Placenta

Measurement of placental zinc content has been infrequently reported and has not been used to assess zinc nutriture. The usefulness of this measurement would, of course, be limited to facilitating a decision as to whether to supplement the newborn with zinc since the placental zinc measurement would only be made after birth. The measurement of placental zinc might be useful in situations in which physiological and clinical evidence suggests zinc supplementation of the mother could improve the outcome of a subsequent pregnancy, e.g., in preeclampsia.[963] Placentae from preeclamptic women have been shown to have significantly less zinc than controls,[196] but these women were not evaluated for other symptoms of inadequate zinc nutriture.

F. Teeth

I am aware of only one report of zinc analysis of teeth, that by Haavikko et al.,[656] who were screening for factors potentially predisposing to atherosclerosis in children. They used proton-induced X-ray emission spectrometry and demonstrated that zinc levels in enamel and dentine were on the order of 130 to 140 μg/g. Since this was done in children and deciduous teeth were analyzed, zinc analysis in teeth may have potential for assessment of childhood zinc status over long periods.

G. Zinc Tolerance Test

The zinc tolerance test is analogous to the glucose tolerance test and is a term used to describe the procedure of giving an oral dose of zinc and monitoring its concentration in the blood over a period of up to 6 hr. The dose usually used is within the range 5 to 50 mg of elemental zinc. In apparently normal humans who have been fasting, the change in plasma zinc is qualitatively similar regardless of the dose within the above-noted range. The blood-

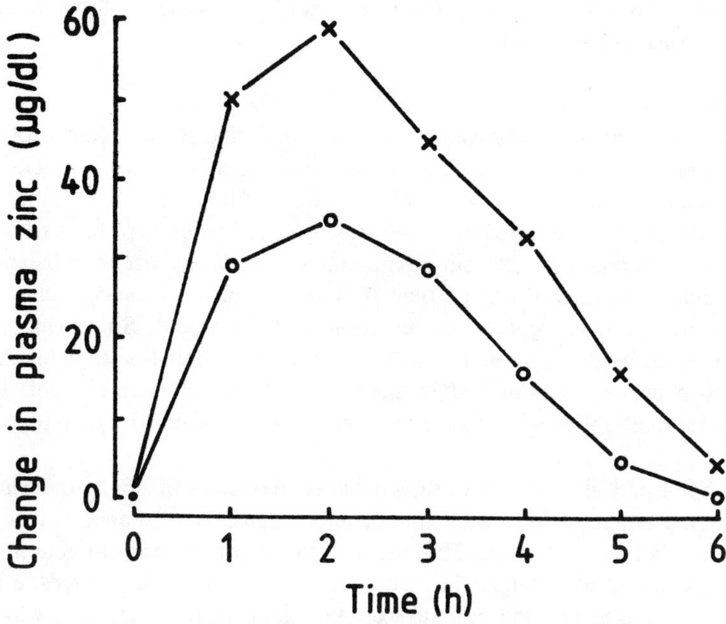

FIGURE 1. The zinc tolerance test measures the change in plasma zinc level from baseline after an oral dose of zinc (5 to 50 mg). The typical change in plasma zinc in an individual with normal zinc nutriture who has been fasting 12 to 18 hr prior to the zinc dose is shown as X——X. Diseases affecting the gastrointestinal tract (celiac, Crohn's, pancreatic insufficiency, and alcoholism) will typically reduce the area under the bell-shaped curve delineating the change in plasma zinc (0 —— 0).

zinc concentration forms a bell-shaped curve with the peak concentration observed 2 to 3 hr after the dose. Normalization of the plasma zinc level usually occurs within 6 hr (see Figure 1). This method has been used to study zinc absorption in clinically normal young[1254,1288] and old adults[95] in clinical conditions such as Crohn's disease,[1084] celiac disease,[329,1199] alcoholic cirrhosis,[1582] pancreatic insufficiency,[160] uremia,[13,65,904] hypertension,[223] jejuno-ileostomy,[47] and after artificial manipulation of the diet.[56,234,516,563] In aging and in the clinical conditions, the bell-shaped curve is usually flatter than in young healthy controls such that the peak zinc concentration attained is lower and the return to baseline is quicker (see Figure 1). The data of Fickel et al.[516] did not support the use of this test to distinguish experimentally zinc-depleted (3.3 mg/day, 8 weeks) from zinc-replete individuals. Nevertheless, the overall data are generally interpreted as indicating that the appearance of zinc in the plasma is impaired and that zinc nutriture is therefore suboptimal. Such an interpretation is usually consistent with other indexes of zinc nutriture.

The effects of various dietary factors on zinc absorption have been studied using the zinc tolerance test. Some foods depress the plasma zinc response,[1254] but many were shown to have no effect.[1216] The prostaglandin synthetase inhibitor, indomethacin, was also without effect.[1568] Iron (300 to 900 mg/day), however, decreased zinc absorption by 40% in controls and 25% in patients with uremia.[11,13] Vitamin D significantly increases zinc absorption measured by the zinc tolerance test.[904]

The method has two recognized limitations:[1502] (1) the dose of zinc is generally pharmacological and (2) differences in gastric emptying time, pH, and osmolarity can significantly affect zinc absorption.[1632] Concern has also been expressed that absorption of zinc unincorporated into food is not necessarily representative of zinc absorbed from a meal.[1502] Valberg et al.[1632] have reported that, in the zinc tolerance test, zinc absorption is similar whether the zinc is given in water or with a turkey meat meal. Thus, as long as conditions for the controls and patients are standardized, the method provides data that is reproducible, simple, and inexpensive to obtain.

H. Zinc Balance

In zinc balance studies, comparison is made of total zinc intake against total excretion (seat, urine, and feces). If losses are greater than intake, the balance is negative and vice versa. Two features of this method of assessing zinc nutriture make it of limited value: (1) in order to make precise measurements, the subjects need to be kept on a metabolic ward where intake and excretion of zinc can be monitored exactly and accurate balance data can be obtained and (2) balance of any nutrient only represents *net* balance without indicating changes in distribution, absorption, or retention of the nutrient. Since zinc excretion is notoriously affected by dietary zinc levels, this is a serious limitation to using zinc balance to assess zinc nutriture. The method is therefore primarily a research tool. It has been especially useful in establishing probable zinc requirements of healthy individuals (10 to 15 mg/day).

Studies by Spencer et al.[1537,1538] have shown that altered intake of zinc, protein and calcium, fasting, and renal failure all influence zinc balance. Thus, zinc balance is readily open to modification by diet or by disease. This method has also been used to determine rates of ''apparent'' zinc absorption, ''apparent'' since zinc from endogenous sources, e.g., bile and the pancreas, is secreted into the gut and excreted along with dietary zinc which may not have been absorbed. In some conditions, e.g., alcoholism, net zinc balance may be negative even though adequate amounts of dietary zinc are still being absorbed.

Because of the restricted conditions under which it can be used, the zinc balance test probably has limited scope in routinely assessing zinc nutriture.

I. Zinc Isotopes

Radioactive and stable isotopes of zinc are available. Both have been used to assess zinc absorption and, indirectly, zinc nutriture. The ease of monitoring the γ-emitting radioactive isotope of zinc, ^{65}Zn, is offset by its radioactive half-life (245 days) and long biological half-life (>500 days). Stable zinc isotopes, mainly ^{70}Zn, ^{68}Zn, and ^{64}Zn, have also been used for the measurement of zinc absorption.[853,906,1380]

For both types of isotope, the question of methodological validity has been raised; extrinsic zinc added to a meal is not necessarily absorbed to the same extent as zinc intrinsic to the meal.[1502] This problem has been overcome in part by feeding the isotope to an animal from which the meal will be derived, e.g., chicken. As such, the isotope becomes an intrinsic label.[853] Flanagan et al.[531] have recently shown that values for ^{65}Zn absorption are the same whether the label is extrinsic or intrinsic. For zinc absorption to be readily monitored by this technique, milligram quantities of zinc are usually required, amounts that are not generally consumed in a single meal. Nevertheless, use of stable isotopes of zinc has considerable potential and, barring the cost and restricted accessibility of the appropriate facilities, should become a good research tool for the measurement of zinc absorption and requirements.

Zinc-65 metabolism has also been studied in conjunction with a zinc loading test (100 mg of zinc per day for 1 year). During zinc loading, Aamodt et al.[1,3] observed that previously injected zinc-65 was removed from thigh muscle and liver, suggesting close regulation of total body zinc to avoid excess.

J. Zinc Uptake In Vitro

In two related conditions, Friedreich's ataxia and Duchenne muscular dystrophy, erythrocyte uptake of zinc was shown to be increased, both in association with hyperzincemia.[1454] Low zinc intake in rats[1376] and pigs[131] has been shown to correlate with increased zinc-65 uptake by erythrocytes in vitro.[1376] Subsequent zinc supplementation of the rats decreased erythrocyte uptake of ^{65}Zn toward the normal range. Although Chesters and Will[269] found that erythrocyte uptake of ^{65}Zn was inversely proportional to plasma zinc, too many other extraneous factors rendered the test ineffective, e.g., stress, infection, and differences in protein intake. Nevertheless, as an in vitro test of zinc metabolism, this simple assay merits further research, particularly with respect to clinical zinc depletion.

K. Postexercise Plasma Zinc

Normally, plasma zinc levels rise after exercise. Lukaski et al.[1029] have suggested that, since the reverse occurs in men previously fed a low zinc diet, this may be a suitable index of zinc status.

L. Response to Zinc Supplementation

The method of assessing zinc nutriture that is considered most reliable is that of clinical evaluation of the individual's response to zinc supplementation.[20,913,1299,1302,1344] Regardless of plasma zinc concentration, enzyme activities, apparent zinc absorption, or zinc balance, if the clinical symptoms suggestive of zinc depletion are alleviated by zinc supplementation, then zinc depletion should be considered to have existed.

Nowhere was this more dramatically proven than in the case of acrodermatitis enteropathica reported by Garretts and Molokhia.[581] The child presented with severe eczema, nail dystrophy, and diarrhea, which had started after weaning. She was diagnosed as having acrodermatitis enteropathica, and diodoquin therapy was partially successful in overcoming the skin lesions and diarrhea. Serum, dermal, and epidermal zinc concentrations were all subsequently determined to have been above normal, as was serum alkaline phosphatase. In spite of the high zinc values, the clinical symptoms were sufficiently suggestive that zinc supplementation (300 mg $ZnSO_4$ per day) replace diodoquin as a treatment. An improvement in the patient's condition was quickly noted. Within 5 months, the child was symptom-free. Discontinuation of zinc therapy (enhanced by supplementation with 1.5 g calcium per day) rapidly reversed the child's condition and symptoms of zinc depletion reappeared. Zinc therapy was restarted 3 weeks later, and the symptoms again disappeared.

This case suggests that a defect in zinc transport can exist in which zinc will accumulate in the target tissues but will not be available to the sites at which it is required. Furthermore, zinc depletion was clinically present in the absence of decreased serum or tissue zinc levels. Two conclusions can be drawn: first, clinical improvement following zinc supplementation is, so far, the best indication of the prior existence of a *functional* depletion of zinc. Secondly, measurement of a variable other than zinc itself, or a zinc metalloprotein may ultimately provide a more reliable index of zinc status. As will be discussed in the next section, such parameters would include functional tests of zinc status, e.g., dark adaptation, taste-smell function, and metabolic tests of other nutrients whose function is dependent on zinc, e.g., vitamin A and essential fatty acids.

III. FUNCTIONAL TESTS OF ZINC NUTRITURE

Functional tests are those physiological tests which current evidence suggests are dependent on zinc status for optimal results. Those that are potentially useful in assessing zinc nutriture are shown in Table 2.

A. Taste/Smell Acuity

Clinical zinc depletion is often associated with disorders of taste (dysgeusia and hypogeusia) and smell (dysosmia and hyposmia).[679,710-712,718-720,1499] Hepatitis, cirrhosis, pregnancy, chronic renal failure, anorexia, and penicillamine therapy are some of the conditions in which zinc and/or copper metabolism is altered and in which abnormalities of taste and

Table 2
FUNCTIONAL TESTS OF ZINC NUTRITURE

Taste/smell
Immune function
Dark adaptation
Clinical response

Table 3
METABOLIC TESTS OF ZINC NUTRITURE

Zinc metalloenzymes
Vitamin A
Essential fatty acids
Cholesterol
Blood ammonia
Blood urea nitrogen
Thyroxine
Growth hormone

smell have been reported.[205,243,1464,1576,1662] In patients with idiopathic hypoguesia, parotid saliva has been shown to contain about 20% of the zinc present in the saliva of people with normal taste acuity.[718] It has been demonstrated that zinc is present in the taste bud and that saliva contains a zinc metalloprotein, gustin.[718]

The correction of abnormal taste and smell by zinc supplementation has also been observed,[712,715] but double-blind trials of zinc evaluation in idiopathic hypogeusia have shown no correlation between taste acuity and plasma zinc,[243] erythrocyte zinc, or hair zinc.[1662] Because of significant placebo effects, the usefulness of defective taste and smell function as reliable indexes of zinc status is not conclusively established.[1499]

B. Immune Function

Golden et al.[612] have shown that topical application of zinc to malnourished children potentiates delayed hypersensitivity reactions and have shown that this response is inversely related to plasma zinc. This change in immune response to zinc application was considered as a possible functional index of zinc status. Smith,[1482] however, has found that delayed hypersensitivity is reduced following topical application of zinc. Further work is evidently required to determine the suitability or restrictions of such a test of zinc status. Natural killer-cell activity has been shown to be decreased in sickle-cell disease (secondary zinc depletion, see Chapter 6) and in human experimental zinc deficiency.[1599] Thymulin levels in human plasma are directly proportional to zinc status and may be increased by zinc supplementation.[1772]

C. Dark Adaptation

Dark adaptation is defective in alcoholics, and zinc supplementation has been shown to correct this condition.[1618] Nevertheless, it appears that defective dark adaptation in alcoholics is not due specifically to zinc depletion[1617] and is not always responsive to zinc supplementation.[1485] The disagreement between the results of Toskes et al.[1618] and Smith[1485] may be due to the longtime course required to restore retinal reductase after zinc depletion in rats.[312] With vitamin A, however, zinc supplementation may be effective.[1086] The usefulness of dark adaptation as an indicator of zinc status must therefore remain speculative.

IV. METABOLIC TESTS OF ZINC NUTRITURE

Except for the measurement of the activity of zinc metalloenzymes, metabolic tests of zinc status are nonspecific, but may be useful secondary tests to assist with the diagnosis of zinc depletion (Table 3).

A. Zinc Metalloenzymes

One of the most frustrating aspects of assessing the function of zinc and, hence, zinc nutriture is that the activity level and protein level of remarkably few of the 200 plus zinc metalloenzymes or zinc-activated enzymes are reliably affected by clinical zinc depletion. This includes the enzymes that contain zinc as a structural component, e.g., alkaline phosphatase and carbonic anhydrase, as well as those enzymes whose activity is acknowledged to be dependent on the presence of zinc, but for which zinc has not been established as a structural component, e.g., collagenase. In addition, there are enzymes whose activities are dependent on zinc intake but do not structurally contain zinc, e.g., linoleic acid desaturase. The activity of some enzymes is inhibited by zinc, e.g., ribonuclease.

A few zinc metalloenzymes have been reported to be affected by zinc depletion in humans. These include decreased serum and neutrophil alkaline phosphatase,[61,371,729,831,1299,1302,1377,1696] decreased erythrocyte carbonic anhydrase,[1299] decreased deoxythymidine kinase in skin collagen,[1302] and increased plasma ribonucleases.[1299]

The activity of zinc metalloenzymes, including intestinal alkaline phosphatase,[898] serum alkaline phosphatase,[909] and thymidine kinase[415] has been shown to be decreased in zinc-deficient rats. In zinc-deficient rats, activity of alkaline phosphatase has been shown to be restored with the in vitro addition of zinc.[909] The affinity of intestinal alkaline phosphatase for zinc is also reportedly reduced in zinc-deficient rats.[1351] The activity of other zinc-dependent enzymes, including malic and lactic dehydrogenase and carbonic anhydrase, does not readily reflect zinc status.[1766] Hence, primary zinc depletion in experimental animals is correlated with altered activity of alkaline phosphatase. However, some reports have also shown that serum alkaline phosphatase is not a reliable indicator of zinc status, both in humans[1174,1370] and in calves with hereditary zinc deficiency,[948] nor does it necessarily correlate with serum zinc.[1084]

It has been proposed that the change in vitro activity of a zinc-dependent enzyme following the addition of zinc could be used as an index of zinc nutriture.[377,1697] The activity of serum alkaline phosphatase has also been shown to be responsive to zinc supplementation in experimentally zinc-depleted adults[728,1316] and in parenterally fed infants.[1377]

Certain difficulties are associated with assessing zinc status using zinc-dependent enzymes:[267] (1) optimal assay conditions for the various isoenzymes of alkaline phosphatase are different so that accurate information about enzyme activity is difficult to obtain and (2) even in the situations in which zinc depletion can be reliable expected to cause reduced activity of certain enzymes, the relevance of such an observation to the etiology of the clinical effects of zinc depletion remains to be determined because most enzymes are not rate-limiting in their respective pathways. Hence, it is unlikely that the altered enzyme activity that may be observed would be directly responsible for a given pathological effect of zinc depletion, e.g., dermal lesions.

B. Vitamin A

An interaction between zinc and vitamin A has been proposed both in humans and animals.[1488,1514] In animals, zinc deficiency causes decreased plasma levels of vitamin A, but the effect appears to be more related to reduced food intake than to zinc deficiency per se.[1485] In humans, the relationship between zinc and vitamin A has been studied in alcoholic cirrhosis in which plasma levels of both vitamin A and zinc have been documented.[1427] However, 11 days of zinc supplementation in cirrhotics have been shown not to affect plasma vitamin A.[1485] In the presence of normal vitamin A intake, zinc supplementation has been shown to correct defective dark adaptation not corrected by vitamin A alone.[1150,1086] Zinc also corrects low vitamin A and low retinol-binding protein in children with protein-calorie malnutrition,[55,1461] but not in cystic fibrosis,[1234] acne,[1641] or vitamin A-deficient children.[55] The effectiveness of zinc seems, therefore, to be limited to situations in which taste and smell were also improved and in which protein-energy intake may be suboptimal; it does not seem to be effective in restoring normal vitamin A levels in conditions of adequate protein-energy intake.

Whether the correlation between plasma zinc and retinol-binding protein levels that has been reported[1514] is sufficiently reliable to be considered as an index of zinc nutriture remains to be further explored. Such a relationship in which a functional as opposed to structural interaction exists between zinc and another protein, e.g., retinol-binding protein, is a promising measure of zinc nutriture.

C. Essential Fatty Acids

The relationship between zinc and essential fatty acids is well-established, both in animals and humans.[341] A number of studies have indicated that this relationship may be predictive of zinc status in humans. In cystic fibrosis, a strong positive correlation was shown between plasma zinc and plasma levels of dihomo-γ-linolenic and arachidonic acids.[687] In cystic fibrosis, it has been shown that abnormalities in percentage composition of stearic acid, oleic acid, and the essential fatty acid, linoleic acid, were corrected with zinc supplementation.[690,1669] In peripheral blood leukocyte from patients with Crohn's disease, lower zinc levels correlated significantly with lower incorporation of tritiated arachidonic acid into leukocyte phospholipids.[345]

In unpublished studies of human experimental zinc depletion by Professor Janet King and colleagues, levels of unesterified arachidonic acid in plasma were shown to be increased, an effect possible due to increased phospholipase A_2 activity. Further studies of this nature might reveal that changes in essential fatty acid levels in various plasma lipid fractions reflect zinc status. Prasad et al.[1316] have observed that, in experimental zinc depletion, subscapular fat thickness was markedly reduced. Essential fatty acid levels were not studied. Since the fatty acid composition of adipose tissue is very stable, fat biopsies analyzed for fatty acid composition might be useful for zinc assessment in human zinc depletion.

D. Cholesterol

In hemodialysis patients, plasma zinc levels have been shown to be significantly negatively correlated with total cholesterol and high-density lipoprotein cholesterol.[1518] In view of the apparent effect of high doses of zinc on serum cholesterol (see Chapter 13), it might be worth studying the possible usefulness of serum cholesterol as a marker of zinc status.

E. Blood Ammonia/Urea Nitrogen

Reding et al.[1344] have recently summarized the data demonstrating that plasma zinc varies directly with blood urea nitrogen and liver ornithine transcarbamylase (which detoxifies ammonia), but does so inversely with blood ammonia. In their study of zinc supplementation in hepatic encephalopathy, plasma zinc and blood urea nitrogen responded positively to 600 mg/day zinc acetate for 7 days. The inverse relationship between plasma zinc and ammonia has been reported[1301,1322,1575] as well as the decrease in plasma ammonia following zinc supplementation.[1302,1318]

F. Thyroxine

Hartoma et al.[698] have observed that in normal volunteers given 50 mg elemental zinc three times daily for 2 months, serum zinc and thyroxine were positively correlated. Morley et al.[1148] have shown that serum zinc levels below 70 μg/mℓ are associated with lower triiodothyronine values.

G. Growth Hormone

Henkin[708] has shown that plasma zinc varies inversely and urinary zinc varies directly with plasma growth hormone levels.

V. SUMMARY

A number of problems still remain in the search for a suitable body fluid or tissue from which to reliably assess zinc nutriture. It seems likely that, with the possible exception of the platelet, all the available body sources from which zinc measurements can be made have been explored to a greater or lesser extent. However, the approach seems to have been largely haphazard. In this respect, three points stand out.

First it is true that the body does not store zinc in the way it stores iron or copper and that zinc can easily reequilibrate from plasma to liver. Postprandial and diurnal changes make standardizing the basic conditions for measuring plasma zinc difficult. Furthermore, although we know that about 95% of plasma zinc is protein-bound, the proteins (albumin and α_2-macroglobulin) are rarely measured when plasma zinc is measured. Plasma zinc levels are therefore based on the most primitive unit (a volume of plasma or serum). Although the laboratories that have reported plasma-total zinc in conjunction with plasma albumin and albumin zinc levels have often found no correlation between these parameters, this relationship has been insufficiently studied for it to be ruled out as potentially useful.

Second, in the nucleated cells (and erythrocytes), zinc has been measured in the total digest of the cells. Recent evidence suggests that we may be overlooking differences in zinc content by not separating the total lipid from the protein. In erythrocytes, for instance. Chvapil et al.[281] observed that although only a small proportion of the total zinc was membrane-bound (in the erythrocyte ghost), 68% of the total membrane-bound zinc was in the lipid fraction. Over 50% of the lipid-bound zinc was associated with phospholipid. Ho et al.[754] have recently shown that the increase in erythrocyte zinc that occurs in multiple sclerosis is due to an increase in phospholipid-bound zinc. Bettger and O'Dell[137] have recently stressed the importance of zinc in membranes. Cunnane[341,342] has reviewed the role of zinc in the metabolism of the major fatty acid components of phospholipids, the essential fatty acids. Thus, not only do membranes and, specifically, phospholipids bind a major proportion of zinc in cells, but this zinc is labile in at least one clinical condition, multiple sclerosis. In view of these observations, it would seem to be time to explore the role of zinc in lipid and long-chain fatty acid metabolism more thoroughly. If this yields useful information about zinc status, that would be a bonus.

Third, measuring zinc itself may not be the most ideal way to assess zinc nutriture, regardless of the tissue or matrix chosen. A functional test is also required. ^{65}Zn uptake by erythrocytes might be appropriate because it meets the requirements of sensitivity to altered zinc status, as well as technical simplicity. Some of the other tests described in this chapter are in their infancy as diagnostic tests of zinc nutriture. They have been included here to expand the range of useful tests of zinc nutriture away from direct zinc assays toward indirect, functional, and metabolic assays that may be equally or, indeed, more valid than zinc analyses per se.

Chapter 3

PRIMARY ZINC DEPLETION

I. INTRODUCTION

An individual whose plasma zinc is significantly lower than the mean value for apparently healthy individuals, as measured in that particular laboratory, may or may not be zinc depleted. A lower plasmic zinc is a physiological response to pregnancy and to acute infection. Nevertheless, clinical zinc depletion does exist, although it is often difficult to diagnose. Since the etiology of low zinc nutriture is rarely sufficiently obvious to indicate whether it is exclusively dietary, the term "zinc depletion" is used in preference to "deficiency" when discussing altered zinc status. The only exception is reduced zinc intake of a defined experimental nature (human or animal) in which the term "deficiency" does apply and is used here in that context.

Manifestations of clinical zinc depletion are shown in Table 4. In babies and young children whose diet is zinc deficient, these symptoms, especially growth retardation, poor appetite, dermatitis, scaly skin, and immunodeficiency, are most severe. The other symptoms, e.g., taste/smell dysfunction or defective dark adaptation, are not always present and may depend on the nature of the zinc depletion, e.g., alcoholism or drug treatment.

Zinc depletion can be subdivided into three basic categories according to etiology: (1) primary, (2) secondary, or (3) acute. Primary zinc depletion is of dietary origin. Secondary zinc depletion involves defective handling of zinc by the individual (absorption, requirement/utilization, or excretion). Acute zinc depletion is usually a physiological phenomenon of no long-term risk to a healthy individual.

Primary zinc depletion in its severest form is a frequent component of childhood protein-calorie malnutrition, two examples of which are kwashiorkor and total parenterally fed children after surgery. Growth retardation, skin lesions, delayed secondary sexual maturity, and diarrhea typically occur, but they do not necessarily all occur simultaneously in the same individual. This is a situation in which zinc depletion is of a *primary* nature, e.g., the diet having inadequate zinc. In these cases, plasma zinc is generally low, and the diagnosis of primary zinc depletion is not difficult to make.

In *secondary* or conditioned zinc depletion, the manifestations of zinc depletion may not be as obvious. In adults, assessment of growth retardation and delayed sexual maturation cannot be applied. The less reliable characteristics such as low plasma zinc, defective taste/smell, male infertility, or reduced dark adaptation (Chapter 2) may then become important in diagnosing zinc depletion.[1381] Secondary zinc depletion is a result of abnormal metabolism of zinc in the presence of potentially adequate dietary zinc intake. Abnormal zinc metabolism includes defective zinc absorption, increased zinc requirement or utilization, increased zinc excretion, or a combination of these symptoms.

Although the etiology of nutrient depletion can be classified as *primary* or *secondary*,[726] in the case of zinc depletion, the etiology is often combined (low zinc intake in the presence of an agent which, for example, enhances zinc excretion). Two examples are subclinical and alcohol-induced zinc depletion. Subclinical zinc depletion is considered to be prevalent in the majority of the North American population.[1397] It probably originates from the combined effect of consumption of foods of low zinc content along with prescription drug abuse (zinc chelation) and alcohol intake. Alcoholic cirrhosis is an example of secondary zinc depletion of multiple etiology in which low food (zinc) intake, defective zinc absorption, and increased zinc excretion both occur as a result of alcohol abuse.[827]

The third category is *acute* zinc depletion. It is not depletion strictly speaking, but rather

Table 4
CLINICAL MANIFESTATIONS OF ZINC DEPLETION

Growth retardation
Poor appetite (anorexia)
Taste/smell dysfunction
Retarded Secondary sexual development and hypogonadism — juvenile males
Infertility — adult males
Delayed onset of menstruation — juvenile females
Amenorrhea — adult females
Alopecia
Dermatitis (predominantly peri-oral and at sites of dermal irritation)
Defective dark adaptation
Stillbirths and low-birthweight infants — during pregnancy
Gastrointestinal distress and/or diarrhea
Impaired wound healing
Immunodeficiency

''redistribution'' of zinc from plasma to tissues and to excretion. It includes conditions that induce a temporary shift in zinc homeostasis, but which, in healthy individuals, do not represent a serious or permanent compromise of zinc balance requiring zinc supplementation to correct. Acute zinc depletion is generally associated with traumatic events, e.g., acute infection, myocardial infarction, and surgery. Plasma zinc is reduced in these conditions, and in some cases urinary zinc is increased immediately subsequent to the event. In myocardial infarction and acute infection, this change in plasma zinc level is sufficiently predictable to be virtually diagnostic of acute trauma. If such a traumatic event occurs in an individual already predisposed to subclinical secondary zinc depletion, e.g., an alcoholic, acute zinc depletion could precipitate secondary zinc depletion. Whereas zinc supplementation is beneficial in most conditions involving primary or secondary zinc depletion, it is not required nor effective in acute zinc depletion.

In many diseases, altered plasma zinc levels have been reported, but the mechanism of the defect in zinc metabolism has not been elucidated or even alluded to. Placing diseases into the aforementioned categories of ''zinc depletion'' in order to clarify the origin of the defect in zinc metabolism may therefore be somewhat arbitrary. Its use here is to provide a framework upon which these diseases can be related to abnormalities of zinc utilization. A discussion of altered zinc metabolism of unknown etiology is the subject of Chapter 6. Conditions described include hypertension, rheumatoid arthritis, and hypothyroidism.

Primary zinc depletion has three possible causes: (1) low intake of food containing adequate amounts of zinc, (2) consumption of food low in zinc, or (3) a combination of low intake of foods containing low amounts of zinc. Examples are given in Table 5.

II. LOW FOOD INTAKE

A. Malnutrition

Malnutrition is a term indicating suboptimal nutrient assimilation of any etiology. It may be caused by low food intake or an inability ot utilize foods of adequate nutritional composition. Primary zinc depletion is implicit in malnutrition whether it be kwashiorkor (protein-energy malnutrition, which also involves secondary zinc losses), failure of any infant to successfully breast-feed, or malnutrition caused by alcoholism, poverty, or starvation. Anorexia nervosa amounts to secondary malnutritiion, but, because there may be a conscientious voluntary component, it is considered separately from malnutrition.

The early reports of human zinc deficiency[1308,1405] were of populations of essentially malnourished adolescents. The malnutrition originated from a combination of the following: (1) consumption of food of low zinc and protein content, (2) high phytate intake, (3) gut

Table 5
CAUSES OF PRIMARY ZINC DEPLETION

- Low food intake
  - Malnutrition
    - Kwashiorkor
    - Fetal growth retardation
    - Prematurity
    - Aging
  - Alcoholism
  - Anorexia
- Intake of food of low zinc content
  - Total parenteral nutrition
  - Food processing
  - Experimental zinc deficiency

microbial infestation causing diarrhea, e.g., with hookworm, and (4) poor zinc absorption. This syndrome has recently been reported in Australian aborigines.[259,301] Infection seems to be a constant companion of such individuals since zinc depletion causes thymic atrophy and depressed cell-mediated immunocompetence.[612]

The specific importance of zinc in malnutrition has been demonstrated by the beneficial effect of zinc supplementation, for example, in Iranian growth-retarded and malnourished dwarfs.[1308] Nevertheless, two cautions need to be expressed. First, "spontaneous" resolution of the symptoms of apparent zinc depletion in a similar group of Middle Eastern adolescent dwarfs to those described by Prasad et al.[1308] has been reported.[292] These dwarfs did not have hookworm or schistosomiasis, suggesting that gastrointestinal losses of zinc, e.g., in the study of Prasad et al.,[1309] may be a factor precipitating zinc losses that are clinically responsive to zinc supplementation. Second, supplementing with zinc *alone* may not be sufficient, as demonstrated by Smith et al.,[1493] who were unable to accelerate weight gain in growth-retarded Australian aboriginal children supplemented only with 20 or 40 mg zinc per day over 10 months. This period of time and amount of zinc given should have produced a growth spurt, suggesting that zinc alone was not responsible for the growth retardation in the study of Smith et al.[1493] and that without additional supplements of energy, protein, essential fatty acids, or vitamin B_6 (for example), these children could not utilize the additional zinc for growth purposes.

1. Kwashiorkor

Childhood kwashiorkor is a severe form of protein-energy malnutrition frequently associated with zinc depletion. A rapid clinical response has been reported in children with kwashiorkor who are supplemented with a combination of zinc and a high-energy diet.[213,608,612,614,899,957,967]

2. Fetal Growth Retardation

Zinc depletion during pregnancy causes fetal malnutrition or intrauterine growth retardation,[955,1099] but it responds well to zinc supplementation.[1675] Fetal alcohol syndrome may be a consequence of primary zinc deprivation of the fetus, but the true relationship between alcohol and zinc with respect to fetal growth is as yet unclear[62] (see also Chapter 4, Section III.B).

3. Prematurity

The growth deficit present in premature infants is more closely associated with inadequate zinc intake than with any other factor, including intakes of protein and energy and gestational age.[570] A number of cases have been reported of premature infants having overt symptoms of zinc deficiency even though they have been breast-fed.[21,25,955,959,1164,1240] This is a condition of primary zinc depletion because the breast milk is usually found to be low in zinc, and the infants respond to zinc supplementation. Breast milk of mothers with premature infants will frequently not contain sufficient zinc to match intrauterine zinc accretion rates; hence, the potential onset of neonatal zinc deficiency.

It has been calculated that to match intrauterine zinc accretion rates, parenterally fed premature babies need to retain at least 25% of the zinc in milk[1109,1110] or from 350 to 440 μg/kg/day.[1768] These estimates agree with those of Lockitch et al.,[1009] who found that at zinc intakes <400 μg/kg/day in parenterally fed low birthweight infants, plasma zinc could not be maintained at a stable level. Tyrala[1630] deduced similar zinc requirements for premature infants; in order to maintain positive zinc balance, 34-week-old infants weighing an average of 1550 g required at least 430 μg/day of zinc. Even the breast-fed premature infant requires at least 300 μg of zinc per kilogram per day.[1572] However, Haschke et al.[700] have reported that premature infants (day 6 to 122 of life) fed a cow's milk formula containing 0.1 or 4.1 mg/ℓ of zinc did not differ in weight gain, although plasma zinc was higher in the zinc-supplemented group. The zinc intake of the infants fed the low zinc formula would have averaged no more than 100 μg/day (at 1ℓ of milk per day and the infant weighing 1000 g). The normal weight gain in these infants is at variance with that predicted from these other studies and awaits further clarification.

4. Aging

Malnourishment in the aged is a cause of zinc depletion, but whether the aged have an increased zinc requirement has not been established.[748,791,1403] Vir and Love[1658] noted that subjects in the 65 to 95-year age range had plasma zinc levels from 72 to 85 μg/dℓ, which correlated positively with plasma albumin levels. Less than 2% of those tested had plasma zinc <50 μg/dℓ. Low plasma zinc is therefore not necessarily correlated with aging but may be dependent on age-related changes in plasma albumin or food intake habits. Beneficial effects of zinc supplementation in the aged have been observed.[420]

B. Alcoholism

The generally suboptimal nutrient intake of alcoholics[1085] predisposes them to dietary (primary) zinc depletion. This may be due to the high percentage of calories derived from alcohol with a proportional reduction in intake of nutrient-derived calories. Alcohol abuse also impairs zinc absorption and increases zinc excretion.

C. Anorexia

The effect of low food intake is associated with zinc depletion in anorexia nervosa.[93,94,237,238,776,1500] Whether zinc depletion initiates the anorexia or vice versa has not been elucidated. Alcoholism has been shown to be a precipitating factor in anorexia nervosa and severe zinc deficiency.[466] The effect of zinc deficiency on food intake may be mediated in part by prostaglandins since "2 series" prostaglandins are increased in the blood of zinc-deficient rats[627] and prostaglandin E_2 is anorexia-inducing.[499]

As in alcoholism, multiple nutrient deficiencies are thought to exist in anorexia nervosa.[1500] In contrast to alcoholism, increased zinc excretion has not been reported so far in anorexia nervosa. However, this could be expected in more severe cases since starvation is associated with increased urinary loss of zinc.[1537]

III. FOODS OF LOW ZINC CONTENT

Low zinc intake due to intake of food of inadequate zinc content arises with the consumption of synthetic diets or highly processed foods. Synthetic diets that may be low in zinc include total parenteral nutrition, liquid weight-reducing diets, synthetic diets used in phenylketonuria, and those designed to be specifically zinc-free for human experimental zinc depletion. Infant milk formulas may also be in this category; their zinc content is generally adequate from a theoretical standpoint, but the zinc is significantly less absorbable than that in human milk.[234,381]

A. Total Parenteral Nutrition

Total parenteral nutrition (TPN) is now considered an iatrogenic cause of zinc depletion.[1302] Up until a few years ago, however, TPN was a frequent cause of zinc depletion in hospitalized patients requiring parenteral feeding. Since the formulas are synthetically prepared, omission of zinc was possible. In fact, the U.S. Food and Drug Administration did not approve its inclusion in TPN formulas until overwhelming evidence was collected documenting zinc depletion arising from low zinc or zinc-free TPN.[41,78,534,536,639,880,1020,1115,1159,1229,1279,1550,1602,16,24,1730,1737,1757]

Because patients receiving TPN are frequently in a catabolic state, and the TPN solutions lack natural dietary zinc ligands, zinc losses can even occur with TPN containing apparently adequate amounts of zinc.[23,913,973] Hence, the zinc requirement is often considerably elevated, particularly in parenterally fed newborn infants.[1767]

Mozzillo et al.[1159] have suggested that the hypertonic glucose present in TPN might also exacerbate zinc depletion or increase the zinc requirement. The free amino acids in TPN formulas, e.g., histidine and cysteine, may also bind zinc and promote its excretion. Feeding TPN solutions might also involve essential fatty acid depletion; glucose absorption is increased in zinc-deficient rats[1530] and, like zinc deficiency, glucose inhibits essential fatty acid metabolism.[87,176,341] Thus, if the effects of zinc deficiency are expressed in part through inhibition of essential fatty acid metabolism, a common link could be excess glucose absorption.

B. Experimental Zinc Deficiency

Buerk et al.[207] were the first to describe the feeding of a semisynthetic zinc-deficient diet to humans. They observed that volunteers fed 0.6 to 1.0 mg zinc per day rapidly developed negative zinc balance. Skin lesions were noted on the joints and in the groin area. Individuals with plasma zinc <80 μg/dℓ were surgically given full-thickness skin wounds, but healing rates were not different from controls.

King and colleagues[89-91,737,1666] and Prasad et al.[1316] have also described the experimental use of synthetically prepared diets depleted of zinc. King's group used a liquid-based formula with emulsification of the solid ingredients. They almost totally depleted zinc from the diets fed to young men. This caused a significant decrease in plasma, urinary, fecal, and seminal zinc. Exacerbation of previously existing acne was observed in one case.[90] This group has also more recently demonstrated that young men fed diets low in zinc (5.5 mg/day) maintain zinc balance and normal plasma zinc levels, suggesting that enhanced zinc absorption occurs in such a situation.[1666]

Prasad et al.[1316] used a soy-based formula that did not totally exclude zinc from the diet. They observed no significant clinical deterioration as a result of feeding adults 3.5 mg zinc per day for up to 40 weeks. Oligospermia, however, was observed.[6]

C. Other Synthetic Diets

Phenylketonuria is managed using totally synthetic diets with protein sources low in phenylalanine. Children fed such diets have been reported to have low hair zinc and, in some, low plasma zinc has also been observed.[1604]

Davies[387] has remarked that other synthetic diets, e.g., for weight reduction or protein restriction, may be a cause of zinc depletion as may some infant formulas. Such special diets have not been reported to be associated with zinc depletion, but such a potential does exist. In the case of infant formulas the zinc content is generally adequate or even high; the problem is that the absorption of zinc from such formulas is much lower than from human milk. In addition, these formulas are usually fortified with other nutrients, e.g., copper and iron, which compete with zinc for absorption.

D. Food Processing

Processed foods include textured vegetable protein, highly refined foods, and canned or frozen vegetables. The latter, especially peas, are treated with ethylenediaminetetraacetic acid (EDTA) to retain their color. This process strips much of the zinc content from these foods.[1114] Consumption of energy-rich processed foods such as white bread and confectionary and fatty snacks, e.g., potato chips, will provide satiation without nutritional value. As such, they too may contribute to long-term suboptimal zinc nutriture.

Chapter 4

SECONDARY ZINC DEPLETION

I. INTRODUCTION

Secondary zinc depletion is a function of zinc *availability*, e.g., the degree to which adequate dietary zinc can be utilized by the body. Conditions may exist in which adequate dietary zinc cannot meet the body's needs because of (1) decreased zinc absorption, (2) increased requirement or decreased utilization, or (3) increased excretion. These factors govern zinc availability.

II. ZINC AVAILABILITY

Zinc availability refers to the degree of efficiency with which zinc is absorbed, transported, and utilized peripherally. Zinc that is present in the diet, but which does not enter peripheral tissues as required, is said to be unavailable. With the exception of massive urinary losses of zinc, zinc availability is the main determinant of whether secondary zinc depletion will develop. Faulty zinc absorption and transport mechanisms both reduce zinc availability. Since the body very efficiently maintains zinc homeostasis, zinc toxicity per se does not occur under normal conditions. Clinically, the problem is therefore not one of zinc excess, but of insufficient availability of zinc. Aside from dietary (primary) zinc deficiency over which the body has no control, two factors in particular determine zinc availability — zinc absorption and transport. Factors that control these processes differ depending on whether one considers the pre- or postweaning infant (or adult).

A. Preweaning Infant

In the absence of substances interfering with zinc transfer across the placenta (alcohol and cadmium) or extremely low maternal zinc intake, the fetus is normally assured of adequate zinc for development. After birth, the neonate must adapt to an oral zinc supply. Development of processes for the absorption of zinc from milk are crucial to maintaining zinc homeostasis in neonates because of (1) the absence of zinc storage mechanisms and (2) the great demand for zinc for growth. In premature and intravenously fed infants, it is even more difficult to maintain zinc accretion.[381,676,1109]

Prior to the availability of milk formulas infants could only receive zinc from breast milk, a medium containing low amounts of zinc, but from which zinc is readily available. Infants that are not breast-fed usually face reduced zinc availability from either cow's milk or milk formulas. Cow's milk usually contains as much or more zinc than human breast milk,[1725] so it is a matter of zinc absorption from the milk rather than its concentration in the milk which is the major determinant of zinc availability to the preweaning neonate.[248,1456,1725] Aspects of zinc availability from breast milk compared to formulas or cow's milk relate to zinc ligands in the milk that stimulate or inhibit zinc absorption (human milk having more of the former while cow's milk and milk formulas have more of the latter — see Chapter 9 for more details). Thus, breast milk substitutes create severe demands on neonatal zinc homeostasis.

B. Postweaning Infant

Zinc depletion in the weanling has diverse manifestations. Many of these are precipitated as a result of concurrent protein-energy malnutrition (reviewed by Hambidge).[677]

1. Zinc Absorption

Regulation of zinc absorption is critical for the maintenance of zinc homeostasis. This has been demonstrated by studies involving suboptimal intake of zinc in humans,[1666] ingestion of zinc-65,[554] and by studies of the effects of zinc supplementation on zinc excretion.[842] These studies have shown that zinc balance in humans appears to be controlled primarily at the intestinal level rather that at an internal tissue store. The result is that if zinc nutriture is low, intestinal absorption is increased and vice versa.[88]

The events that take place during the transfer of zinc from the intestinal lumen to the plasma transport proteins have been elucidated to a great extent by Cousins and colleagues (reviewed by Cousins[315]). Briefly, zinc is transported across the intestinal mucosal brush border by an ATP-dependent process. Binding of the metal to metalloproteins and/or metallothionein within the mucosal cell facilitates the transfer of zinc to the plasma exchange sites at the serosal surface of the intestinal cell. Once there, zinc is exchanged to the plasma carrier proteins. (See Chapter 9 for more complete details of this process as it is currently understood).

What is important to understand is that the process of zinc absorption is susceptible to inhibition or blockage by a large variety of substances. In most instances, their mechanism of action is not understood. The importance of the interplay between factors promoting and inhibiting zinc absorption is illustrated by the fact that impaired zinc absorption is a leading cause of secondary zinc depletion. Thus, adequate intake of zinc by no means ensures optimal zinc nutriture. Metals such as copper and calcium compete with zinc for absorption and ligands such as phytate remain bound to zinc and prevent its absorption. Gastrointestinal disease and infection significantly reduce zinc absorption. Alcohol and other drugs induce net loss of zinc, partly through effects on absorption and partly by altering its excretion. These factors are discussed in greater detail in Chapters 5 and 9.

The mechanism of zinc absorption and transfer to the blood is, as yet, poorly understood even under optimal conditions. Intestinal ligands are important. Some are derived from pancreatic secretions; others are present in the diet. Some compounds which form complexes with zinc either promote (diiodohydroxyquinoline) ethylenediamine tetraacetic acid or inhibit (EDTA) zinc absorption.

2. Zinc Transport

The second major determinant of successful postweaning utilization of zinc is the blood transport system. As with defective zinc absorption, defective zinc transport mechanisms play a major role in the expression of clinical zinc deficiency or depletion.

Two proteins, albumin and α_2 macroglobulin, are the major carriers of zinc (in terms of mass of zinc carried, but not necessarily in terms of biological importance, e.g., ease of exchangeability). Together, they account for 90 to 95% of zinc measured in plasma.[548,601] Of the two, albumin is considered to more readily exchange zinc with peripheral sites.

Conditions altering serum albumin concentration will significantly alter zinc levels in plasma. Examples of hypoalbuminemia are malnutrition and total parenteral nutrition (TPN). The zinc-binding capacity of albumin may be optimal in both, but if albumin is the main carrier of zinc to peripheral sites and if its serum level is low, tissue zinc availability will be decreased. Reestablishment of serum albumin to normal levels is crucial to successfully restoring normal zinc nutriture in both malnutrition[608] and TPN.[106] The physiological importance of the amino acids in blood, e.g., histidine and cysteine, which are thought to bind the zinc not bound to albumin or α_2 macroglobulin, is not understood. These amino acids (and other minor zinc carriers, e.g., lipids and immunoglobulins) may not be quantitatively important zinc carriers but, biologically and ultimately pathologically, they may be very important. Drugs that bind zinc also fit into this category. Chronic treatment with steroids, for example, may severely limit zinc exchange from serum to peripheral sites (see Chapters 6 and 18).

Table 6
ETIOLOGY OF SECONDARY ZINC DEPLETION

Decreased zinc absorption
- Dietary factors
- Absence of appropriate absorption ligands
- Gastrointestinal dysfunction

Increased zinc requirement or utilization
- Surgery
- Burns
- Dermatological disorders
- Pregnancy/lactation
- Malignancy
- Chronic infection/inflammation
- Growth hormone therapy

Increased zinc excretion
- Muscle catabolism
- Alcohol
- Renal disease
- Muscular dystrophy
- Porphyria
- Thyrotoxicosis
- Hyperparathyroidism
- Sickle-cell disease
- Gastrointestinal infestation

III. SECONDARY ZINC DEPLETION

The etiology of secondary zinc depletion is shown in Table 6.

A. Decreased Zinc Absorption

Factors associated with decreased zinc absorption are shown in Table 4 (Chapter 3). Decreased zinc absorption is caused by many foods, depending on their composition.[1420] Competitive inhibition by specific dietary components is well documented, e.g., calcium, copper, or iron, and binding agents preventing absorption, e.g., phytate, fiber, or chelating agents. Other causes include pancreatic dysfunction, immature or defective absorption sites (gut surgery or Crohn's disease), and inadequacy of appropriate ligands.

1. Dietary Factors

Dietary factors influencing zinc absorption are listed in Table 7.

a. Calcium

Most of the data suggesting that calcium competitively inhibits zinc absorption are from animal studies (see Chapter 9). In humans, dietary calcium *alone* has not been shown to inhibit zinc absorption.[1399,1539,1540] Only as a complex with phytic acid has calcium been demonstrated to inhibit zinc absorption in humans.[385] Geophagia or pica, the practice of eating clay (particularly observed in Iran where human zinc depletion was first definitively demonstrated), may contribute to zinc depletion because of the high calcium content of the clay.[1300]

b. Copper

Solomons[1502] has suggested that the competitive interaction of zinc and copper for absorption sites in the gut, which is well documented in animals (reviewed by Cunnane[341]), may only be a pharmacological effect. This is because studies that have demonstrated such

Table 7
FACTORS ASSOCIATED WITH DECREASED ZINC ABSORPTION

Dietary factors
- Calcium
- Copper
- Iron
- Fiber/phytate
- Alcohol
- Chelating agents

Absence of appropriate absorption ligands
- Acrodermatitis enteropathica
- Cystic fibrosis
- Pancreatic dysfunction
- Breast milk vs. milk formulas
- Phenylketonuria
- Hypothyroidism

Gastrointestinal dysfunction
- Intestinal mucosal damage
- Malabsorption syndrome
- Gastrointestinal surgery

an interaction in animals have used copper levels well in excess of those encountered by humans. At more physiological concentrations, copper does not affect zinc absorption in rats.[1219] Nevertheless, in Wilson's disease, <50 mg supplemental zinc effectively reduces copper absorption (see Chapter 8).

c. Iron

In pregnant women, zinc absorption has been shown to be reduced by oral iron supplements[680,1099] (reviewed by Solomons et al.[1504]) or to be unaffected by iron supplementation of up to 240 mg ferrous fumarate per day.[1459] In a zinc tolerance test, a ratio of iron to zinc increasing from 0:1 to 3:1 given in aqueous solution (zinc kept constant at 25 mg) caused a progressive decrease in the plasma response to the ingested zinc in healthy nonpregnant subjects.[1503] The total number of ions as well as the iron to zinc ratio seem to be critical because at an iron to zinc ratio of 2.5:1, zinc absorption from a water vehicle in fasting individuals is not different from controls.[1409]

In uremic patients, 300 mg iron given with 25 mg zinc in a zinc tolerance test caused a 40% decrease in peak plasma zinc in controls and a 25% decrease in the patients.[11] The apparently decreased zinc absorption was associated with lower-fasting plasma zinc and was exacerbated by aluminum.[13] Since aluminum poisoning is not uncommon in hemodialyzed patients, these interactions with zinc metabolism are probably of long-term relevance to the prognosis of such patients.

In contrast to the situation in adults, including pregnant women, infants do not appear to be as prone to the inhibitory effects of iron on zinc metabolism. Low birthweight infants (800 to 1200 g) at 6 to 12 months of age were fed a formula containing iron at 1 or 2 mg/kg/day. All infants in both groups had plasma zinc levels > 75 μg/dℓ.[1392] Even in 3-month-old infants receiving 30 mg iron daily, no effect on serum zinc or copper was seen.[1754] Hence, in healthy infants in which zinc depletion is not evident, iron supplementation at <30 mg/day does not appear from current evidence to affect zinc nutriture.

d. Fiber and Phytate

Phytate (phytic acid, myoinositol 1,2,3,4,5,6-hexakis dihydrogen phosphate) is a component of plant protein. It has been implicated as a factor exacerbating the zinc deficiency present in the Iranian dwarfs documented by Prasad et al.[1308] Others have corroborated these initial findings.[958,979,1205,1254,1502,1505,1506] Morris and Ellis,[1149] however, have reported no effect of phytate on zinc absorption unless calcium levels are also manipulated. Dietary fiber may also be a factor inhibiting zinc absorption. Negative zinc balance has been demonstrated in some studies of the effects of fiber supplementation.[974,1215,1350,1627] However, the effect has not been consistently observed in humans or in animals,[1502,1620] which may be due to different effects of soluble and insoluble fiber.

Since phytic acid and fiber are generally found in the same foods (whole-grain cereals, breads, and legumes), the issue of their relative contribution to inhibition of zinc absorption is not as important as that of their combined effect on net zinc absorption. In vegetarians, phytate and fiber intake is significantly higher than in individuals eating an omnivorous diet. In males, plasma zinc was shown to vary inversely with total fiber intake in both vegetarians and nonvegetarians.[974] However, no sign of zinc depletion could be detected by Anderson et al.,[46] King et al.,[907] or by Swanson et al.[1592] who studied pregnant women who consumed exclusively vegetarian diets. Therefore, a degree of zinc depletion may have to arise from another source before phytate or fiber significantly affects zinc nutriture.

The question of the importance of these dietary factors (calcium, copper, iron, phytate, and fiber) is twofold: (1) in reality, are they a deterrent to zinc absorption in humans and (2) is a zinc-deficiency syndrome associated with their consumption? It appears that only in situations of extreme excess intake of these substances or in periods of vulnerability to their excess will zinc depletion be induced. Thus, in the Iranian dwarfs consuming clay containing >15% calcium as well as unleavened bread rich in phytate in a diet already marginally deficient in zinc, an effect on zinc status was observed.[1308] Likewise, during pregnancy, zinc absorption may be more susceptible to competitive inhibition by iron than in typical volunteers (young healthy males). Thus, in situations of limited zinc availability or increased requirement, supraoptimal intake of calcium, copper, iron, phytate, or fiber may adversely affect zinc status.[1399]

e. Alcohol

Alcohol decreases zinc absorption in the rat[68,1465,1582] (reviewed by McClain and Su[1085]). In human alcoholics, the evidence is equivocal. Using a zinc tolerance test, Sullivan et al.[1578] observed that zinc absorption was decreased by concurrent alcohol consumption. Absorption of zinc-65 was recently shown to be lower in alcoholic cirrhosis.[1632] In alcoholics consuming a standard meal, absorption of 50 mg but not 25 mg zinc was decreased.[401] However, zinc absorption, turnover, and excretion have been shown to be increased in alcoholics.[653,1131,1132] The study of Mills et al.[1131] was a base line study (alcohol not ingested with zinc), thus not necessarily indicating that alcohol does not inhibit zinc absorption.

Whether the effects of alcohol are predominantly on zinc absorption or excretion, the net result is generally decreased plasma zinc concentration[191,442,699,1044,1132,1148,1224,1582,1746] and leukocyte zinc concentration.[886] Occasional alcohol consumption, therefore, does not appear to threaten zinc homeostasis, but its use on a regular basis is one of the most common causes of secondary zinc depletion.

Spencer et al.[1537] have observed that following alcohol withdrawal, zinc balance is positive, suggesting a possible reason for the discrepancy between the results of Sullivan et al.[1582] and Mills et al.[1131] Whether zinc absorption is decreased in alcoholics does not alter the fact that they are generally zinc depleted. The cause may be related to reduced absorption or to increased excretion of zinc.[1537,1577,1580]

f. Chelating Agents

EDTA has been shown to reduce zinc absorption in humans.[1506,1539] In the study of Spencer et al.,[1539] the decrease in zinc absorption did not affect zinc balance. Since EDTA is used

Table 8
CONDITIONS IN WHICH THERE APPEARS TO EXIST AN ABSENCE OF APPROPRIATE ZINC ABSORPTION LIGANDS

Acrodermatitis enteropathica (AE)
Cystic fibrosis
Pancreatic dysfunction
Milk formulas
Phenylketonuria
Hypothyroidism

to remove zinc from vegetables during processing,[1114] it appears to have a doubly negative effect — both on zinc content of the final product and on its absorption. As with alcohol, the effect of chelating agents on overall zinc homeostasis may very much depend on the frequency and quantity of their use.

2. Absence of Appropriate Absorption Ligands

Conditions in which decreased zinc absorption may reasonably be attributed to an absence of appropriate absorption ligands are shown in Table 8.

a. Acrodermatitis Enteropathica (AE)

AE is the classical human example of zinc depletion caused by absence of an appropriate absorption ligand (general review by Walravens[1674]). It is an autosomal recessive disease with onset usually after weaning from breast milk. If untreated, it is fatal. Symptoms include low plasma zinc, alopecia, diarrhea, and dermatitis of the extremities and perioral, perianal, and genital regions. Mood disturbances, symptoms of visual dysfunction including color blindness and lack of cone vision,[1156] photophobia,[1151] and deficient cellular immune function[250,460] are also present. In 1973, Moynahan and Barnes[103,1157] reported that a patient with AE under their care responded to zinc supplementation. Since their initial report, unequivocal evidence has been presented of zinc depletion in AE and the unique effectiveness of zinc in preventing the symptoms of AE[44,946,1120,1155,1184,1185,1563,1570] immunodeficiency.[216,1711,1734] Whether zinc excretion in AE is also altered is uncertain; Aggett and Harries[23] have reported that it is, whereas others have shown it to be unchanged.[838,1012]

Up until the association with zinc, AE was treated with drugs such as diodoquin (diiodohydroxyquinoline). The reason for their effectiveness was not understood until after the successful use of zinc supplementation. It was then observed that diodoquin enhanced zinc absorption and might also act as a zinc ionophore.[22]

The proportion of dietary zinc absorbed by zinc-supplemented AE patients has been shown to be similar to that in unsupplemented AE patients.[84] Zinc is therefore only effective in AE because the total zinc available is increased. Hence, in order for zinc supplementation to be effective in AE, saturation of the mucosal uptake mechanism appears to be necessary, thus suggesting that the defect is ligand-related.[84] The defect in the intestinal mucosa is not fully understood, but the result, in most cases, is dramatically reduced zinc absorption.[84,1012] Casey et al.[231] have shown that the binding of zinc to duodenal secretions is reduced in patients with AE. Piletz and Ganschow[1284] have suggested that absence of a specific ligand is not the only cause of reduced zinc absorption in AE, arguing that the casein-associated zinc ligands are found in both human and cow's milk.

Weaning from human to cow's milk appears to be the precipitating event in the onset of AE. This appears to be due to an absence of ligands in cow's milk that are capable of binding zinc in the intestine and promoting its absorption.[231,479] Differences in ligands may be important between the types of milk, but other differences between cow's and human milk also exist that may be related to AE.[339] Significant among these is the essential fatty acid (EFA) content; in human milk it is six to eight times higher than in cow's milk.[857] Furthermore, in human milk, the fat binds about 30% of the total zinc,[562,1016] whereas in cow's milk, the fat only binds 14% of the total zinc.[561]

Cunnane[339] has shown that the EFA, including linoleic acid (18:2n-6), γ-linolenic acid (18:3n-6), and dihomo-γ-linolenic acid (20:3n-6), which are present in human milk, significantly increase zinc absorption in neonatal rats. Arachidonic acid (20:4n-6), although present in human milk, did not affect zinc absorption. The only n-6 EFA in cow's milk is linoleic acid. These results are relevant to the defect in zinc absorption in AE because EFA metabolism has been shown to be defective in AE.[236,357,1719] Cottonseed oil (45% linoleic acid) given intravenously in three patients has been shown to partially alleviate the symptoms of AE while arachidonic acid had no effect.[236]

These clinical results are similar to the experimental results of an effect of EFA on zinc absorption and suggest that the EFA may be important in zinc absorption. Furthermore, since EFA ameliorated the symptoms of AE in the absence of supplemental zinc, the primary defect in AE may be of EFA, not zinc metabolism. Because zinc is so important in EFA metabolism (see Chapter 13), defective zinc absorption in AE may be masking a defect in EFA metabolism.

Variant forms of AE have been reported in which the clinical symptoms were indistinguishable from those of AE, but in which there was a disparity between serum or tissue zinc levels and clinical symptoms. Thus, zinc in serum has been shown to be in the normal range[945] or to be elevated.[390,581] These cases are further discussed in Chapter 6.

b. Cystic Fibrosis

Cystic fibrosis has been associated with zinc depletion.[404,673,844,1509] Although plasma zinc levels may be normal in cystic fibrosis,[1233,1234,1501,1509] other parameters of zinc depletion, including low hair zinc and increased taste threshold have been observed.[1509]

In view of these studies indicating zinc depletion in cystic fibrosis, it is disconcerting to see a lack of clinical response to zinc supplementation.[1233,1234] What may be crucial in tying together these various observations is the suggestion that plasma zinc levels in cystic fibrosis appear to be dependent on the degree of growth retardation and pulmonary disease. If these are not severe, plasma zinc may be normal[673,1187] and there may be a lack of response to zinc supplementation.

c. Other Forms of Pancreatic Dysfunction

In unspecified exocrine pancreatic insufficiency, Dutta and Iber[430] have observed a reduction in zinc absorption and fecal zinc excretion but increased urinary zinc. Ligation of the pancreatic duct in the rat has been shown not to affect serum zinc, but to cause a decrease in liver zinc.[9] Pancreatitis subsequent to alcoholism causes reduced zinc concentration in pancreatic secretions.[1730] These secretions are normally an important component of the enterohepatic circulation of zinc.[1581] Alcoholic pancreatitis associated with zinc depletion is reversible with zinc supplementation.[1730]

During the passage of a meal through the gut, the exocrine pancreas is known to secrete endogenous zinc, sometimes in amounts equivalent to the amount of zinc in the consumed meal.[56,1069,1502] These data provide clinical and experimental data suggesting that, on the whole, intact exocrine pancreatic function is necessary to maintain zinc absorption.

d. Breast Milk vs. Milk Formulas

The long-running controversy over the relative merits of infant feeding via breast or bottled milk (based on cow's milk or soy formula) is particularly applicable to the issue of neonatal zinc depletion. The availability of zinc from breast milk is greater than from cow's milk or formulas,[234,327,859] even though in breast milk, the zinc content is similar to[1034] or less than[1725] it is in cow's milk. Male bottle-fed infants have lower hair zinc[1033] and lower plasma zinc[685] than do male breast-fed infants. Human milk therefore appears to have a zinc ligand that is not present in similar amounts in cow's milk or synthetic formula milks. The nature of this ligand is a matter of considerable controversy and may or may not be one of a combination of the following: lactoferrin, EFAs, prostaglandins, citric acid, or picolinic acid (see Chapter 9).

e. Phenylketonuria

Phenylketonuria is treated by feeding semisynthetic diets low in phenylalanine. Low plasma and very low hair zinc have been reported in phenylketonuria[14] and might be due to the nature of the diet.

f. Hyopothyroidism

Hypothyroidism has been associated with decreased bidirectional transport of zinc across the gut mucosa, an effect completely reversible with supplemental thyroxine.[1088] Low triiodothyronine may therefore be a factor contributing to zinc depletion in alcoholism[1148] and starvation.[1147]

3. Gastrointestinal Dysfunction

a. Intestinal Mucosal Damage

The mucosal surface of the gut is the initial site of zinc absorption. It may be damaged in various conditions including AE, Crohn's disease, and anorexia nervosa as well as with the use of TPN. Each of these is associated with zinc depletion partly because of impaired zinc absorption.[33,1324] Inflammation of the mucosal cells of the intestine may be partly responsible, as may diarrhea/steatorrhea.

There seems to be little doubt that zinc absorption is impaired in Crohn's disease: (1) plasma concentrations are lower than normal,[535,630,953,971,1404,1508,1511] (2) plasma zinc correlates inversely with disease activity,[1426] (3) the zinc tolerance test produces a below average plasma zinc response,[1084] (4) absorption of a stable zinc isotope is reduced,[1569] and (5) i.v. zinc supplementation in Crohn's disease is associated with increased body weight, skinfold thickness, and serum albumin.[1043] Nevertheless, there was no relationship between serum zinc and zinc intake at zinc infusion values <220 μg/day. Main et al.[1043] concluded that since zinc intake was positively correlated with urinary zinc, zinc was not efficiently utilized by Crohn's disease patients when administered as an i.v. infusion.

Bloomfield et al.[153] reported that, in Crohn's disease, arachidonic acid levels in serum and mononuclear cells were 50% of control values. This situation may be due, at least in part, to impaired arachidonic acid synthesis due to the inhibitory effect of zinc depletion on linoleic acid desaturation.[87,343]

b. Malabsorption Syndrome

Malabsorption syndrome is typically characterized by incomplete absorption of most nutrients, along with diarrhea, protein depletion, and symptoms indicative of specific mineral or vitamin deficiency, e.g., iron-deficient anemia and peripheral neuritis (vitamin B_6 deficiency). Not surprisingly, plasma zinc has been reported to be low in malabsorption syndrome[2,306,1081,1668] and in celiac disease.[1180,1366] Zinc supplementation has also been shown to improve wound healing and normalize erythrocyte zinc in patients with malabsorption.[1095] Diarrhea of any etiology, including malabsorption appears associated with net losses of zinc from the intestine.[1737]

Table 9
CONDITIONS IN WHICH INCREASED ZINC REQUIREMENT OR UTILIZATION APPEAR TO EXIST

Surgery
Burns
Dermatological disorders
Pregnancy/lactation
Malignancy
Chronic infection/inflammation
Growth hormone therapy

c. Gastrointestinal Surgery

Negative zinc balance has been reported in patients having undergone surgical removal of sections of intestine.[42,487,580,731,966] Its origin may be twofold: (1) reduced mucosal surface for zinc absorption or (2) increased zinc excretion due to muscle catabolism, typically occurring after major surgical procedures.[505,1537] In the latter case, if the patient was otherwise healthy, plasma zinc would be decreased temporarily, e.g., only acute zinc depletion would be present (see Chapter 6). This is supported by the findings of Engels et al.,[461] who reported a normal zinc balance in "short-bowel" patients 5 years after surgery. In rats, the intestinal mucosal mass also increases after resection, allowing net zinc uptake to be unchanged as compared to presurgery values.[1631]

B. Increased Requirement for or Utilization of Zinc

Zinc depletion may arise in any situation in which the body's demand for zinc is increased in the presence of static zinc intake (see Table 9). These conditions represent potential zinc depletion occurring in the presence of suboptimal dietary zinc and zinc absorption. The cause of the increased demand for zinc is thought to be partly related to synthesis of new protein that involves a number of zinc-dependent enzymes, notably DNA and RNA polymerase. In addition, zinc excretion via the urine may also be increased as a stress response, e.g., after surgery. This reduces available zinc and contributes to acute zinc depletion.

1. Surgery

Zinc metabolism is altered following surgery. At least three changes have been documented: (1) reduced serum zinc independent of albumin, (2) zinc redistribution within the body, particularly toward the liver, and (3) increased urinary zinc losses (for reviews see Van Rij and Pories[1649] and Van Rij[1648]). Negative zinc balance may enhance the risk of infection and decrease the rate of wound healing. It is particularly severe in parenterally fed newborn infants after a surgical operation.[1236] However, it is doubtful whether surgical procedures in previously healthy individuals represent a potential cause of zinc depletion (see Chapter 6).

The decrease in plasma zinc levels during, or shortly after surgery, is well documented.[541,669,1236] However, only in infants has the postsurgical drop in plasma zinc subsequently led to clinical zinc deficiency.[1236] This suggests that a preexisting zinc depletion or relatively high risk of zinc depletion, e.g., in young infants, is a prerequisite for surgery-related zinc deficiency. This is supported by the observations of various investigators[277,541,661,670,1142] who have shown that supplemental zinc is only beneficial in surgical patients whose presurgical serum zinc levels were below normal. In patients with normal serum zinc levels, supplemental zinc was of no additional benefit. Similar data are available from studies with rats.[1731] Nevertheless, it is evident (from rat studies) that zinc does accumulate at the wound site and, in zinc-deficient rats, the amount of zinc accumulated at the wound site is reduced.[1447]

The equivocal results of the effect of zinc on wound healing (reviewed by Van Rij[1648]) may therefore be partly duc to differences in the zinc status of the patients prior to surgery. Thus, in the healthy individual, surgery itself only represents a temporary insult to zinc balance (see Chapter 5) and is not a risk of chronic zinc depletion. Conditions related to surgery may promote the onset of zinc depletion. These include TPN and protracted hospitalization.[215,1648,1649]

2. *Burns*

Parallel effects on zinc homeostasis occur in burn patients as occur in surgical patients. Zinc is redistributed from tissues, particularly muscle, via the blood to the liver and may also be excreted in the urine due to tissue catabolism.[293,369] Zinc is also mobilized to the wound site partly as a function of the immune system and partly for protein synthesis during tissue rebuilding. Zinc losses may also occur in the exudate from the burn. Depending on the severity of the burn, the individual's age, growth rate, and preexisting zinc status, hypozincemia and hyperzinuria may be persistent.[972,990,1294]

If preburn plasma zinc levels are within the normal range and this level can be regained during epithelialization of the burned area, burns do not seem to be a cause of chronic zinc depletion. As in surgery, in healthy individuals only very severe burns involve a risk of inducing secondary zinc depletion.

Factors such as preexisting subclinical zinc depletion or prolonged hospitalization, anorexia, heavy use of antibiotics, or infection occurring as a result of severe burns do appear to be a significant cause of zinc depletion and hence increased zinc requirement in burn patients.[723,990,1193,1407]

3. *Dermatological Conditions*

The skin contains about 20% of total body zinc with about 75% of that in the epidermis,[1142] and zinc is very rapidly transported to the skin from the gut.[411] The possibility has been discussed that conditions involving epidermal lesions may therefore be caused by zinc deficiency or may, through inducing zinc depletion, increase zinc requirements. Under normal conditions, epidermal desquamation does not cause significant zinc loss from the body. However, conditions involving epidermal scaling, e.g., dandruff and psoriasis, cause significant zinc losses by this route (70 to 100 μg/g) compared to the normal epidermal values of about 50 μg/g.[1142,1423]

Equivocal results have been reported for serum zinc in relation to psoriasis: no change,[1296] increased,[1621] or decreased.[636,1423] Although Portnoy and Molokhia[1296] and Tsambaos and Orfanos[1621] have suggested that there is no correlation between the degree of skin involvement and serum zinc levels in psoriasis, McMillan and Rowe[1097] did find such a correlation. Drug treatments may be a factor determining whether zinc depletion will develop in psoriasis (see Chapter 6).

Other skin conditions reported to be associated with low serum zinc include acne,[1121] AE,[103] eczema,[382,1231] erythematous lesions,[1603] leg ulcers due to vascular insufficiency[635] or sickle-cell disease,[1448] skin lesions in kwashiorkor,[608] leprosy,[124] recurrent vulvovaginal candidiasis,[447] and cutis laxa following penicillamine therapy.[693]

Patients with atopic eczema have been reported to have low serum zinc levels.[382] They have also been shown to have an abnormal pattern of EFAs in plasma phospholipids[1049] (Figure 2). The defect in EFA metabolism is indicative of impaired desaturation: the substrate/product ratios for each of the desaturases (Δ 6, Δ 5, and Δ 4, in order) were increased. In the zinc-deficient rat, each of these desaturase reactions has been documented by various laboratories to be impaired (see Chapter 13). It is therefore suggested that zinc depletion in

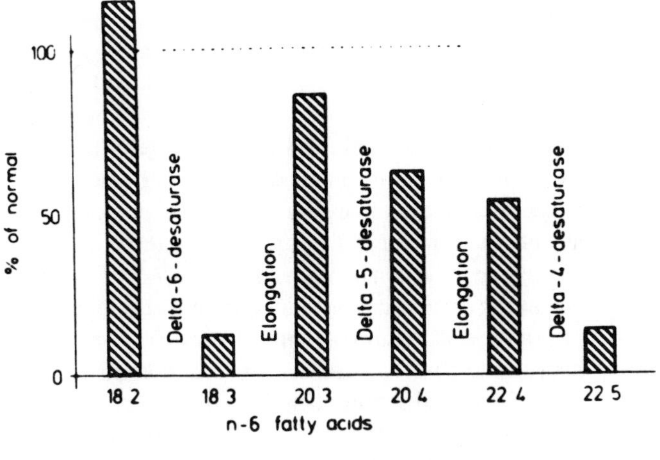

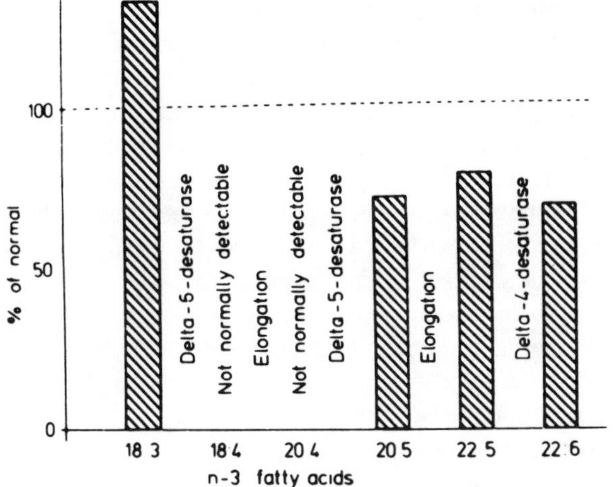

FIGURE 2. Levels of the fatty acids in both families of EFAs in the serum phospholipids in a study of patients with atopic eczema. Values are shown for the linoleic acid family (18:2n-6, upper) and for the α-linolenic acid family (18:3n-3, lower) as a percentage of the values in a normal control population. Both primary substrates (18:2n-6 and 18:3n-3) are above normal (100%), whereas the subsequent products are below their respective normal values. In addition, the desaturase substrate fatty acids (20:3n-6, 22:4n-6, and 22:5n-3) are not as decreased as their immediate products (20:4n-6, 22:5n-6, and 22:6n-3). These data indicate that the desaturases metabolizing EFAs are inhibited in patients with atopic eczema, a situation analogous to that observed in animals made experimentally zinc deficient. The defect in EFA metabolism in atopic eczema may, therefore, be related to an abnormality in zinc metabolism. (From Manku, M. S., Horrobin, D. F., Morse, N., Wright, S., and Burton, J. L., *Br. J. Dermatol.*, 110, 643, 1984. With permission.)

atopic eczema may bear a metabolic relationship to the altered EFA composition of the plasma phospholipids.

Although these associations between low serum zinc and various skin lesions have been made, it is only in those that respond to zinc supplementation, e.g., oral ulcers,[1113] venous leg ulcers,[637,670] acne vulgaris,[1652] and kwashiorkor,[608] that a causal relationship between zinc depletion and epidermal pathology is implied. In none has an increased requirement for zinc been demonstrated.

4. Pregnancy/Lactation

The recommended dietary allowance for zinc uptake by American adults has been set at 15 mg/day. For pregnant women, the value is 20 mg/day and for lactating women, 25 mg/day as set by the National Research Council in 1980.[1178] By Canadian standards,[212] the standards of the National Research Council (U.S.) are high (see Chapter 10). Regardless of the discrepancies between these recommendations, the requirement for zinc is higher in pregnancy because of fetal and placental development[1397] (reviewed by Solomons et al.[1504]) and in lactation because of zinc transfer to the newborn via the milk. In human pregnancy, zinc absorption has been shown to be nonsignificantly increased.[1592] In spite of the postulated increase in the requirement for zinc during lactation, normal development has been observed in infants breast-fed by mothers consuming only 30 to 40% of the recommended zinc intake.[1154] Increased capacity to absorb or retain zinc must therefore exist in pregnancy and lactation to overcome the increased requirement posed by the developing fetus. Various indexes of lower zinc status, e.g., lower zinc levels in plasma and hair,[678,1592] are present in normal pregnancy. This, however, is a physiological response to (1) a higher zinc requirement, (2) hemodilution due to plasma volume expansion, and perhaps to (3) increased circulating steroids. That the nature of the shift in zinc distribution is probably physiological is indicated by the fact that these indexes usually return to normal following delivery. Plasma zinc is lower than normal in pregnant low-income women, an effect reversible with zinc supplementation.[805] Thus the degree of the decrease in plasma zinc in pregnancy is dependent on zinc nutriture. Another factor that may impinge on the zinc status of a pregnant woman is gestational diabetes, although with good control this need not be the case.[1724]

If the increased requirement for zinc cannot be met by the mother, maternal, fetal, and neonatal complications characteristic of chronic secondary zinc depletion may arise. These include low birthweight of the infant, intrauterine growth retardation, fetal malformations, spontaneous abortion, uterine atony, and pregnancy-induced hypertension (see Table 4) (Chapter 3). Postnatally, transient hypogammaglobulinemia has been associated with maternal zinc depletion during pregnancy.[991]

Even without apparent zinc depletion, pregnant women have been clearly shown to benefit from zinc supplementation. Age and parity-matched women received either no supplement or 20 mg zinc aspartate per day from 25 weeks of pregnancy to term. Zinc-supplemented women had less blood loss at delivery, more appropriate-for-gestational-age babies, shorter labor, less toxemia, and fewer fetal complications or malformations.[963] This study, if confirmed elsewhere, suggests that the conventional indexes of zinc status, particularly in pregnancy, do not adequately indicate the difference between genuinely zinc replete individuals and those who will clinically benefit from zinc supplementation in spite of no *apparent* zinc depletion. This study also suggests that the recommended zinc intake for pregnant women set by the National Research Council[1178] of 20 mg/day may still not allow for optimal fetal development and parturition.

Fetal alcohol syndrome has a high association with maternal zinc depletion,[82,242,245,427,540,806,1161,1656] although the relationship is not considered conclusive.[58,62,686] Coexisting zinc depletion of a different origin, e.g., malnutrition, may have to be present in addition to excess alcohol intake in order for fetal alcohol syndrome to develop.

It is important to note that much of the evidence relating birth defects and other feto-maternal complications to zinc depletion has been based on the finding of low tissue plasma zinc levels. As discussed in Chapter 3, this can create a misleading impression; in fact, the relationship between low maternal zinc status and low birthweight is considered tentative by some researchers,[227] while others have reported that maternal plasma zinc levels are not at all related to fetal birthweight.[222,262,417,593,822] Some preterm babies have been shown to have normal plasma zinc levels[595] and their mothers have been shown to have breast milk containing a similar concentration of zinc as that of mothers with full-term babies. Increased amniotic fluid zinc has been found to be associated with spinal tube defects occurring in the absence of any change in fetal serum zinc.[1241] In mothers of infants with spina bifida, hair zinc has been shown to be above normal.[127]

It is therefore evident that if these data have been obtained under reliable and controlled conditions, tissue zinc levels do not necessarily represent zinc *availability*. Furthermore, the interpretation of low plasma zinc levels hinges on protein status (Chapter 2); enteric losses of protein can be the *cause* of low plasma zinc levels, yet have been interpreted as the *result* of zinc depletion in conditions such as cow's milk intolerance, congestive heart failure, and immunodeficiency.[1704]

What is fundamental, therefore, is to know whether the babies, although preterm, are of appropriate weight for their gestational age at birth or whether they were growth-retarded. It is only in the latter case that zinc depletion has been implicated.[1099,1100,1470,1471] The potential for zinc depletion in the breast-fed or parenterally fed premature infant is discussed in Chapter 3.

5. Malignancy

Two aspects of zinc metabolism are potentially affected by malignancy: (1) the role of zinc in the immune system and (2) the demand by the malignant cells for zinc for growth. Both aspects are thought to increase the body's requirement for zinc. Thus, in the face of unchanged zinc intake, zinc depletion is likely to manifest itself. Other factors will contribute, such as anorexia and tissue catabolism, both of which increase urinary zinc excretion. Nevertheless, serum zinc cannot be predicted to be decreased in all conditions of malignant growth.

Serum zinc has been reported to be decreased in acquired immunodeficiency syndrome (AIDS),[235] Hodgkin's disease,[246] liver metastasis,[1653] acute lymphoblastic leukemia,[393] squamous carcinoma of the esophagus,[1107,1613] squamous cell lung cancer,[834] carcinoma of the bronchus,[48,383] bronchogenic carcinoma,[40] and metastatic osteosarcoma.[526] However, serum zinc is unchanged in malignant lymphoma[921] and benign or malignant breast tumors[579] and increased in primary osteosarcoma.[526] Zinc content of lymphocytes has also been shown to be lower in children with leukemia.[228]

No doubt some of these differences in plasma zinc levels are real and depend on the type of malignancy, but they may also be due to differences in sampling, e.g., at different stages in the growth of the malignant tissue as well as effects on levels of plasma proteins, etc. Since protein is increased in ascites fluid in patients with neoplasia, and this correlates with increased ascites zinc, part of the hypozincemia observed in malignant conditions may be due to the mobilization of plasma proteins to ascites fluid.[373]

In comparison with normal tissue, zinc in malignant tissue is frequently increased, e.g., in the breast,[1433] liver,[1745] and prostate.[372] Habib et al.[657] have reported decreased zinc in carcinoma of the prostate but increased zinc in benign prostatic hypertrophy.[658,977] Therefore, in general, zinc levels in neoplastic tissue are higher than in the host tissue with the consequence that zinc requirement will be increased.

6. Chronic Infection

Hypozincemia and hyperzincuria are characteristic of infectious conditions whether acute[122,1257,1261] or chronic.[120,121]

The question is whether hyperzincuria and hypozincemia are physiological responses observed in all individuals or an indication of a condition requiring zinc supplementation, e.g., conditioned zinc depletion. The answer seems to depend on the zinc status, age, and growth rate of the individual prior to the infection as well as the severity and duration of the infection, i.e., its effect on normal food intake and, hence, zinc availability and excretion. Long-term, debilitating infection requiring hospitalization, e.g., pulmonary tuberculosis,[157]

Table 10
CONDITIONS ASSOCIATED WITH INCREASED ZINC EXCRETION

- Muscle catabolism
  - Starvation
  - Anorexia
  - Surgery
  - Burns
- Alcoholism
- Renal disease
- Muscular dystrophy
- Porphyria
- Thyrotoxicosis
- Hyperparathyroidism
- Sickle-cell disease
- Gastrointestinal infestation

could seriously compromise zinc status and lead to zinc depletion. It therefore represents a situation in which the zinc requirement is undoubtedly increased. This is especially true in children.

In conditions such as childhood gastroenteritis in which fecal zinc losses are high due to mucosal damage and diarrhea, zinc depletion predictably exists.[163,1179,1262] Chronic zinc depletion, e.g., in malnutrition, causes cell-mediated immunodeficiency and enhanced susceptibility to infection.[250,368,556,614,621,849] Zinc supplementation readily stimulates cell-mediated immunity and corrects the immunodeficiency.[614,1260,1685] infection, if there is a sustained stress on cell-mediated immunity, the zinc requirement will undoubtedly be increased.

7. Growth Hormone Therapy

Treatment of hypopituitary dwarfism with human growth hormone has been suggested to increase the zinc requirement because of growth stimulation.[111] Nevertheless, it has also been reported that growth hormone therapy does not significantly alter zinc status.[1513]

It is worthwhile to note that growth retardation of endocrine origin, e.g., hypopituitarism, is not necessarily associated with altered zinc status,[1512] whereas growth retardation of dietary origin, e.g., malnutrition, usually is.

C. Increased Zinc Excretion

At this stage, it is probably evident that the etiology of secondary or conditioned zinc depletion cannot be packaged into discrete categories, e.g., dietary deficiency, decreased absorption, increased requirement — all of which are mutually exclusive. Although some conditions of zinc depletion do neatly fit into these categories, e.g., AE, they are more the exception than the rule. Most of the complicated conditions causing clinical zinc depletion such as alcoholism, TPN, or surgery involve altered zinc intake, absorption, and excretion.

Nevertheless, it is still useful to distinguish those conditions inducing increased zinc excretion, particularly if this is well-established (see Table 10). Broadly speaking, increased zinc excretion occurs for two reasons: (1) in association with increased muscle catabolism and (2) proteinuria or because of drug effects on zinc absorption, metabolism, and excretion. In both, it is the change in urinary zinc excretion that is most easily noted because this is generally a minor route of zinc excretion — generally about 500 μg/24 hr, equivalent to <5% of total daily excretion.[18] Although changes in urinary zinc excretion may be useful diagnostically, it is doubtful whether they contribute significantly to negative zinc balance since the differences with normal zinc excretion via this route rarely represent more than

10% of total zinc excretion. Increased zinc excretion has also been documented, but generally in association with diarrhea.[1262]

1. Muscle Catabolism

a. Starvation/Anorexia

Prolonged starvation is recognized to cause increased urinary zinc excretion,[1537] but during a short-term fast (72 hr) in healthy volunteers, plasma levels were shown to be significantly *increased* over base line.[722] Whether the rise in plasma zinc is a short-term response to starvation unrelated to increased urinary zinc excretion or a change that occurs concurrently with increased zinc excretion has not been established.

Anorexia is another cause of increased zinc excretion due to starvation and tissue catabolism. This has been described in an anorectic patient with systemic sclerosis.[718]

b. Surgery/Burns

Topics under this heading have been discussed in detail earlier in this chapter (see Section III.B).

2. Alcohol

Alcohol induces hyperzincuria in humans[164,598,1131,1224,1313,1575,1577,1580,1640] and in rats.[26] The cause of alcohol-induced hyperzincuria is still unknown, but may involve increased muscle catabolism and increased zinc losses in association with proteinuria.[505,1575] Alternatively, it may be due to reduced hepatointestinal extraction of absorbed zinc.[887]

3. Renal Disease

Changes in zinc metabolism in renal disease are complicated (reviewed by Agarwal and Agarwal[18]). Uremia has many of the characteristics of zinc deficiency including skin lesions, poor wound healing, hypogonadism, and impotence. Plasma, leukocyte, and hair zinc levels are generally decreased,[307,781,1041] but this is not always the case.[956] In children with renal failure,[1464] researchers have documented abnormal taste acuity, decreased hair and erythrocyte zinc, and increased urinary zinc excretion. In uremic patients, hyperzincuria may be correlated with proteinuria,[566] but this is not always the case.[300,1052,1349] Thus, although zinc deficiency is widely associated with chronic renal disease,[1302,1440] it is not necessarily manifested by enhanced urinary zinc excretion. Hyperzincuria in uremia is likely to be determined by the degree of muscle wasting.[128] Zinc may also be a determinant of heme synthesis in uremia since it is a structural component of aminolevulenic acid dehydratase.[1750] Hence, zinc status in uremia may ultimately determine the amount of supplemental iron required and its effectiveness in overcoming anemia.

The increase in urinary zinc excretion in uremia depends on a number of factors, including the degree of polyuria and use of aluminum hydroxide during hemodialysis.[13] In polyuria of early remission from nephrotic syndrome, urinary zinc has been reported to be increased five times, but was otherwise not different from controls.[1349] The use of aluminum hydroxide during hemodialysis has also been associated with lower plasma zinc in patients with chronic renal insufficiency.[1769,1770]

In renal disease, it is important to distinguish patients according to whether they are receiving peritoneal dialysis or are on artificial kidney machines. In the former, plasma zinc may be normal[233] and erythrocyte zinc elevated,[307] but in the latter, both plasma zinc and erythrocyte zinc have been shown to be elevated because of zinc contamination from the disposable filter coils used in artificial kidneys.[1373] It may therefore be hemodialysis itself that is partly responsible for altered zinc metabolism in renal disease.

Erythrocyte zinc levels seem consistently raised in renal patients whether or not they are on dialysis.[116,1543] The location of the increase in erythrocyte zinc requires further investigation particularly in view of the findings of Dore-Duffy's group[753,754] that raised erythrocyte zinc in multiple sclerosis is confined to the membrane lipid of the erythrocyte.

4. Muscular Dystrophy

Although plasma zinc is generally normal in Duchenne muscular dystrophy, due to muscle catabolism, urinary zinc is increased.[839,1454]

5. Porphyria

Increased zinc excretion in the urine has been reported in acute intermittent porphyria[1269,1368] and attributed to the formation of zinc-porphyrin complexes.[1269] In acute intermittent porphyria, zinc depletion due to excess urinary losses of zinc has been suggested to account for the muscle pain experienced in that condition since it is reversible with zinc supplementation. In cutaneous porphyria, however, plasma and urinary zinc levels have been reported as normal.[1368] Histidine treatment, although reducing prophyrin excretion, has been shown to increase urinary zinc excretion.[719,998]

6. Thyrotoxicosis

Zinc excretion via the urine has been shown to be increased in thyrotoxicosis, an effect thought to be due to protein catabolism.[175] Erythrocyte zinc levels have also been shown to be lower in hyperthyroidism, a change correlated with lower plasma albumin and retinol-binding protein.[28]

7. Hyperparathyroidism

Untreated hyperparathyroidism is associated with hyperzincuria, which further increases after surgery.[1046]

8. Sickle-Cell Disease

Hyperzincuria has been observed in patients with sickle-cell disease.[1070,1319,1605] Matustik et al.[1070] noted that increasing dietary sodium from 20 to 140 mg/day significantly decreased urinary zinc excretion in sickle-cell disease. Prasad et al.[1319] found an inverse correlation between erythrocyte zinc and urinary zinc in sickle-cell disease. Neill et al.[1192] reported that sickle-cell patients in the steady state (symptomless) had higher plasma zinc than those in crisis. They suggested that this might be due partly to an acute stress response (see Chapter 6) in the patient during the sickle-cell crisis, similar to that occurring in other traumatic conditions.

9. Gastrointestinal Infestation

Gut infestation with nematodes causing fecal blood loss is a cause of zinc depletion. This situation is most common in tropical countries with endemic malnutrition.[1308]

IV. SUMMARY

Defining the specific causes of secondary zinc depletion is frequently difficult because they may be masked behind the effects of alcoholism, absorptive disorders, or renal disease. The purpose in following Herbert's[726] system of defining the etiology of nutrient deficiency is to demonstrate that, for instance, zinc depletion associated with diuretics (see Chapter 6) is not caused by the same mechanism as zinc depletion induced by surgery, AE, or sickle-cell disease. Some may say that the etiology is irrelevant if zinc therapy will cure all three. Zinc therapy may cure drug-induced zinc depletion and AE, but, in a healthy person undergoing surgery, zinc therapy is unnecessary and may be detrimental in terms of potential immune system suppression (see Chapter 8). Also, with diuretics, zinc supplementation may cause side effects, whereas in AE, this is unlikely. If zinc depletion is drug-related, removal of the drug will generally cause remission of the symptoms of zinc depletion. Therefore, understanding the etiology of zinc depletion can help demonstrate similarities between diseases that might facilitate the therapeutic use of zinc where it might not otherwise be used and prevent its use where it is unnecessary.

Chapter 5

ACUTE ZINC DEPLETION

I. INTRODUCTION

Stress due to acute trauma or injury invariably induces hypozincemia[494] and hyperzincuria (reviewed by Agarwal and Agarwal[18]). Examples include acute infection, surgery, burns, total parenteral nutrition (TPN), myocardial infarction, and acute accidental injury[1153] (see Table 11). The increase occurs in the context of the injury and may, in part, represent the "overflow" from the metabolic response to redistribute zinc to the liver. Tissue catabolism also probably contributes to stress-related hyperzincuria. What distinguishes acute zinc depletion from primary or secondary zinc depletion is that in healthy individuals it is a transient event: (1) zinc levels in plasma and urine will return to normal after the injury is repaired and (2) zinc supplementation will not affect the outcome or time course of the trauma response.

II. ACUTE INFECTION

The decrease in serum zinc in response to acute infection is a physiological process involving the mobilization of zinc to the liver and an increase in zinc absorption, both of which are stimulated by leukocytic endogenous mediator (LEM).[122,874,1259,1263,1675] The process of zinc mobilization to the liver occurs in conjunction with increased metallothionein synthesis by the liver.[172,1497] That the decrease in serum zinc is a necessary physiological response to infection is suggested by the study of Chvapil et al.[286] who showed that this decrease maximized the phagocytic function of leukocytes.

III. DRUGS

A. Alcohol

As discussed earlier (see Chapter 4), hyperzincuria is associated with chronic use of alcohol. Hyperzincuria is also a consequence of *acute* alcohol consumption; it is a temporary phenomenon and does not compromise zinc nutriture.

B. Chelators

Chelating agents, including ethylenediaminetetraacetic acid (EDTA)[75] and diethylenetriaminepentaacetate,[294] significantly increase urinary zinc excretion in rats and humans. Penicillamine increases copper excretion, hence its use in Wilson's disease. However, it also increases zinc excretion,[919,1079] which may be partly responsible for the report of cutus laxa[693] and for autoimmune complications[1443] following penicillamine therapy.

C. Diuretics

Diuretics increasing zinc excretion are shown in Table 12). In the case of furosemide, urinary zinc levels were normalized 2 hr after furosemide was given.[1549] Wester[1714,1715] has distinguished between the *concentration* of zinc in the urine and *24 hr zinc excretion* in patients on diuretics. Although diuretics do increase the 24 hr zinc excretion, this is partly due to diuresis. Urinary zinc concentration is also increased in diuretic users, but to a lesser extent. Thus, part of the effect of diuretics on zinc excretion must be attributed to diuresis, but part is also due to active tubular zinc excretion.[1714,1715] Captopril binds zinc[803] and has been shown to cause taste loss, alopecia, dermal lesions, and nail dystrophy, which can be

Table 11
CAUSES OF ACUTE ZINC DEPLETION

Acute infection
Drugs
  Alcohol
  Chelators
  Diuretics
  Steroids
  Other
Myocardial infarction
Surgery
Burns
Parenteral nutrition

Table 12
DIURETICS THAT HAVE BEEN SHOWN TO INCREASE ZINC EXCRETION

Diuretic	Ref.
Hydrochlorthazide	1232, 1356, 1713—1715
Furosemide	1549
Bumetamide	1714, 1715
Triamerene	1714, 1715
Chlorthalidone	1356
Captopril	1480

corrected by 400 mg/day oral zinc sulfate.[1480] Chlorthalidone (10 to 15 mg/day) over at least 6 months has been associated with impaired sexual function in men, but this was not associated with decreased testosterone; in fact, serum and hair zinc were higher than in controls.[584]

D. Steroids

Classically, corticosteroid therapy is considered to decrease plasma zinc[189,455,494,1758] and to increase zinc excretion.[31,542,708] was especially evident in women also consuming a low-zinc diet (0.2 mg zinc per day); plasma zinc decreased from 81 to 45 μg/dℓ.[737] The positive effect of glucocorticoids on liver zinc uptake and stimulation of metallothionein synthesis[315] may be relevant to their effects on plasma zinc levels. The mechanism of steroid-induced hyperzincuria is thought to be due to tissue catabolism, although an increased glomerular filtration rate may also be a factor.[18]

In diseases of corticosteroid deficiency, e.g., Addison's disease, urinary zinc is usually decreased,[716] although exceptions have been noted.[554] In corticosteroid excess, e.g., Cushing's syndrome, urinary zinc excretion is increased.[704,717] The use of oral contraceptives has been associated with increased zinc excretion, a factor that might predispose such users to anorexia.[94]

In spite of the generally well-accepted effect of steroids on zinc metabolism, some reports have not been able to confirm the majority view (preceding paragraphs). In asthmatic children with or without prednisone treatment, plasma zinc was found to be in the normal range.[615] Also, hospitalized patients receiving prednisone (40 to 50 mg/day) for skin diseases had no demonstrable change in plasma zinc levels over 2 weeks of steroid therapy and were not given zinc supplementation.[1698] Long-term (>6 months) oral contraceptive users who subsequently became pregnant did not have plasma zinc levels significantly different from controls, and fetal and noenatal health was unaffected, suggesting no long-term impairment of zinc homeostasis.[1298] It is interesting that in apparently healthy menstruating women, whether in the luteal or follicular phase, plasma zinc does not vary appreciably, suggesting that *endogenous* steroids do no significantly alter zinc status.[189] This suggests that the effects of corticosteroids on zinc excretion are very much dose-dependent.

E. Anticonvulsants

In animals, anticonvulsant therapy is associated with symptoms similar to that of zinc deficiency, e.g., anorexia, teratogenic effects during pregnancy, and mood changes. In humans, no differences in plasma zinc were reported in either hospitalized or well-controlled ambulatory epileptics on phenytoin and/or phenobarbitone.[1430] Recently, however, Simpson and Bryce-Smith[1472] have shown that anticonvulsants can be responsible for cutaneous symptoms of zinc deficiency in humans.

F. Other

6-Azauridine, which is used in the treatment of psoriasis, has been shown to increase urinary zinc excretion.[1479]

The antitubercular drug, ethambutol, has been associated with visual failure in animals due to its effects on the retina and dismyelinating effects on the optic nerve. However, in humans, its use at the therapeutic dose (>25 mg/kg) has been shown to have no effect on plasma zinc.[220]

The anticancer drugs methotrexate and 6-mercaptopurine have been reported to decrease appetite and cause hypogeusia and dermal lesions, all of which were resolved with 220 mg/day zinc sulfate.[370] 6-Mercaptopurine and its analogs, including azothioprine, are purine derivatives with sulfhydryl groups that might complex with zinc. The immunosuppressive effects of these drugs[622] might therefore be attributable to zinc chelation and excretion.

Histidine has been shown to increase zinc excretion in humans and induce a syndrome of zinc deficiency characterized by anorexia and taste and smell dysfunction.[719] Schechter and Prakash,[1419] on the other hand, found no effect of histidine on zinc metabolism or appetite for food.

The decrease in plasma zinc subsequent to a myocardial infarction was first described by Wacker et al.[1665] Zinc in the injured tissue has also been shown to decrease after a myocardial infarction.[1712] It is one of the classical examples of trauma-induced hypozincemia[1019,1290,1769] (reviewed by Lindeman et al.[1004]). The transient nature of this phenomenon and its possible diagnostic usefulness have been discussed.[1019]

V. SURGERY/BURNS

As discussed in Chapter 4, the trauma of surgery or burns usually precipitates hypozincemia and hyperzincuria. This is a *physiological* response to the trauma and is probably elicited in part by increased corticosteroid release and induction of metallothionein. In healthy individuals, it is a transient event and does not pose a threat to long-term zinc homeostasis.

VI. SUMMARY

Acute zinc depletion is not clinically important unless subclinical secondary zinc depletion is also present, e.g., in alcoholism or other chronic diseases (Chapter 4). Acute zinc depletion caused by acute infection, temporary drug use, or surgery will disappear spontaneously without requiring zinc therapy. Should the condition or drug use become chronic, however, secondary zinc depletion could arise, e.g., after prolonged hospitalization, diuretic, or alcohol use.

Chapter 6

ALTERED ZINC METABOLISM OF UNKNOWN ETIOLOGY

I. INTRODUCTION

Based on our current knowledge, the etiology of some conditions in which zinc metabolism is altered cannot readily be categorized according to the scheme outlined in Chapters 3, 4, and 5. Nevertheless, the association between hypozincemia and a certain condition, e.g., rheumatoid arthritis, may be sufficiently well known that mention of it here is warranted. This chapter deals both with hypozincemia and increased tissue zinc levels whose etiology is currently unknown.

II. HYPOZINCEMIA

In view of the accepted relationship between stressful conditions and hypozincemia, it may be that the hypozincemia associated with cardiovascular, endocrine and central nervous disease, and rheumatoid arthritis is due to increased steroid levels and zinc mobilization to the liver. However, this has not actually been established in any of the following disease conditions.

A. Cardiovascular

Blood pressure regulation is apparently connected with zinc metabolism. In young normotensive adults, plasma zinc levels have been reported to vary inversely with blood pressure.[1103,1104,1608] In essential hypertension, Thind and Fischer[1608] showed plasma zinc levels were normal, but in patients with renal artery stenosis or renal parenchymal disease, plasma zinc was significantly decreased. Zinc and blood pressure have been linked through cadmium; an increased plasma cadmium to zinc ratio[1609] as well as increased zinc excretion[1094] have been found in hypertensives.

In the vascular diseases, atherosclerosis obliterans, thromboangitis obliterans, and Takayasu's disease (low pulse in the upper torso due to the obliteration of major arteries), serum zinc levels have been reported as below normal.[85] In patients in whom post-morten diagnosis of peripheral vascular disease was made, the zinc concentration of the aorta was shown to vary inversely as the degree of atherosclerosis. The aorta zinc levels did not correlate with serum zinc levels.[1333] In view of the chronic and often terminal nature of these vascular diseases, the alteration in zinc metabolism is undoubtedly multifactorial.

B. Endocrine Disease

A possible relationship between the glucagonoma syndrome and zinc depletion was suggested by Horrobin and Cunnane.[776] This was based on the similarities between them, including diabetes, weight loss, psychiatric disturbance, and skin rash. However, Amon et al.[45] could not detect zinc depletion in this syndrome.

C. Central Nervous Disease

Serum zinc levels have been reported for various central nervous disorders including Down's syndrome, autism, schizophrenia, multiple sclerosis, and Sjogren-Larsson syndrome. In Down's syndrome, plasma zinc depletion has been reported,[673] but that has been more recently contested.[1068,1186] In Sjogren-Larsson syndrome, a single report of zinc measurement has shown a lack of change with respect to healthy and neurological controls.[848] No change in brain zinc was found by Greiner et al.[641] in a study of schizophrenia. Plasma zinc levels have been reported to be normal[410,1694] or low[1235,1738] in multiple sclerosis.

In childhood autism and hyperkinesis, zinc levels have been reported as unchanged[840] or decreased.[947] The beneficial effect of supplemental zinc in autism[947] suggests that the lack of change in plasma zinc may be misleading.

Low serum zinc levels have been reported in treated epileptics.[101] Anticonvulsant drugs induce zinc deficiency in animals (see Chapter 5) and have also been reported to be responsible for dermatological symptoms of zinc deficiency in humans.[1472] It is therefore possible that low serum zinc in epileptics may be a result of drug treatment.

D. Arthritis

Plasma zinc levels have been reported to be low in rheumatoid arthritis[1191] and to be related to the degree of osteoporosis.[895] Synovial fluid zinc levels have been shown to differ significantly in three types of arthritis (higher in rheumatoid than psoriatric arthritis, but lower in osteoarthritis than in the other types). The synovial fluid values did not correlate with plasma zinc.[37]

Low plasma zinc in arthritis may be a reflection of (1) low plasma albumin,[107] (2) steroid treatment, or (3) chronic inflammation.[894] Cimmino et al.[288] claim that no study to date has clearly demonstrated zinc depletion in rheumatoid or psoriatic arthritis. This may be due in part to the occurrence of spontaneous remissions. That spontaneous remissions in rheumatoid arthritis would affect plasma zinc is suggested by the normal plasma zinc levels also reported in this disease.[99] Longitudinal studies of plasma zinc would clarify this possibility.

E. Diabetes

Altered zinc metabolism in diabetes has been reported, but the findings have not been uniform, hence its classification here (reviewed by Donaldson and Rennert[406]). Diabetes mellitus has been associated with hypozincemia,[18,1065,1282] hyperzincemia,[1065] and normal plasma zinc levels.[274] In noninsulin-dependent diabetes mellitus, Kinlaw et al.[908] reported 25% of the patients they studied had hypozincemia and hyperzincuria related to proteinuria.

F. Inherited Diseases

Klinefelter's syndrome is a sex-linked syndrome that is characterized by hypogonadism, fibrosis of the seminiferous tubules, and impaired Leydig cell function. Konczewska[925] has suggested the possibility of zinc depletion in such individuals. Children with phenylketonuria have been reported to have low plasma zinc, which may be a function of the semisynthetic diets containing low zinc or marginal zinc nutriture.[14] Aspartylglucosaminuria is a disease of impaired glycoprotein metabolism and reduced elasticity in connective tissue. Copper has been shown to be elevated in hair and zinc and low in plasma and urine.[1175]

III. INCREASED TISSUE ZINC LEVELS

It is unusual that tissue zinc levels are elevated in the absence of increased zinc intake, although this has been reported in a sufficient number of conditions to warrant their discussion.

A. Variant Acrodermatitis Enteropathica (AE)

Variant forms of AE have been reported in which the symptoms were indistinguishable from those of AE except for tissue zinc levels. In one case, zinc levels in serum have been reported to be normal[945] and in another case, zinc in hair, serum and skin were significantly elevated.[581] In both forms, the response to zinc supplementation was an improvement in clinical symptoms and in the latter case tissue zinc decreased toward normal. In spite of the normal or elevated zinc levels, Krieger et al.[946] have classified the cases they have seen as variant AE since, without the zinc supplementation, clinical symptoms of AE persist. These

Table 13
DISEASES IN WHICH ERYTHROCYTE ZINC HAS BEEN SHOWN TO BE SIGNIFICANTLY INCREASED

Pernicious anemia
Chronic pancreatitis
Retinitis pigmentosa
Essential hypertension
Hypothyroidism
Multiple sclerosis
Uremia
Duchenne muscular dystrophy

cases suggest that tissue zinc levels are not necessarily an index of zinc availability and that intracellular or transport ligands are vital to maintain zinc availability.

B. Multiple Sclerosis

In multiple sclerosis, zinc has been reported as increased in erythrocytes,[410,753,756] whole blood,[1359] and brain.[325] The possibility has not yet been discussed, but it may be speculated that multiple sclerosis involves localized zinc toxicity in neural tissue.

C. Genetic Hyperzincemia

A case of familial benign hyperzincemia has been discribed in a black American family. In the family members, serum zinc levels were in the region of 300 μg/dℓ in the absence of obvious exogenous zinc contamination or toxicity.[1483,1490] It was speculated and later confirmed[490] that increased binding of zinc to albumin, a major zinc transport protein, may have been partially responsible. The cause of such increased binding should be investigated; it might reveal basic mechanisms of peripheral zinc availability from albumin.

D. Increased Erythrocyte Zinc

An increase in brain, erythrocyte, and urinary zinc has been observed in Pick's disease.[302] The atrophy of the brain in this disease might account for the increase in brain zinc, but would not necessarily have a direct bearing on erythrocyte or urinary zinc.

Increased erythrocyte zinc has been reported in association with other diseases as well (see Table 13). In only one of these diseases (multiple sclerosis) has the increase in erythrocyte zinc been localized. In multiple sclerosis, the increase in erythrocyte zinc is exclusively in the membrane lipid.[753] It would be of considerable value to establish whether this is also the case in the other diseases with elevated erythrocyte zinc and would also help establish the usefulness of erythrocyte zinc measurements in the assessment of zinc status (see Chapter 3).

One observation that may have a possible bearing on the increase in erythrocyte zinc in the conditions shown in Table 6 (Chapter 4) is the effect of oleic acid (18:1n-9) on erythrocyte zinc uptake; Kruckeberg et al.[952] reported that 75 m*M* oleic acid increased 65-zinc uptake by erythrocytes in vitro. Although no relationship between the erythrocyte content of oleic acid and diseases such as multiple sclerosis has yet been reported, the role of altered lipid or fatty acid metabolism in altering erythrocyte zinc metabolism should be considered a distinct possibility.

E. Fetal Malformations

The zinc content of umbilical cord serum has been shown to be nearly twice the control values in cases of spina bifida and anencephaly. In addition, a higher affinity of zinc for α_2

macroglobulin was also noted.[1765] The possibility was considered that folate may be protective in neural tube defects, in part by increasing zinc excretion, a possibility already experimentally supported in humans.[1134]

Significantly elevated zinc in the amniotic fluid has been reported in association with neural tube defects.[1241] In these cases, amniotic fluid zinc and α-fetoprotein were highly and significantly correlated. Fetal serum zinc levels were not correlated with fetal outcome.

F. Other

Henkin et al.[716] recently reported elevated uptake of zinc-69m in the liver and erythrocytes of patients with adrenocortical insufficiency in whom steroid treatment was used. The increase in liver zinc may have been due to induction of metallothionein by the steroid treatment.

Aitken[30] showed that the zinc-to-calcium ratio in bone increased with age and suggested that because this ratio is also increased in osteoporosis, it might be a disease characterized in part by relative zinc accumulation in the bone.

At present, the most likely explanation for elevated levels of zinc in serum or other body fluids (excluding urine) is an increase in the affinity of albumin for zinc.[490] The possibility also exists that changes in lipid or fatty acid metabolism may contribute to elevated zinc in tissues, particularly the erythrocytes.

One possible exception is the apparent association between ''fifth day fits'' and acute zinc depletion.[607] Goldberg and Sheehy[607] noted lower zinc in the cerebrospinal fluid (CSF) of neontes dying of convulsions of unknown etiology than in infants with fits of known etiology. All cases of fifth day fits had been breast-fed and were apparently normal.

IV. ALTERED RESPONSE TO ZINC

In the presence of added zinc, homogenates of human prostate from patients with benign prostatic hypertrophy compared to controls have been shown to produce significantly more 5 α-reduced metabolites of testosterone.[1475] Since testosterone increases zinc retention,[241] increased levels of zinc in the prostate[1474] may be related to the greater production of testosterone metabolites in patients with benign prostatic hypertrophy.

V. SUMMARY

One of the most interesting aspects of altered zinc metabolism is that of increased erythrocyte zinc. It occurs in endocrine disease, CNS disease, uremia, and hypertension. The mechanism has not been explored, nor has the localization of the increased zinc within the erythrocyte. Peripheral tissue zinc depletion may be present in these conditions as exemplified by variant AE; tissue zinc levels are normal or increased, but clinical zinc depletion exists and responds to zinc supplementation. More information is therefore required to understand abnormalities of zinc utilization and mechanisms causing the peripheral sequestration of zinc.

Chapter 7

THERAPEUTIC USES OF ZINC

I. INTRODUCTION

While it is generally accepted that zinc supplementation will only work in cases of demonstrable *preexisting* zinc deficiency or depletion,[1414] that situation presumes that zinc depletion is always demonstrable when it is present. As discussed in Chapters 3 and 4, providing definitive evidence of zinc depletion can sometimes be a tall order. Clinical response to zinc supplementation is therefore still the most reliable indicator of whether preexisting zinc depletion may have been present. Such a clinical response may have no relationship to the biochemical indexes of zinc status. A classic example was the clinical improvement in a case of acrodermatitis enteropathica (AE) in which skin, hair, and plasma zinc levels were *elevated*.[581] The diagnosis and decision to supplement with zinc had been made on the basis of clinical symptoms not, tissue zinc levels. Had the reverse been true, zinc might never have been tried. This case is relatively extreme, but illustrates the point that clinical response is the most reliable index of true zinc availability.

The following conditions/diseases are representative of the spectrum of zinc's clinical usefulness.

II. ACRODERMATITIS ENTEROPATHICA

The completely successful treatment of this otherwise lethal disease characterized by skin lesions, alopecia, chronic infection, irritability, and gastrointestinal distress (in short, the symptoms predictive of zinc deficiency) using zinc was probably crucial to the acceptance of the clinical importance of zinc. This condition demonstrated that a clinical syndrome of apparently pure zinc deficiency could exist independently from the association of zinc depletion with chronic infection, alcoholism, or malnutrition, in all of which the zinc depletion is of multiple etiology. The role of zinc in AE was first described by Moynahan and Barnes,[1155-1157] but subsequently by many others.[647,682]

Not only are the clinical symptoms alleviated completely by zinc, including the skin lesions, diarrhea, alopecia, and gaze aversion,[947] but the biochemical defects are also corrected: disappearance of lysosomal inclusion bodies in the intestinal epithelium[864,891] and abnormalities in fatty acids, e.g., linoleic acid and serum lipids.[357,682,1148,1669] The latter example supports the observations made prior to those of Moynahan that EFA metabolism is defective in AE[236] (see Chapter 13). The dose of zinc used in the treatment of AE must be individually titrated because copper-dependent normocytic anemia has been reported in a man receiving zinc (45 mg/day) for AE.[767]

III. DERMATOLOGICAL CONDITIONS

Consistent with the effectiveness of zinc in curing the skin lesions in AE are its effects in other dermatological conditions (reviewed by Norris[1201]) including the dry, atrophic eczematous skin in kwashiorkor,[613] leg ulcers and bed sores,[637,1054,1231,1567] oral ulcers,[1113] acne vulgaris,[333,527,747,1121,1652] Lines of Beau on the fingernails,[1692] complexed with pyrithione for dandruff,[1056] skin lesions in leprosy,[1066,1067] herpetic keratitis,[395,441] and dermatitis in both the aged[1702] and in alcoholics.[466] Part of the beneficial effect of zinc in acne might be attributable to its effect in reducing sebum secretion.[394] This, in turn, may be related to zinc's inhibition of bacterial lipase, thereby reducing free fatty acids in sebum and on the skin surface.[1340]

It should be recognized that in the majority of conditions just described, the response to zinc supplementation may be due to chronic zinc depletion of multiple etiology. Hence the lesion itself does not necessarily specifically benefit from the additional zinc. Rather, the zinc supplementation helps to restore normal zinc nutriture and cell-mediated immunity. As a consequence of this, zinc contributes to healing skin lesions.

Although alopecia caused by AE or penicillamine treatment[919] are both corrected by zinc supplementation, Ead[435] showed no beneficial effect of 100 mg, zinc per day for 3 months in a double-blind trial in patients with alopecia areata. Zinc (100 mg elemental zinc per day for 10 to 65 days) was not found to be of any benefit in acute tropical ulcers, even though serum zinc levels were initially low.[1683] Perspiration odor has been reported to be significantly reduced by 20 mg of zinc per day (as zinc sulfate).[1439] Zinc was also not found to be of any benefit in epidermolysis bullosa.[1693] As discussed earlier (Chapter 4), the reported beneficial effect of zinc in enhancing the rate of wound healing may be indirect. In healthy individuals of normal zinc status, zinc supplementation has no effect on the rate of wound healing.

IV. WILSON'S DISEASE

Brewer and Hoogenraad and their respective colleagues have separately demonstrated the therapeutic effectiveness of zinc as an alternative treatment to penicillamine in Wilson's disease.[179,180,183,184,745,764,766,769-772] Both groups have demonstrated that the effectiveness of zinc in enhancing copper excretion (200 to 600 mg of zinc sulfate per day) was generally without significant side effect. Their results suggest that copper toxicity in Wilson's disease is partly related to its inhibitory effect on zinc metabolism. The beneficial and nontoxic effect of zinc in Wilson's disease is particularly helpful in those patients who react adversely to penicillamine, a chelator which, in addition to removing copper, also binds zinc.

Walshe,[1676] who observed no beneficial effect of zinc supplementation in three cases of Wilson's disease, has recently cautioned that zinc supplementation cannot always be considered effective due to the variable nature of Wilson's disease. This caution has been echoed byVan Caille-Bertrand et al.[1642] who nevertheless had success using 100 to 150 mg zinc per day in a Wilson's disease patient intolerant of penicillamine.

V. GASTROINTESTINAL DISORDERS

Gastric ulcers have been reported to heal significantly more rapidly in patients treated with 220 mg zinc sulfate three times daily as compared with a placebo.[573,1113,1172] These initial observations have been supported by three more recent publications. In a double-blind crossover trial, zinc acexamate (1800 mg/day for 30 days) was shown to heal duodenal ulcers[36] and to be as effective as ranitidine (300 mg/day).[1651] Zinc acexamate has also been shown to inhibit the occurrence of reserpine-induced ulcers in rats.[1276]

Zinc was not shown to be of any additional benefit to established treatment in ulcerative colitis.[418] In celiac disease, patients not responding to the removal of gluten from the diet were noted to respond positively after zinc was given orally (dose not specified).[1018] Improved retinal function in chronic pancreatitis has been demonstrated following zinc treatment.[1618]

VI. ALCOHOLISM

Zinc sulfate has been shown to reverse[1150] or to have no effect on[1695] night blindness in cirrhotics. In view of the longtime course required to reestablish retinal reductase in zinc-deficient rats,[312] the discrepancies noted above may depend on the time period of the studies. Taste acuity in alcoholics has been reported to be improved by zinc supplementation.[1695]

Reding et al.[1344] have recently shown that the enzyme defects in hepatic encephalopathy caused by alcoholism are partly corrected by zinc supplementation. Zinc also helped to normalize blood ammonia. McClain and Su[1085] have reviewed the role of zinc deficiency in alcoholism and noted its beneficial effect on the skin lesions in alcoholics. Dermal lesions associated with alcohol-induced malnutrition have been reported to be cured by zinc.[442,466] In view of the chronic zinc depletion frequently present in alcoholics, dose and period of zinc administration are probably crucial in determining its effectiveness.

VII. SICKLE-CELL DISEASE

The therapeutic assessment of zinc in sickle-cell anemia was based on (1) its ability to increase the oxygen affinity of erythrocytes,[1218] (2) its enhancement of erythrocyte filterability (both effects shown in vitro), (3) erythrocyte survival (in a rat model),[1429] and (4) the fact that zinc depletion through increased urinary excretion has been reported in sickle-cell disease.[187,1302]

The effectiveness of zinc in sickle-cell disease has been with regard to (1) reduction of pain during crisis,[186,187] (2) reduction of plasma bilirubin and lactic dehydrogenase (indication of reduced hemolysis), (3) increased erythrocyte filterability,[182,185] (4) decreased hyperammonemia.[180,1302,1318] (5) improved growth,[1306] and (6) improved immune function.[1047] In adolescents with sickle-cell anemia, 15 mg zinc acetate (three times daily for 1 year) has been shown to increase weight gain.[1306]

VIII. ARTHRITIS

Effects of zinc supplementation have been studied in two types of arthritis: rheumatoid[1466-1468] and psoriatic.[291] In both types, 220 mg zinc sulfate three times daily for 4 to 6 weeks was effective for relief of stiffness, joint pain, and swelling, and also reduced walking time and use of analgesics. These effects have been suggested to involve the stimulation by zinc of the antiinflammatory prostaglandin, prostaglandin E_1.[780] Cimmino et al.[288] have argued that zinc is not an effective antirheumatic agent and that no studies to date have demonstrated that either rheumatoid or psoriatic arthritis are conditions of zinc depletion.

IX. EHLERS-DANLOS SYNDROME

Ehlers-Danlos syndrome is genetically inherited and presents with skin fragility and hyperelasticity and loose-jointedness. Low plasma zinc has been reported.[904] A case of Ehlers-Danlos syndrome has also been reported as responding to zinc supplementation.[459] In view of the role of zinc in collagen cross-linking (see Chapter 13), zinc depletion was thought of as a possible complication in spite of normal zinc in the serum. Lenard and Lombeck,[989] in a study of two cases of Ehlers-Danlos syndrome, found neither low plasma zinc nor a beneficial effect of zinc supplementation.

X. PORPHYRIA

Zinc excretion in the urine is increased in acute intermittent porphyria. Zinc supplementation has been reported to alleviate the muscle pain present during relapse.[1368,1369] The mechanism by which this occurs has been suggested to be due to removal of the lactic acid in the tissue by the zinc-dependent enzyme, lactate dehydrogenase.[1368] In erythropoeitic porphyria, zinc is protective against radiation-induced erythema and hemolysis.[203]

XI. INFERTILITY

Zinc depletion in males is associated with both reduced sperm count and motility and with impotence. Since sperm motility is directly correlated with semen zinc concentration, zinc supplementation has been tested as a means of reversing male infertility. Zinc has been demonstrated as an effective treatment for restoring sperm motility and count.[697,1283]

For impotence associated with chronic renal failure, reports of the effectiveness of zinc are conflicting; Rodger et al.[1365] report no benefit while others have found that 50 mg zinc per day for 6 months significantly reduces uremia-induced impotence.[66,1040]

For intentional female infertility (contraception), intrauterine devices containing copper or zinc are considered highly effective.[1766]

XII. HYPOGEUSIA

Zinc has been reported to improve hypogeusia originating in association with cysteinuria,[715] uremia,[1543] anorexia nervosa,[1387] Weber-Christian disease,[1364] pica,[683] chronic pancreatitis,[1616] and treatment of systemic sclerosis with the zinc-binding amino acid, histidine.[721]

XIII. GROWTH RETARDATION

Dietary zinc deficiency is a major component of growth retardation and malnutrition both in the developed[684] and underdeveloped[611] countries. The importance of zinc as part of the nutritional therapy for growth-retarded children cannot be overemphasized. It improves growth, protein assimilation, energy utilization, immunocompetence, and dermal condition.[610,611,967,1675] Alcohol-induced malnutrition is also responsive to zinc supplementation.[466] It should nevertheless be pointed out that even in an apparently obvious situation for zinc supplementation in growth retardation, alone it is not always effective: growth-retarded Australian aboriginal children with low plasma zinc did not increase weight or height in relation to supplementation with 20 or 40 mg zinc per day over 10 months.[1493] Therefore, where energy or essential nutrients other than zinc are limiting, zinc supplementation *alone* cannot be expected to stimulate growth.

Growth retardation in premature babies has been documented and associated with low zinc levels in breast milk. Such cases have been shown to respond to zinc supplementation,[21,25,955] but the zinc must be added to the milk; zinc supplementation of the mothers does *not* increase the zinc content of the milk.[503,943] In constitutionally short children (growth-hormone deficient) oral zinc (220 mg/day) also significantly increases growth.[297,588]

XIV. IMMUNE FUNCTION

The functional role of zinc in the immune system is not understood. However, its importance for adequate cell-mediated immunity is universally accepted (reviewed by Cunningham-Rundles,[368] Fraker et al.,[558] Good et al.[621]). Thymic function is especially sensitive to zinc nutriture. Three aspects of immune function appear to benefit from zinc supplementation: (1) clinically obvious chronic immunodeficiency, e.g., in malnutrition, (2) subclinical chronic immunodeficiency, e.g., in the elderly, and (3) acute infection.

Thymic atrophy is a feature of childhood malnutrition and rapidly responds to zinc supplementation (4 mg/ℓ in a high-energy liquid diet).[612,614] Reduced natural killer cell activity in experimental human zinc deficiency is restored to normal after zinc supplementation.[1599] Inflammatory nodules, panniculitis and low serum gamma globulins in Weber-Christian disease all respond to zinc supplementation.[1364]

Decreased immunocompetence in conjunction with zinc depletion in Down's syndrome has been reported to respond to zinc supplementation. Decreased lymphocyte responsiveness, skin hypersensitivity, and neutrophil chemotaxis were all significantly improved after 2 months of treatment with 135 mg zinc per day.[147] In vitro, 1 mol zinc per liter can restore the depressed serum thymic factor activity seen in Down's syndrome and in the aged.[488]

Individuals with recurrent furunculosis (boils) have been shown to have low serum zinc.[193] Given 135 mg zinc per day, serum zinc became normalized, existing lesions regressed, and new ones did not appear. Chronic inflammatory conditions, including granulomas and pilonidal cysts have been shown to respond to zinc supplementation.[165]

The high zinc content of prostatic fluid has been suggested as one reason why males are less susceptible than females to urinary tract infection.[491] Zinc supplementation in cases of bacterial prostatitis was shown to increase plasma zinc, but not to change prostatic fluid zinc levels.

Alcoholics have been shown to have a decreased delayed hypersensitivity response to skin antigen challenge which indicates impaired cellular immune function. Zinc supplementation (200 mg/day for 2 months) has been recently reported to augment the delayed hypersensitivity response by 50% in alcoholics.[965]

In a study of the potential need for zinc supplementation of the elderly, Duchateau et al.[420] supplemented asymptomatic volunteers (over 70 years of age) with 220 mg zinc sulfate twice daily for 1 month. After this period, the number of circulating lymphocytes, delayed skin hypersensitivity, and IgG response to tetanus vaccine were all increased. Lymphocyte mitogen response, however, was unchanged compared to basal levels. Duchateau et al.[420] concluded that the elderly would benefit from zinc supplementation even if they were in apparently good health. It was their opinion that since the subjects did not have overt zinc deficiency (the only criterion assayed was plasma zinc), the effect of zinc as an immunostimulant was pharmacological. In view of the inadequacy of plasma zinc measurement in the diagnosis of clinical zinc deficiency, this conclusion remains debatable,[60] i.e., since there was a beneficial effect of zinc supplementation on the immune system, this response was a better indicator of zinc status than those conventional indexes used, e.g., plasma zinc level.

In a double-blind trial, zinc gluconate lozenges were shown to be an effective treatment for the common cold.[440] Zinc supplementation in tablet form was not effective, but the sucking of zinc-containing lozenges that released zinc into the oral cavity was effective. Zinc may be effective against rhinoviruses because of its ability to prevent viral replication.[585,1455]

In acute lymphoblastic leukemia, the use of immunosuppressive drugs such as azothioprine and methotrexate is associated with increased bacterial and viral infection. Zinc supplementation (0.02 mg/kg for 8 days) was shown to reduce these infections and to increase T-cell count in such patients.[1685] In Hodgkin's disease patients not responding adequately to skin antigen challenge were shown to have lower plasma zinc than controls,[247] indirectly confirming similar observations seen by others.

XV. LIPID METABOLISM

Controversy exists as to the effect of zinc supplementation on cholesterol levels in healthy subjects (further details in Chapter 13). Hooper et al.[773] have reported that, in males, 400 mg zinc sulfate per day for 5 weeks causes a significant decrease in serum high-density lipoprotein (HDL) cholesterol from pretreatment values of 40.5 mg/dℓ to post treatment values of 30.1 mg/dℓ. They found no change in low-density lipoprotein cholesterol. Since it is considered desirable to *increase* the level of HDL cholesterol, this effect of zinc supplementation was interpreted as detrimental. Goodwin et al.[623] have recently implicated exercise as an additional variable influencing the effect of zinc on HDL cholesterol. In individuals >60 years old, HDL cholesterol varied with the amount of exercise. In individuals taking 15 mg zinc per day, the correlation between exercise and HDL cholesterol no longer existed, but on discontinuation of zinc, HDL cholesterol rose and was again correlated with exercise.

In a similar study, but in women given 100 mg zinc per day (same as 440 mg zinc sulfate) for 8 weeks, Freeland-Graves et al.[565] found no change in HDL cholesterol. Since the dose was the same as that used by Hooper et al.,[773] and it was given over a longer period in the study of Freeland-Graves et al.,[565] a sex difference may be invoked to account for the discrepancy in these results.

Conceptually, however, the need for supplementation of "healthy" individuals with 100 mg zinc per day is hard to justify. Thus, the clinical relevance of a drop in HDL cholesterol due to zinc supplementation at pharmacological doses is not clear. That free-living individuals may voluntarily consume such an extreme amount of zinc is another issue.

XVI. VASCULAR DISEASE

Henzel et al.[724,725] have reported on the therapeutic use of zinc in atherosclerosis. Zinc was apparently beneficial for improving circulation in the limbs. Since zinc has also been shown to correct venous leg ulcers resulting partly from poor circulation,[637] its use for this purpose should be further investigated.

Venous leg ulcers have been reported in association with secondary hypozincemia.[635] These ulcers are usually a complication of prolonged hospitalization which, in itself, can lead to zinc depletion. Nevertheless, zinc sulfate (220 mg three times daily for 1 month) has been shown to completely heal leg ulcers.[661,820]

XVII. SCHIZOPHRENIA

Pfeiffer and Cott[1273] have reported that, in combination with manganese, zinc has a beneficial effect on the EEG in schizophrenics. Decreased plasma copper, increased urinary copper, and increased plasma zinc were also observed.[1274] Zinc alone (50 mg/day) reduced the abnormally high coefficient of variation and mean amplitude of the EEG in schizophrenics.[616]

XVIII. UREMIA

Zinc depletion associated with uremia has been shown to be reversible by zinc supplementation (25 mg zinc three times daily for 6 months). Symptoms corrected included impotence, defective taste, low plasma zinc, high plasma ammonia, and improved lymphocyte function and viability.[64,65,1040,1042,1197,1543] Hyperprolactinemia in uremic men is also considerably reduced by 50 mg zinc per day.[1039]

XIX. PRIMARY BILIARY CIRRHOSIS

In one case of primary biliary cirrhosis, liver copper was reduced and decreased histological abnormalities in the liver were observed 18 months after treatment with 200 mg zinc sulfate three times daily.[768] Enzymes suggestive of liver function (serum glutamic-oxaloacetic transaminase (SGOT) and alkaline phosphatase) were not significantly changed after zinc. Olsson[1227] found no beneficial effect of zinc in primary biliary cirrhosis.

XX. OTHER

Dental plaque growth has been reported to be inhibited by zinc.[695] Mouthwashes containing

17 to 31 mM zinc, as the sulfate or phenolsulfonate, have been demonstrated to inhibit plaque growth. Zinc is bactericidal and accumulates in the plaque.[644]

Zinc supplementation has been shown to be of benefit in the treatment of senile cataract.[704]

In a study of childhood hyperkinesis, Krischer[947] observed that 90% had elevated serum copper, that serum zinc was generally decreased, and that zinc supplementation was dramatically effective in correcting the symptoms.

Radiation-induced tissue damage in cancer patients has been reported to be reduced by zinc supplementation.[1732]

Collipp[296] has reported that obese children have lower plasma zinc than nonobese children and that they lose weight when given 100 mg zinc per day for 3 months followed by 100 mg zinc per week.

In a double-blind, crossover trial of zinc supplementation in healthy adults (135 mg/day for 14 days), muscle strength was shown to be significantly increased, an effect suggested to be related to a change in glucose metabolism or lactic dehydrogenase activity.

XXI. SUMMARY

Zinc has a wide range of therapeutic uses, many of which are not understood. Many of its effects are in conditions in which zinc depletion has not been demonstrated, but in which there is an abnormality of zinc utilization. The wide range of the apparent therapeutic effectiveness of zinc is understandable in view of evidence accumulating to the effect that it has an important role in the structure and function of membranes. Nevertheless, the lack of good controls in most of the studies reported here requires that caution be used in interpreting the data. The point in presenting this spectrum of information about the effects of zinc is that much of it has never been reported outside the primary literature; by reviewing it at least once, further evidence may be sought which will help solidify or refute these results.

In considering the possible mechanism of the therapeutic effects reported here, one is reminded of the fact that the best evidence suggests that homeostatic regulation of zinc metabolism is primarily at the level of the gut (see Chapter 9). The therapeutic effects of zinc may therefore involve making available additional zinc for peripheral utilization. Variant AE is one example of such a possibility in which variables indicating zinc nutriture may be normal, but in which peripheral zinc availability is inadequate.

Chapter 8

ZINC TOXICITY

I. INTRODUCTION

Zinc toxicity occurs at two levels: (1) as "side effects" of zinc supplementation and (2) during toxic intake due to industrial or accidental exposure.

II. ZINC SUPPLEMENTATION

Of increasing clinical significance are the side effects of zinc when it is given as a supplement for therapeutic reasons. The symptoms generally include nausea and gastrointestinal distress, but may also include bleeding gastric ulcers.[332,648,1145] Zinc is well-known to compete with copper for gut absorption sites and blood transport proteins (reviewed by Cunnane,[341] Chapter 15). As such, it is not surprising that supplemental zinc decreases plasma copper in humans and has been shown to shift the copper-to-zinc ratio in plasma from about 1.2 to 0.5 to 0.7.[8] Anemia due to copper depletion has been reported as one of the consequences of zinc therapy.[251,767,1249,1275,1295,1304,1541] The dose of zinc required to produce this effect varies from 150 to 5000 mg/day.

Zinc given in combination with other substances has also been reported to induce toxic effects. The toxic effects of the dandruff shampoo containing zinc-pyrithione, e.g., paralysis and neuropathy, have generally been attributed to the pyrithione, but zinc may have facilitated its toxicity.[112,1388,1496] Whitehouse et al.[1720] have observed that a zinc-penicillamine complex was lethal when administered to rats (50 mg/kg i.p. for 4 days). Caution was therefore advised concerning the concomitant use of zinc with penicillamine.

Diabetic patients have been reported to show a relatively high (56%) allergic reaction to complexes of zinc with insulin, whereas zinc-free insulin is generally without side effect.[504]

Hydralazine given for high blood pressure has been shown to cause a syndrome similar to systemic lupus erythematosis with symptoms including leg ulcers and arthritis. Elemental zinc given at 135 mg/day to patients on hydralazine caused a facial eczematous rash, fever, and gastrointestinal distress, which was relieved when the hydralazine was discontinued.[528]

Chandra[251] has shown that 150 mg zinc three times daily for 6 weeks reduced lymphocyte response to phytohemagglutinin (PHA) and decreased phagocytosis by polymorphonuclear leukocytes. Natural killer cell activity in mice has also been shown to be decreased by zinc supplementation,[1558] suggesting that the immunological reactions observed in individuals given high zinc levels may be due to the zinc itself.

These case reports have so far been relatively rare and therefore support the concept that zinc is generally nontoxic in amounts up to about five times the daily requirement (15 mg/day).[1178] Nevertheless the incidence of inadvertent zinc toxicity will undoubtedly increase as we become more aware of the symptoms.

In those individuals who cannot tolerate modest therapeutic doses of zinc (about 50 mg elemental zinc per day), zinc depletion may not be the cause of the symptoms for which the zinc was given. Their intolerance may, therefore, be indicative of very sensitive regulation of zinc balance or excretion easily upset by excess zinc.

In view of the postulated relationship between zinc and prostaglandins,[776] it is interesting that symptoms of zinc and prostaglandin excess are similar, e.g., gastrointestinal distress, diarrhea, nausea, hypotension, fever, and muscle pain. Part of the effect of excess zinc may therefore relate to stimulation of prostaglandin synthesis.

III. INDUSTRIAL/ACCIDENTAL EXPOSURE

Typically, industrial or accidental exposure to zinc causes gastrointestinal distress, diarrhea, nausea, vomiting, muscle pain, and fever. These symptoms have been reported as a consequence of "metal fume fever" which is due to the inhalation of zinc oxide fumes[51,1299] (reviewed by van Reen[1647]) or as a consequence of accidental exposure to zinc i.v.[192] or orally.[1165] Intravenously, zinc toxicity has been reported due to zinc contamination from dialysate during hemodialysis.[18,604] Zinc chloride in the form of welder's flux, when splashed in the eye, is extremely toxic to the lens and cornea and produces an effect similar to that of angle-closure glaucoma.[782] In spite of these well-established toxic effects of zinc, it is considered to be nonmutagenic, noncarcinogenic and nonteratogenic (reviewed by Leonard et al.[992]).

IV. SUMMARY

There is an increasing need to be aware that zinc is not completely nontoxic even in the "therapeutic" dose range (50 to 300 mg/day). Frequently, zinc causes gastrointestinal side effects. It has biphasic effects on many pathways (see Chapter 18) and on the immune system. Its suppression of copper utilization may also be detrimental in the long run.

Part II — Biochemistry

INTRODUCTION

The clinical significance of zinc was described in Part I. Aspects of zinc metabolism and biochemistry of a fundamental nature not specifically related to the clinical role of zinc is discussed in Part II. This includes zinc metabolism, zinc enzymes, zinc deficiency in animals, the relation of zinc to protein, lipid and carbohydrate metabolism, its interactions with the macroelements of vitamins, other trace elements and hormones, and the physiological and pharmacological effects of zinc.

The primary emphasis is on the human aspects of zinc biochemistry, but, in contrast to the clinical half of the book, liberal reference to animals studies will be made. The function of this part of the book is to provide equally a general and relatively up-to-date basis for what is known about the biochemistry of zinc and to bring to light some aspects of the interactions of zinc with other nutrients that are currently underrated but may be of considerable importance for the ultimate understanding of the role of zinc in physiology and pathology.

Chapter 9

ZINC HOMEOSTASIS

I. DIETARY SOURCES

Sources of zinc in some selected foods are shown in Table 14. The primary sources are red meats, seafood, and cereals. Further details on the zinc content of foods can be obtained from the publication *Zinc* by the National Research Council,[1766] *McCance and Widdowson's The Composition of Foods*[1253] by Paul and Southgate, and from Food Surveillance Paper Number 5 by the Ministry of Agriculture, Foods and Fisheries (MAFF).[1036] It is important to remember that the zinc content of raw vegetables, legumes, cereals, and even meat is not retained after cooking. Furthermore, availability of the zinc in various foods may be limited by ligands preventing zinc absorption, e.g., phytate. Hence, it is difficult to estimate the actual absorbed amounts of zinc on the basis of zinc intake calculated from food tables.

II. REQUIREMENT

A. Humans

The National Research Council's (U.S.) Recommended Dietary Allowances (RDA) standard for zinc is one of the most widely cited reference guides to indicate the zinc requirement of humans.[1178] It recommends that adults (male and female) consume 15 mg/day of zinc. Other government advisory bodies have set different recommendations for zinc intake. The Canadian Bureau of Nutritional Sciences[212] has recommended that a lower zinc intake (9 mg/day for adult males and 8 mg/day for females) is safe and adequate. The full range of U.S.- and Canadian-recommended values for zinc intake are shown in Table 15. The World Health Organization Expert Committee on Trace Elements in Human Nutrition has estimated that between 5.5 and 11 mg zinc per day is adequate for normal adults.[1723]

The American values (adults — 15 mg/day) are sometimes viewed as controversial on the basis that amongst an ostensibly healthy population, only a small percentage of individuals achieves that recommended intake of zinc,[1397,1399] particularly vegetarians.[939] The argument therefore is that, *if* the population is healthy, its zinc requirement cannot be as high as is recommended. The lower Canadian, British, and WHO standards would concur with the argument that a zinc intake of 10 mg/day in "normal" adults is sufficient. In Britain, MAFF has determined that the average British diet contains 10.5 mg zinc per day, an amount considered adequate.[1036]

B. Animals

Zinc requirements differ according to the species and sex[1006] and to the type of diet fed. Soy-based diets which contain sufficient phytate to limit zinc absorption increase the zinc requirement. Interactions with other minerals such as calcium[755] and copper[341-343] may also increase zinc requirements.

Environmental factors also affect zinc requirement.[113] Rats maintained in a "germ-free" environment have been reported to have a lower zinc requirement than those in conventional housing with the usual microflora.[1489] As in humans, periods of stress and/or rapid growth, e.g., pregnancy and lactation, represent a greater zinc requirement. The zinc requirement of various animal species is shown in Table 16.

III. TISSUE LEVELS

Zinc is a component of all cells. Its distribution is widely variable depending on the tissue.

Table 14
ZINC CONTENT OF VARIOUS FOODS OR BEVERAGES

	mg zinc per 100 g
Meat	
Beef	
Steak	6.4
Hamburger	4.7
Liver	5.5
Chicken	
White	1.1
Dark	2.8
Heart	4.3
Gizzard	4.1
Pork	3.8
Veal	3.9
Seafood	
Clams	1.7
Crab (steamed)	4.6
Haddock	1.1
Oysters (Atlantic)	79.0
Tuna (canned)	1.1
Dairy products	
Milk	0.3
Cream (50%)	0.4
Cheese	4.0
Eggs	
White	<0.03
Yolk	1.2
Bread	
White	0.6
Rye	1.3
Whole wheat	1.0
Vegetables	
Peas	
Raw	3.2
Boiled	1.0
Potatoes	0.3
Green beans	0.2
Carrots	0.3
Tomatoes	0.2
Rice	
Brown, cooked	0.7
Spinach	1.0
Fruit	
Apricots	0.1
Peaches	0.1
Pears	0.1
Apples	0.05
Bananas	0.3
Seeds/nuts/legumes	
Common beans	
Raw	2.7
Boiled	0.9
Chickpeas	
Raw	2.7
Boiled	1.4

Table 14 (continued)
ZINC CONTENT OF VARIOUS FOODS OR BEVERAGES

Cowpeas	
Raw	3.7
Boiled	1.1
Cereals	
Oatmeal (raw)	3.0
Wheat	3.9
Beverages	
Juices	
Orange	0.1
Apple	0.1
Grapefruit	0.1
Tea	0.02
Coffee	0.03

Adapted from Halsted, J. A., Smith, J. C., Jr., and Irwin, M. I., © *J. Nutr.*, 104, 345, 1974, American Institute of Nutrition. With permission.

Table 15
RECOMMENDED DIETARY ALLOWANCE FOR ZINC INTAKE BY HUMANS

	American[a]		Canadian[b]	
	Age (years)	**mg/day**	**Age (years)**	**mg/day**
Infants	<6 months	3	< 3 months	2
	6—12 months	5	3—12 months	3
Children	1—10	10	1—3	4
			4—6	5
			7—9	6
			10—12	7
Male	>11	15	12—13	8
			>13	9
Females	>11	15	>13	8
Pregnant		20		
Lactating		25		

[a] Data from Reference 1178.
[b] Data from Reference 212.

At present, zinc is typically measured in the whole tissue. The value of such measurements must, however, be questioned. A few studies (see Chapter 2) have described the subcellular distribution of zinc and demonstrated that various organelles, particularly microsomes and nucleoli, are very rich in zinc. Hence, although zinc levels in soft tissues are not markedly decreased in zinc deficiency, subcellular zinc distribution might be significantly altered. Such changes might also be dependent on the ratio of extracellular to intracellular zinc, which is changed in zinc deficiency.[142]

Zinc levels in tissues of humans and two animal species (rat and pig) are shown in Table 17.[674] Values for zinc levels in human blood cells and body fluids are shown in Table 18. Bone appears to be one of the few tissues to consistently have lower zinc content in zinc deficiency. McBean et al.[1076] have reported similar values.

Table 16
ZINC REQUIREMENTS (mg/kg DIET) OF VARIOUS ANIMAL SPECIES

	Protein source	Zinc requirement
Laboratory animals		
Rat	Egg white or casein	12—13
	Soy	19
Mouse[a]		>3
Rabbit		>3
Guinea pig	Casein	12
	Soy	20
Dog	Egg white	>100
Monkey	Casein	15
Ruminants		
Cattle[a]	Egg white	10—14
Sheep[a]	Egg white	15
Pig	Casein	14—20
	Soy	50
Poultry		
Chicken	Casein	12
	Soy	19
Japanese quail		25

[a] Species not extensively studied, so accurate information not available.

Table 17
TISSUE ZINC IN THE HUMAN, RAT, AND PIG[a]

	Human[b]	Rat	Pig
Liver	141—245	101 ± 13	151 ± 12
Kidney	184—230	91 ± 3	98 ± 3
Lung	67—86	81 ± 3	—
Muscle	197—226	45 ± 5	—
Pancreas	115—135	—	140 ± 4
Heart	100	73 ± 16	—
Bone	218	168 ± 8	95 ± 2
Prostate:		—	—
Normal	520	—	—
Hyperplastic	2330	—	—
Malignant	285	—	—
Eye (retina)	571	—	—
Testis	—	176 ± 12	54 ± 2
Esophagus	—	108 ± 17	88 ± 3
Brain	50—65[c]	—	—
Hair	150—250	—	—
Feces (mg/24 hr)	5—10	—	—

[a] Mean ± SD, mg/kg dry wt adapted with permission from Reference 674.
[b] Range.
[c] Adapted from Donaldson, J. T., St. Pierre, J. L., Minnich, L., and Barbeau, A., *Can. J. Biochem.*, 51, 87, 1983.

Table 18
BODY FLUID AND BLOOD CELL LEVELS OF ZINC IN HUMANS

Fluid	Zinc[a]	Refs
Plasma/serum	90—100	1653
Erythrocyte	10—12	893
Leukocyte (μg/g dry)	5	886
Urine (μg/24 hr)	150—650	—
Milk	1.2—3.6,	561
	3—12,	232
	0.1—4	1281
Bile	171 ± 106	1565
Sweat (meq/ℓ)	63	1449
Seminal plasma	692 ± 24	1428
Cerebrospinal fluid	0.03 ± 0.02	19

[a] μg/mℓ (mean ± SD) except as noted.

Levels of zinc in organs of women have been shown to be higher than in males[49] and appear to decline with age.[1742] Tissue levels in various species have been shown to be seasonably variable.[334,539,654,823,824,1243] Accounting for the tissue mass as a percent of the total body weight, percentage organ distribution of total body zinc can be approximated as follows: 60% — muscle, 29% — bone, 2% — liver, 1% — gastrointestinal tract, 1% — skin, 1% — kidney, 1% — brain, 1% — lung, 1% — prostate, and <1% each — other organs.[1766] More complete details on tissue levels of zinc in humans and other species are available elsewhere.[1766]

IV. ABSORPTION

Much of the information concerning the events involved in zinc absorption is limited to that which can be obtained from research in animal models or pathological conditions in humans, e.g., acrodermatitis enteropathica (AE) (see Chapter 5). One of the most widely used models has been the rat intestinal segment, either isolated but perfused *in situ*[384,1492] or isolated and studied as an in vitro preparation.[131,384,1435] In addition, preparations of intestinal mucosal vesicles are attractive because of the possibility of total control of their environment[1108,1163] and the opportunity to differentiate between the fast and slow phases of zinc absorption and their kinetics.[148]

In humans, zinc absorption has typically been studied by measuring its kinetics, following oral ingestion of cold zinc or zinc-65[531,1681] (see also Chapter 4 regarding use of other isotopes). More recently, recovery of intestinal contents at various positions in the gut with the use of a gastroesophageal cannula[1069] has permitted the assessment of the interplay between exogenous and endogenous zinc.

The events involved in zinc absorption have been the subject of several reviews.[113,315,316,318,319,473] Zinc uptake by high molecular weight proteins in the intestinal mucosa is an active process requiring ATP.[384,937]Zinc uptake by low molecular weight proteins, e.g., metallothionein, may be passive.[1442] Zinc uptake by the intestinal cells (enterocytes) is bidirectional (from the intestinal lumen or from the blood supply, the former predominating). In the rat, zinc absorption appears to occur throughout the small intestine. There does not appear to be any agreement on which segment absorbs zinc maximally — the ileum[67,863] or the duodenum.[113,384] Zinc-binding molecules or ligands determine net zinc absorption. Some ligands, e.g., phytate, reduce zinc absorption, while others, e.g., histidine, increase zinc absorption.

Table 19
FACTORS AFFECTING ZINC ABSORPTION

Stimulatory	Inhibitory
Citrate	Alcohol
Picolinate	Phytate
EFAs	Calcium
Prostaglandins?	Oxalic acid
Vitamin D	Copper
Histidine	Iron
Lactoferrin	
Immunoglobulins	
EDTA	
D-Penicillamine	
Zinc deficiency	
Pregnancy	
Wine	
Histamine	

The process of zinc uptake by enterocytes is saturable, and zinc transfer from the enterocyte to the circulation is concentration dependent; both factors may contribute to regulating zinc absorption and homeostasis. The carrier proteins removing zinc at the vascular-enterocyte interface are albumin and/or transferrin.

Four major factors determine the net amount of zinc which will be absorbed at any one time: (1) ligands — since zinc is a metal ion, it will be bound to one or more ligands, some of which will impede and others of which will enhance zinc absorption, (2) zinc status — zinc absorption tends to be increased during zinc deficiency and decreased during zinc excess, (3) the active transport mechanism in the intestinal epithelium — the uptake of zinc complexes from the intestinal luman and their turnover to the portal circulation is an active process under metabolic control, and (4) endogenous zinc secretion — significant amounts of zinc are secreted into the intestinal lumen via the epithelial cells, bile, and pancreatic secretion. Factors affecting zinc absorption are shown in Table 19.

A. Ligands

During the digestive process, zinc is released from its dietary ligands (predominantly proteins) and becomes associated with intestinal low molecular weight ligands,[132,321,423,663,812,1435,1441] which make zinc available to the intestinal microvilli. Some of these ligands are of dietary origin, e.g., amino acids (histidine), and others are thought to be of endogenous origin, including metallothionein.[1525] The identity of these ligands has been the subject of intense research (see Table 19). The list was recently headed by citric acid and picolinic acid (putative ligands in milk), but may also include immunoglobulins[1177] and lactoferrin[32,149] and, in human milk, an unidentified protein of mol wt 12,500.[443] Although most studies have examined zinc absorption in the small intestine, a recent report demonstrated that amino acids significantly increase zinc absorption in the *colon,* a site not previously regarded as absorbing either amino acids or zinc.[1680]

Zinc absorption[339,1492] and intestinal prostaglandin levels[1523] are both increased in zinc deficiency. Prostaglandin E_1 has been shown to increase zinc absorption[339] and there is a positive correlation between gut contents of zinc and prostaglandin E_1[1117] in zinc-deficient rats. On the average, 29% of the total zinc in human milk is bound to the fat fraction.[1016] Since 15% of human milk fat is essential fatty acids (EFAs), the potential role of the EFAs, and even prostaglandins, in zinc absorption should not be underestimated.

Cottonseed oil was shown to improve the clinical condition of three cases of AE before the defect in zinc absorption was established.[236] Since cottonseed oil contains no appreciable amounts of zinc, citric acid, or picolinic acid, but does contain 54% linoleic acid, the observation in rats that EFAs, excluding arachidonic acid, increase zinc absorption very significantly[339] may be relevant to humans. Furthermore, linoleic acid and γ-linolenic have been recently reported to be increased in phospholipids of intestinal mucosa from zinc-deficient rats.[344] As with the prostaglandins, the point is not that the EFAs necessarily bind zinc, but that they may facilitate the absorption of zinc complexes through an as yet unknown mechanism.

Some components of the diet compete with zinc during absorption or form complexes with zinc that prevent its absorption. Calcium, copper, and iron compete with zinc for absorption (discussed in relation to humans in Chapter 4). Although vitamin D influences calcium absorption, it has a disputed effect on zinc absorption.[258,927] Oxalic acid (present in spinach) strongly complexes zinc and prevents its absorption.[892]

Phytate-zinc complexes are largely unabsorbed. Thus, plant proteins, such as soy, increase zinc requirement in comparison with proteins of animal origin, e.g., casein.[113,552,1015,1208,1451,1627] In spite of the acknowledged inhibitory effect of phytate on zinc absorption in experimental situations in humans, it does not always appear to have this effect.[1408,1451]

B. Zinc Status

Zinc absorption is increased in zinc-deficient rats and decreased in rats fed excess zinc.[339,474,532,787,1492,1689,1690] Zinc absorption is also increased in pregnant rats,[386] an effect abolished after parturition.[1425] The apparent conservation of zinc balance by increasing zinc absorption has also been suggested by Wada et al.,[1666] who found no change in plasma zinc in humans, fed 5.5 mg zinc per day. In view of the apparent lack of tissue storage sites for zinc, such a mechanism would contribute to maintaining zinc homeostasis in the face of dietary deficiency or increased demand. Increased zinc absorption in zinc-deficient rats is not related to increased uptake through defective intestinal mucosal tight junctions.[1146]

C. Intracellular Transport

In spite of the research into the identity of intestinal zinc ligands, the mechanism by which zinc is transferred to or across the mucosal surface of the microvilli is completely unknown. Once in the intestinal cell, zinc becomes associated with metalloproteins, including metallothionein. This process appears to be dependent on protein synthesis, since cycloheximide and actinomycin D inhibit mucosal zinc uptake.[1357] Although metallothionein is important in the hepatic extraction of zinc from the blood, the role of intestinal metallothionein in zinc absorption is not understood (see Chapter 12). The complexing of zinc with the intracellular metalloproteins is an energy-dependent process, requiring ATP and DNA synthesis.

The release of zinc from intracellular protein ligands and its transfer to the portal blood is likewise poorly understood. Both transferrin and albumin[316,474] have been proposed as likely serum proteins for zinc transport subsequent to its absorption.

D. Endogenous Secretion

Although there is endogenous secretion of zinc from the pancreas, it has been shown that zinc exchanged from the blood to the intestinal mucosa is *not* secreted into the lumen.[158] The secretion of endogenous zinc into the intestinal lumen in pancreatic secretions has been established in animal studies.[113,384] Clarification of the magnitude of this process in humans came from the ingenious studies of Matsesche et al.,[1069] who demonstrated that even under "normal" conditions nearly as much zinc could be endogenously secreted from the pancreas as was absorbed. The amount of "enteropancreatic" circulation[1502] of zinc appears to depend on the origin of the dietary protein. If it is of plant origin, more endogenous zinc is secreted, but less is secreted if the predominant protein in the meal was of animal origin.[1069]

V. TRANSPORT

A. Blood

Quantitatively, two major zinc ligands carry >95% of the zinc in blood: albumin and α_2 macroglobulin. Quantitatively, minor ligands account for the remainder. These minor ligands are collectively grouped as ultrafilterable (mol wt <50,000) and include amino acids such as histidine and cysteine. The term "minor ligands" may be a misnomer since the biological importance of the amino acids in the process of zinc exchange from the plasma to peripheral sites has not been fully evaluated.

Albumin is quantitatively and qualitatively the most important zinc ligand in blood. Zinc is considered to be bound primarily to the histidine molecules of albumin. Albumin-bound zinc is in equilibrium with zinc bound to the ultrafilterable carriers, but not with α_2 macroglobulin. The importance of albumin is illustrated by the fact that conditions that cause hypoalbuminemia, e.g., malnutrition, will, of necessity, reduce the capacity of the blood to carry zinc. As a result, it is important that plasma albumin be determined in cases of idiopathic hypozincemia. Nevertheless, it is interesting to see that in analbuminemic rats, zinc is carried by other unspecified proteins, but the amount carried by α_2 macroglobulin remains similar to that in normoalbuminemic rats.[1462]

α_2 macroglobulin incorporates zinc in the liver and liberates it there as well. In the blood, there appears to be little correlation between total zinc, α_2 macroglobulin-bound zinc, and zinc nutriture.[601,1078] Thus, as a measure of zinc availability, α_2 macroglobulin appears to be of little value. Its role in the hepatic utilization of zinc is also not currently understood.

B. Milk

In considering the zinc ligands in human milk, it is typical to centrifuge the milk, remove the fat fraction (cream), and assess the zinc ligands in the whey fraction (aqueous). This process has led to detailed research on the components of milk to which zinc is bound both before and after its ingestion. Dominant among these ligands have been citric acid and picolinic acid.

Whether picolinic acid or citric acid is the predominant low molecular weight zinc ligand in human milk has been controversial.[476,814,863] The controversy has arisen because, although human milk generally contains less zinc than cow's milk, its availability from human milk is significantly greater.[234] Some research indicates that a specific protein ligand is present in human milk that is not present in sufficient amounts in cow's milk.[443,446] The possibility also exists that the association of zinc with citric or picolinic acid is an artifact of isolation procedures.[321,1017] For both citric acid and picolinic acid, the general consensus is that they both significantly enhance zinc absorption. However, the question is one of physiological relevance. Do they, in fact, exist as such in human milk at concentrations sufficient to augment zinc absorption? At present, the answer is uncertain.

Other compounds in the whey fraction of milk, which may or may not be ligands per se, also facilitate zinc absorption. Some, such as histidine,[1585,1679] ethylene diaminetraacetic acid (EDTA),[113] and D-penicillamine[1699] are known to chelate zinc. Others such as EFAs[339,482] and prostaglandins[339,482,1520-1522] may facilitate other aspects of the zinc absorption mechanism rather than binding to zinc directly.[339]

The fraction of milk that has been completely overlooked with respect to the content and availability of zinc (and all other essential metals) has been the fat fraction. Although this fraction generally averages no more than 4% (w/w) of the milk, it contains 20 to 40% of the total copper, zinc, and iron in milk.[562] Most of these metals are located in the milk fat globule membrane[1252] which only represents 1% of the milk fat (w/w). Hence, an average of 1/3 of the total content of the essential trace metals in milk is in a component which represents 0.04% (w/w) of the milk. The bioavailability of zinc from this fraction of milk is completely unknown.

In lactation, efficient control of the zinc content of milk seems to be present, because zinc supplementation at 60 mg/day for 2 weeks did not affect milk zinc concentration.[503,1144] This has implications for the breast-feeding of premature infants because it indicates that zinc supplementation of the lactating mother is probably ineffective to increase neonatal zinc intake.

VI. PERIPHERAL UTILIZATION

Apart from studies of zinc uptake by the liver,[489,1250,1297,1691] very little seems to be known about the utilization of zinc by peripheral tissues once it is absorbed. Cousins,[316] has reviewed the mechanisms governing zinc uptake by the liver as they relate to metallothionein (see Chapter 12). Uptake of zinc-65 by isolated rat hepatocytes in culture has a rapid initial phase, which does not seem to be carrier-mediated, and a slower second phase. Neither phase is affected by cyanide,[1546] prostaglandins, or sex steroids,[489] suggesting that active transport is not involved. High (65,000) and low (metallothionein, about 6000) molecular weight proteins are involved in zinc uptake by hepatocytes. The lower-weight proteins are favored when zinc is available in excess.[1138]

In pregnancy, peripheral utilization of zinc by the feto-placental unit and liver[1425] is increased, as reflected by reduced maternal fecal zinc excretion.[1591]

Phillips[1280] has shown that the uptake of transferrin-bound zinc by human lymphocytes can be stimulated in vitro by a variety of agents including prostaglandin E_1, epinephrine, glucagon, histamine, and serotonin. Prostaglandin $F_{2\alpha}$, however, was inhibitory. The mechanisms were not elucidated, but if they are at all similar to those in the intestinal enterocyte, these data would give credibility to the reports suggesting that prostaglandins may stimulate zinc absorption.

Statter and Krieger[1548] have studied zinc metabolism by human diploid fibroblasts and shown it to be cyanide sensitive. Both citric acid and picolinic acid inhibited fibroblast uptake of zinc, an interesting effect in view of their proposed stimulatory effect on zinc absorption from the intestine.

Horrobin and Morgan[777] have suggested that the peripheral utilization of zinc is abnormal in myotonic dystrophy, thereby causing localized zinc depletion in cardiac and skeletal muscle. More recent studies support the role of muscle as a regulatory site governing zinc homeostasis. Kinetic analysis of metabolism of zinc-65 in humans showed that muscle, along with erythrocytes and active secretion by the gut, were secondary sites governing the handling of *excess* zinc.[1681] Muscle catabolism is also an important mechanism by which zinc can be released to maintain fetal growth in zinc-deficient pregnant rats.[1063]

VII. EXCRETION

Zinc excretion is primarily via the gastrointestinal tract and the feces. Daily values in healthy individuals are usually in the 5 to 10 mg range and depend on the dietary zinc uptake. In pathological conditions, such as chronic diarrhea, this can represent all of the consumed zinc and may rapidly result in negative zinc balance (see Chapter 5). The relative contribution of endogenous (bile, pancreas, and intestinal mucosa) and exogenous (diet) zinc to fecal zinc content is variable. It depends on dietary ligands inhibiting zinc absorption, e.g., phytate, and on pancreatic function. As a result of the dual origin of fecal zinc, it has always been difficult to determine the full extent of absorption of exogenous zinc.

Zinc is also excreted via the urine in the range of 200 to 600 μg/24 hr. It is excreted bound to amino acids and porphyrins. The metabolic significance of this route of zinc excretion is not fully understood. On the one hand, 500 μg/day represents $<10\%$ of that normally excreted via the feces; on the other hand, urinary zinc appears to be quite sensitive to major alterations in zinc status, e.g., experimental zinc deficiency in both humans and animals.[89] It is also sensitive to acute changes in zinc balance, e.g., infection (see Chapter 5).

VIII. HOMEOSTASIS

With the possible exception of bone, there is no known capacity by mammals to store zinc in the true sense. Its homeostasis is therefore governed by the balance between absorption and excretion; when zinc status is low, zinc excretion is decreased and vice versa. This has been amply demonstrated in animals[303] and recently confirmed in humans fed diets containing suboptimal zinc — 5.5 mg/day.[1666] Zinc homeostasis has been shown to be related to the basal metabolic rate; hypothyroid rats have decreased zinc turnover and higher tissue zinc levels.[1749] In periods of increased demand for zinc, its absorption is increased and excretion decreased, e.g., pregnancy,[492,1435] infection,[1256] and diabetes.[590]

In severe, experimental zinc deficiency in rats, zinc excretion via both urine and feces can be almost totally eliminated.[1256] In addition, zinc redistribution from bone into muscle also occurs.[645,841] In pregnant rats, muscle catabolism in the dam releases zinc which can be utilized by the fetus.[1063] Conversely, in experimental zinc supplementation, secretion of endogenous zinc into the intestinal lumen helps maintain zinc homeostasis.[478,1681]

IX. SUMMARY

The paucity of information regarding how zinc homeostasis is maintained is second only to that concerned with *effectively* assessing zinc nutriture. Metallothionein is rapidly gaining importance in regard to zinc absorption and tissue redistribution and probably has a major role in the shift in zinc homeostasis during acute stress (see Chapter 12). Our original concept that zinc homeostasis was mostly regulated at the intestinal level is being challenged by data from radioisotope studies and computer modeling in humans which indicates that there are multiple zinc ''pools'' and from animal studies of zinc availability from muscle. Milk zinc levels appear very closely regulated, making those cases in which critically low milk zinc concentrations have been reported in association with overt neonatal zinc deficiency all the more significant and worthy of investigation.

Chapter 10

ENZYMES

I. INTRODUCTION

Nowhere is the enigma of defining the biological role of zinc more apparent than in its role in enzymes. Numerous enzymes are either zinc metalloenzymes or zinc-enzyme complexes. However, the relationship between the effects of zinc depletion and altered zinc enzyme activity is tenuous at best. Even those enzymes whose activity has been conclusively demonstrated to be reduced in zinc depleted humans or animals have not so far been related to the clinical symptoms of zinc depletion. Furthermore, zinc depletion in both humans and animals (reviewed by Kirchgessner et al.[910]) does not appear to be reliably associated with altered levels of zinc in tissues other than plasma and bone (see Chapter 11). Hence, in zinc depletion, altered activity of a zinc enzyme such as alkaline phosphatase is not associated with altered tissue zinc levels, let alone the pathology of zinc depletion.

II. ZINC METALLOENZYMES

Zinc metalloenzymes are catalytically active enzymes which, on isolation and purification, have been found to contain stoichiometric amounts of zinc.[1362] The activity of these enzymes is usually specifically dependent on the presence of zinc. The first zinc metalloenzyme to be discovered was carbonic anhydrase. Since then, numerous others have been added to the list (for reviews, see Vallee[1634] and Riordan and Vallee[1362]).

If the conditions of stoichiometry and specificity are not met, the enzyme is not a zinc "metalloenzyme" per se. The function of zinc in such enzymes is one of maintaining structural integrity or one of participation in the enzyme reaction itself. Often these functions are combined. Enzymes that have multiple subunits are typical of those for which zinc would have the function of maintaining structure. Alcohol dehydrogenase from horse liver, for instance, has four zinc ions per molecule and two active sites. Two of the zinc ions are known to be required for the activity of the enzyme, as demonstrated by the inhibitory effect of zinc chelators. The other two zinc ions do not interact with chelating agents and are probably structural.[267] The function of zinc in such enzymes is as a Lewis acid or proton donor. A list of zinc metalloenzymes of known zinc content is shown in Table 20; those enzymes of unspecified zinc content are shown in Table 21.

Some zinc metalloenzymes can have the zinc removed and replaced by other divalent cations, such as cobalt. One such example is alkaline phosphatase from *Escherichia coli:* the enzyme activity is lost when the zinc is removed, but it can be reactivated by the addition of cobalt, which occupies the structural sites normally occupied by zinc and also restores the activity of the enzyme.[267]

It would appear that, although a particular enzyme has been identified as a zinc metalloenzyme, there may be conditions under which it can be fully active in the absence of zinc. For instance, although DNA polymerase is a recognized zinc metalloenzyme (in *E. coli,* see Table 10) (Chapter 4), Walton et al.[1677] have shown that a DNA polymerase I enzyme isolated from *E. coli* is also fully active in the structural absence of zinc.

Both RNA and DNA polymerase from bacteriophage T7 have been reported not to be zinc metalloenzymes; the activity of the DNA polymerase is, in fact, inhibited by supplemental zinc,[1478] whereas the activity of RNA polymerase is unaffected by exogenous zinc.[905] Whether the absence of zinc in DNA and RNA polymerase of malignant or transformed cells is significant in relation to their propagation is an issue of potential importance.[266]

Table 20
ZINC METALLOENZYMES

Enzyme	Source	No. of zinc ions
Adenosine monophosphate aminohydrolase	Muscle	2
Alcohol dehydrogenase	Human liver	2—4
	Horse liver	2—4
	Yeast	4
Aldolase	Yeast	2
Alkaline phosphatase	*Escherichia coli*	2
	Human placenta, bone	0.15%
	Calf intestine	0.20%
Alkaline protease	*E. freundii*	
Aspartate transcarbamylase	*E. coli*	6
Carbonic anhydrase	Erythrocyte, various species	1
Carboxypeptidase A	Pancreas, various species	1
Carboxypeptidase B	Pancreas, various species	1
Carboxypeptidase C	*Pseudomonas stutzeri*	
3′-Dehydroquinate synthease	*Neurospora crassa*	1
Dipeptidase	Porcine kidney	1
DNA polymerase	*E. coli*	2
Glutamic dehydrogenase	Bovine liver	2—4
D-Glyceraldehyde phosphate		1
Porcine kidney dehydrogenase		
Lactate cytochrome reductase	Yeast	
Leucine aminopeptidase		2
Malic dehydrogenase	Bovine heart	1
Mercaptopyruvate sulfur transferase	*E. coli*	1
Neutral protease		1—2
5′-nucleotidase	*E. coli*	1
Phosphoglucomutase	Yeast	
Phosphomannose isomerase	Yeast	1
Protease	Snake venom	1
Pyruvate carboxylase	Yeast	4
Reverse transcriptase	Avian myoblastosis virus	
RNA polymerase	*E. coli*	2
Sulfur transferase	Bovine liver	2
Superoxide dismutase	Erythrocyte, various species	2
Thermolysin		1
Transcarbamylase	*P. shermanii*	4

Conversely, the potential exists that zinc supplementation would inhibit malignant cell growth in a manner analogous to its inhibitory effect on the activity of DNA polymerase in bacteriophage.

III. ZINC-ENZYME COMPLEXES

Zinc-enzyme complexes are enzymes that are known to be activated or inhibited by zinc, but for which a specific content of zinc or absolute requirement for zinc has not been established. A list of these enzymes has been compiled[334] and is reproduced in Table 22, along with recent additions.

IV. ZINC METALLOPROTEINS

Proteins which are not necessarily enzymes but which have been shown to bind zinc to

Table 21
ZINC METALLOENZYMES OF UNSPECIFIED ZINC CONTENT

Enzyme	Source	Ref.
ACP-ribose polymerase	Calf thymus	1760
5-Aminolevulenic acid	Bovine liver	1733
dehydratase	Bovine erythrocyte	389, 1071, 1622
Collagenase	*Clostridium histolyticum*, rabbit bone	1445, 1590
Cyclic phosphodiesterase	Rat liver	434
Gluconolactonase	Bovine liver	229
β-Lactamase	*Bacillus cereus*	1383
Lactic dehydrogenase	Rabbit muscle	1665
α-D-Mannosidase	Jack bean	1495
Neutral protease	*B. cereus*	502
Nucleopyrophosphatase	Rat liver	304
Nucleoside phosphorylase	Lymphocytes	—
Phospholipase C	*B. cereus, Pseudomonas aureofaciens*	961, 1007, 1230
Sorbitol dehydrogenase	Sheep liver	856
Thymidine kinase	Rat liver	422

high affinity sites are zinc metalloproteins. They include myoglobulin,[98] 7S nerve growth factor,[1251] and mammary estrogen-binding protein.[1463]

V. SIGNIFICANCE OF ZINC METALLOENZYMES IN RELATION TO ZINC DEPLETION

Although the lists of enzymes in Tables 20 to 22 illustrate the ubiquitous nature of the distribution of zinc in enzymes, we can at present draw no relationship between this role and the pathological consequences of zinc depletion. Others have pointed out this dilemma previously.[137,341,346,776,910,1173] We must search either for the role of zinc in relation to membrane function and composition[137,346] or for sites at which zinc is associated with a rapidly metabolized substrate.[910] Hence, the role of zinc in metalloenzymes is one which is relatively immune to assault by zinc depletion, and we must look elsewhere to relate zinc physiology and pathology.

Table 22
ZINC — ENZYME COMPLEXES

Enzyme	Source	Ref.
Enzymes Stimulated by Zinc		
Adenosine triphosphatase	*E. coli*	1583
	Rabbit skeletal muscle	155
Adenylate cyclase	Rat testes	1222
Angiotensin converting enzyme	Rat lung, horse lung, rat serum	463, 514, 1346
Collagenase	Rabbit cornea	129
	Acromobacter	730
Deoxythymidine kinase	Human connective tissue	1307
Dihydropyrimidine aminohydrolase	Bovine liver	195
Enderopeptidase		1251
Fructose biphosphatase	Rabbit liver	1291
Phosphodiesterase	Yeast	1014
Pyridoxal phosphate kinase	Rat brain	391
Zinc Inhibits		
Adenosine deaminase	Rat brain	1755
Adenosine triphosphatase	Rabbit skeletal muscle	155
	lymphocytes	1444
	erythrocytes	950
Adenylsuccinate lyase	Rat skeletal muscle	194
Adenylosuccinate synthetase	Rat skeletal muscle	194
4-Aminobutyrate-2-oxyglutarate aminotransferase	Rat brain	391
Cytochrome oxidase		421
DNA polymerase	T7 bacteriophage	1478
	herpes simplex virus	568
Glutamine decarboxylase	Rat brain	391
Heme oxygenase	Rat liver	491
NADPH oxidase	Rat liver	279, 280
Phospholipase A_2	*Crotalus adamanteus*	1705
	human pancreas	1038
Succinate semialdehyde dehydrogenase	Rat brain	391
Thromboxane synthetase	Human platelets	752
Xanthine oxidase	Rat liver	324

Chapter 11

ZINC METABOLISM IN ANIMALS

I. INTRODUCTION

The majority of this chapter refers to zinc deficiency, since this is the commonest method for studying processes that might be zinc dependent. There are three types of zinc deficiency in animals: (1) experimental omission of zinc from the diet, (2) diets naturally low in zinc or from which zinc is not readily available (applicable to grazing animals), and (3) genetic strains characterized by zinc deficiency, e.g., the *lm/lm* — lethal milk mouse and the lethal trait calf (A-46). By far the greatest literature is concerned with experimental induction of zinc deficiency by dietary omission of zinc. Among the numerous species in which zinc deficiency has been demonstrated, studies on the rat greatly exceed all others.

The experimental dietary induction of zinc deficiency has been the means by which many of the known functions of zinc have been elucidated. Therefore, the literature on functions of zinc in various organ systems overlaps to a great extent with the literature on zinc deficiency. Since it is my intention to review, in separate chapters, the roles of zinc in relation to proteins, carbohydrates, lipids, and its interactions with other nutrients, the effects of zinc deficiency in relation to these subjects are only discussed briefly here. The primary purpose of this chapter is to outline the breadth of work on experimental zinc deficiency and to point out findings that may be useful in relation to clinical observations. In no way should the reference list be considered comprehensive, particularly in areas referring to domestic animals. An additional objective is to demonstrate where the findings must be considered as limited to the respective models, e.g., the limitations of extrapolation to human zinc deficiency. Where possible, the relationship of the pathological findings in zinc deficiency to biochemical functions of zinc are discussed.

II. RAT

A. Comparative Methods

The commonest means of inducing zinc deficiency in the rat is to feed it a semisynthetic diet, the protein of which is usually spray-dried egg white. Such a diet, fed to weanling male rats, interferes with the normal food intake pattern within a few days, and growth retardation is usually present within 1 week. Normal growth curves can usually be maintained in rats fed egg white-based protein and a zinc content of as little as 6 to 8 mg/kg. Below this value, normal growth cannot be maintained and the accompanying symptoms develop, e.g., alopecia, dermal lesions, and swelling of the joints.[910]

Less commonly used are the diets based on casein that has been ethylenediaminetetraacetic acid (EDTA)-washed.[75] The EDTA removes zinc, and potentially other metals as well, and its presence in the diet is an unnecessary contamination. The use of parenteral feeding for inducing zinc deficiency has recently been described.[498,529]

B. Tissue Zinc Levels

One of the contentious issues in research on experimental zinc deficiency is the degree to which tissue zinc depletion can be demonstrated. What is clear, however, is that zinc is highly conserved in zinc-deficient rats.[645] Apart from a decrease in zinc in plasma and bone, there does not appear to be sufficient evidence to indicate that any other tissue loses significant amounts of zinc, even after prolonged zinc deficiency.[645,1594] Isolated cell types, e.g., peripheral blood leukocytes, do tend to reflect zinc status in humans, but, in the rat, do not lose zinc in response to even severe zinc depletion.[1136] Total zinc in muscle is increased in zinc deficiency, suggesting zinc redistribution from bone to muscle.[645]

It should also be made clear that the majority of the analysis on which this statement is based has been of *whole* tissue analysis; subcellular organelles or cell membranes[135] may very well lose zinc during zinc deficiency.

C. Enzymes

Two problems exist in relating the effects of zinc deficiency to effects on zinc metalloenzymes: (1) has it been definitively established that the activity of any zinc metalloenzyme is reproducibly affected by zinc deficiency and (2) in the event such a change does occur, is it relevant to the pathology associated with zinc deficiency? Species- and tissue-specific effects may also exist which make it difficult to make blanket statements about the relationship of zinc deficiency to the activity of zinc-dependent enzymes.

Prasad's group have been strong proponents of an effect of zinc deficiency on zinc metalloenzymes and zinc-dependent enzymes such as alkaline phosphatase[1311,1312,1315] and deoxythymidine kinase.[1307] Prasad has also noted that ribonuclease activity is increased in zinc deficiency.[1312] Zinc deficiency has also been reported to inhibit the activity of glutathione peroxidase,[1718] carboxypeptidase,[792] and carbonic anhydrase.[830] Others have found no changes in the activity of lactic dehydrogenase, malic dehydrogenase, or carbonic anhydrase[811] (see also Chapter 2).

D. Organ Systems

1. Blood

The hematocrit has been shown to be increased in zinc-deficient rats,[1032,1248] an effect possibly due to transepidermal losses of water and reduced extracellular fluid volume.[142] Platelet aggregation has also been shown to be impaired in zinc deficiency, resulting in longer bleeding times.[625,626,1211] West et al.[1708] have confirmed that prolonged bleeding occurs in zinc-deficient pregnant rats at term, but maintain that the effect is not due to impaired platelet aggregation.

2. Gastrointestinal Tract and Pancreas

The buccal mucosa becomes hyperplastic in zinc deficiency.[81,941] The submandibular salivary gland has been reported to have decreased alkaline phosphatase activity in zinc-deficient rats, an effect suggested to be related to altered taste perception.[257] The esophagus of zinc-deficient rats develops parakeratosis.[104] This may impair swallowing and be a physical limitation to food intake. Koo and Turk[932] have described in detail the effects of zinc deficiency on the pancreas, including the reduction of zymogen granules, lipid, and lysosome accumulation, and defects in ribosomes and endoplasmic reticulum.

Morphological and functional changes in the intestine of zinc deficient rats have been described, including (1) dense inclusion bodies and cellular remnants in Paneth cells,[456,457,1587] (2) increased villus density, but no effect on intestinal flora,[1528,1534] and (3) decreased mucosal protein and disaccharidase activity.[1761] Zinc deficiency has also been shown to increase the susceptibility of the rat duodenum to the lesions induced by colchicine, an effect prevented by supplemental zinc.[399]

The pancreas of rats fed 4 mg/kg zinc (marginally deficient) contains lower amounts of lipase; zymogen granule size and secretion rate is decreased; and acini are reduced in size. Protease secretion, however, is increased.[1264]

3. Liver

No specific lesions in the liver have thus far been attributed to the effects of zinc deficiency. Zinc deficiency is, however, associated with reduced metabolism of various drugs by the liver, including pentobarbital, aminopyrine, and *p*-nitrobenzoic acid.[115] This effect may be associated with a reduction in microsomal cytochrome P-450.

4. Special Senses

Henkin has proposed a definite role of zinc in the maintenance of adequate taste[713] (see also Chapter 2). Taste tolerance for HCl, quinine, and NaCl is higher in the zinc-deficient rat,[244,850,1089] suggesting that taste acuity is not normal. This observation has recently been challenged in a report showing that quinine tolerance was unaffected by zinc deficiency.[156] Jakinovich and Osborn[850] have also shown that the electrophysiological response of the taste buds are normal in zinc-deficient rats and concluded that defective taste perception in zinc deficiency must be of central nervous system (CNS) or endocrine origin. Altered taste in zinc-deficient rats does not appear to be related to zinc levels in saliva which have been shown to be normal.[484]

Chesters and Will[269] maintain that the primary defect caused by zinc deficiency in the rat is a "failure to grow". This reduces energy expenditure and, in turn, may be related to the reduced and cyclic food intake by zinc-deficient rats.[268,269] They maintain that appetite per se is not affected. Miller et al.,[1125] in studies with the pig, have also shown that decreased growth occurs before decreased food intake. The endogenous opiate peptide, dynorphin, which has a role in appetite regulation, has been measured in zinc-deficient rats and been found to be elevated in the cerebral cortex, but decreased in the hypothalamus.[467] In addition, reduced receptor affinity for endogenous opiates involved in appetite control may be one of the factors disposing toward anorexia in zinc-deficient rats.[468-470]

Evidence from the zinc-deficient cat suggests that zinc deficiency increases the threshold for rod but not cone response.[847] However, there is little evidence of a direct effect of zinc deficiency in the rat on retinal function per se.[995] Rhodopsin regeneration after bleaching the eyes of zinc-deficient rats has been shown to be impaired by 50%.[408] Night blindness is associated with zinc deficiency in human alcoholics[1381] (see Chapter 4). Retinal reductase in the retinas of zinc-deficient rats has been shown to be decreased and to vary as tibial zinc concentration.[312] After zinc supplementation, retinal reductase activity returned to normal slowly, an effect that possibly accounts for the slow reversibility of defective dark adaptation.

A recent paper has made the interesting observation that 5 to 7 weeks zinc deficiency in the rat is associated with neovascularization of the cornea, a pathological event not seen in the eyes of zinc-replete rats.[994]

5. CNS/Behavior

Zinc deficiency in the rat is associated with impaired neuronal development in the cerebellum, both biochemically and histologically.[416,431-433,738,938] Decreased brain weight has been associated with decreased incorporation of labeled DNA into the brain and low brain DNA levels in zinc-deficient rats,[860,1402] as well as decreased total brain lipid and myelin lipid.[860,1334] ^{65}Zn uptake, however, is increased in zinc deficiency, suggesting a degree of homeostatic control.[876]

Intracerebral injection of zinc is epileptogenic in the rat[101,835] and in the rabbit.[1255] The effect is blocked by γ-amino butyric acid and may be related to decreased activity of glutamic acid decarboxylase in the hippocampus[835] or to inhibition of sodium-potassium ATPase.[101] Since prostaglandin E_1 is also epileptogenic[774] and zinc appears to stimulate synthesis of prostaglandin E_1,[776] the epileptogenic effect of zinc may be mediated in part through prostaglandin (PG) E_1.

Zinc-deficient rats have lower body temperature and impaired thermoregulation at cold temperatures.[1615] However, they also recover more quickly from nicotine-induced hypothermia.

Behavioral changes in rats induced by zinc deficiency have also been described[665,739] and are reviewed by Halas.[664]

6. Skeleton

Bone from zinc-deficient rats has been shown to have lower synthesis of DNA, collagen, and glycoprotein and decreased resistance of the epiphysis to shearing.[988] Proline content and mineralization are not affected.[198] Because of the large decreases in total zinc and zinc concentration of the femur of zinc-deficient rats, bone would appear to be a major source of zinc during zinc depletion.[52]

7. Immune System

One of the systems most affected by zinc deficiency is the immune system. Thymic atrophy, reduced number of thymocytes, and decreased thymic hormone levels are characteristic in zinc-deficient rats and may be due in part to raised levels of circulating steroids.[224,644,1112,1327] In spite of decreased cell-mediated immunity, growth of various tumors has been shown to be inhibited by zinc deficiency.[1098,1129,1130,1293] Forestomach tumors induced by *N*-nitrosodimethylamine, have recently been reported to occur only in rats that were zinc deficient, compared to zinc-adequate controls.[1188]

8. Endocrine

The secretion of steroids and other pituitary-mediated hormones has been shown to be altered by zinc deficiency, but in general these effects have not been adequately distinguished from effects of reduced food intake. Reeves et al.[1345] have shown that zinc-deficient rats release less corticosterone in response to adrenocorticotropic hormone (ACTH). In adult and immature male rats, plasma-luteinizing hormone has been shown to be increased, but testosterone is decreased in zinc deficiency.[986,1372] Adrenal size is usually increased in zinc-deficient rats, and its incorporation of total lipid, especially cholesterol, is increased in zinc deficiency.[1378] Increased cholesterol uptake by the adrenal would be consistent with higher circulating corticosteroid levels frequently observed in zinc-deficient rats.

Effects of zinc deficiency on the prostate, testes, and sperm appear to be more related to protein synthesis than to androgen binding.[275,400,1106,1390] McClain et al.[1082] have related hypogonadism in the rat specifically to Leydig cell failure to synthesize testosterone.

Circulating triiodothyronine and thyroxine are decreased in zinc deficiency, as is hypothalimic thyroid-releasing hormone.[624] Insulin secretion in response to glucose is decreased in zinc-deficient rats.[801,1330] The peptide hormone, somatomedin-C, is decreased in zinc-deficient rats.[309] The growth retardation of zinc deficiency has been suggested to be related to growth hormone resistance, as well as impaired effects of somatomedin.[1228] Zinc metabolism is markedly altered in streptozotocin-induced diabetes mellitus, such that tissue zinc levels tend to increase,[326] an effect suggested to be partly related to reduced zinc excretion via the gut.[862] Chemicals that induce diabetes, including 8-hydroxyquinoline and dithizone,[462,631] are zinc chelators.

9. Pregnancy/Fetal Development

Zinc deficiency during pregnancy affects both fetal development and the successful termination of pregnancy. Dietary zinc deficiency per se or zinc depletion induced by copper,[1352] cadmium,[27] or alcohol[1382] (see Chapter 17) are all effective. The two main consequences are fetal malformations and delayed and prolonged parturition. Zinc deficiency affects normal development of the preimplantation egg.[816] Whether as a consequence or independent of this effect, fetal malformations also occur in zinc deficiency[123,396,429,444,553,810,817,1093,1170,1341,1343,1401,1595,1659] (reviewed by Adeloye and Warkany[15]).

Zinc deficiency, which need only be present in the final days of pregnancy, causes delayed and prolonged parturition, resulting in stillbirths and early postnatal losses.[72-74,208,340,428,1211,1728] The effects of zinc depletion on parturition have been suggested to be related to defective uterine contractility[335] and to a 90% reduction in utero-placental blood flow near term.[359]

Both impaired uterine contractility and reduced utero-placental blood flow may be related to altered synthesis of prostaglandins by the uterus[336] and/or placenta.[359] A prostaglandin-related effect is further implicated in view of the similar effects of zinc deficiency and aspirin toxicity on pregnancy outcome[29,1211] and the exacerbation of the effects of marginal zinc deficiency by aspirin.[659] Altered prostaglandin metabolism has been suggested to be the mechanism by which progesterone withdrawal is delayed in zinc deficient rats.[208] This would prolong uterine quiescence and delay the onset of uterine contractions. Oxytocin metabolism does not appear to be abnormal in zinc deficient parturient rats.[728]

10. Skin

Hyperkeratosis of the skin and effusion of serum are characteristically seen in young zinc-deficient rats fed diets containing <2 mg/kg zinc.[798] In spite of the hyperkeratinization, incorporation of amino acids into skin proteins is reduced in zinc-deficient rats.[790]

E. Nutrients

Much of the effect of zinc deficiency on organ systems is probably related to effects on the metabolism of other nutrients, e.g., protein synthesis and lipid metabolism (further details in Chapters 12 and 13).

1. Protein/Nucleoproteins

Defective protein synthesis in zinc deficiency is considered to center primarily on inhibited activity of the zinc metalloenzymes related to nucleoproteins, e.g., DNA and RNA polymerase and thymidine kinase.[512,1031,1087,1406,1659] *Euglena gracilis* grown on zinc-deficient media has altered the base composition of RNA and increased mRNA.[496] Methionine incorporation into the proteins of blood, kidney, liver, and muscle has been shown to be significantly decreased in zinc deficiency.[797] This may be related to enhanced oxidation of amino acids in zinc deficiency.[1607] The growth-promoting effects of increasing dietary protein from 4 to 20% are zinc dependent.[1204] Sulfur-35 incorporation into skin proteins is decreased in zinc deficiency.[793]

Inconsistent with the general impairment of protein synthesis in zinc deficiency is the increase in cysteine and methionine incorporation into pancreatic proteins.[793,797] Impaired collagen cross-linking has also been described in zinc deficiency, an effect related to reduced salt-soluble collagen and increased acid-soluble collagen.[511,794,795,1087,1303]

2. Carbohydrate

A relationship between zinc deficiency and reduced glucose tolerance in the rat has been demonstrated.[707,1325] The effect is dependent on the carbohydrate source in the diet; starch caused a greter impairment than glucose. Insulin-induced convulsions and coma are delayed and reduced in zinc-deficient animals.[1325]

Increased absorption of hexose has been recently reported in zinc-deficient rats,[1531-1533] an effect rapidly reversed by zinc supplementation.[1529] In view of the inhibitory effect of both excess glucose and zinc deficiency on essential fatty acid (EFA) metabolism,[87,176] some of the effects on EFA metabolism attributed to zinc deficiency may be due to excess uptake of glucose.

3. Lipid

The relationship between zinc deficiency and lipid metabolism is complex and is discussed in greater detail in Chapter 13. Four main aspects are involved: (1) effects on EFAs, (2) cholesterol transport, (3) triglyceride absorption, and (4) lipid stability in membranes. Zinc deficiency in rats inhibits desaturation of linoleic (18:2n-6) and dihomo-γ-linolenic acid (20:3n-6) in liver[289,518] and testes.[87] Plasma levels of cholesterol are decreased in zinc deficiency.[1245] Triglyceride absorption through the intestinal mucosa is impaired in zinc deficiency, possibly through defective chylomicron formation.[933] Zinc deficiency is associated with increased formation of malonaldehyde.[1412,1579] As far as malonaldehyde production represents lipid peroxidation and instability of lipids in membranes, zinc deficiency can therefore be considered to favor membrane instability.

4. Minerals/Vitamins

Interactions of zinc and zinc deficiency with metabolism of calcium, copper, iron, selenium, cadmium, and lead are described in Chapter 15. Of the vitamins, vitamin A has been most widely described as dependent on zinc status, since vitamin A levels in plasma are decreased in zinc deficiency[197] and retinene reductase (alcohol dehydrogenase) is a zinc metalloenzyme.[50,1487,1491] Eckhert and Hurley[445] found no interaction of high vitamin A and zinc deficiency with respect to teratogenesis. Carney et al.[226] felt that, although zinc deficiency decreased plasma and liver vitamin A in rats, metabolism of newly ingested vitamin A was not affected. Hence, zinc deficiency does not truly interfere with vitamin A metabolism, except by reducing its requirement due to growth inhibition.

Folic acid has been reported to be lower in zinc deficiency.[1729] Pyridoxal phosphokinase, the enzyme-activating pyridoxal, pyridoxine, or pyridoxamine has been shown to be decreased in zinc deficiency.[1593]

F. Therapy

In principle, the deficiency of an essential nutrient, such as zinc, cannot be corrected except by its replacement. However, some conditions have been described in which the effects of zinc deficiency can be considerably alleviated. Nonsteroidal antiinflammatory drugs including aspirin, indomethacin, and phenylbutazone, and unrelated compounds such as chloroquine, histamine, and histidine block the effect of zinc deficiency in the chick on hock swelling.[1195,1196,1348,1710] The antiinflammatory drugs and chloroquine block the actions or synthesis of PGs, suggesting that the hock swelling in zinc-deficient chicks may be due to PG excess, a possibility with support elsewhere (see Chapter 13).

EFAs reduce parakeratosis in zinc deficient swine,[691,1289] as does histidine.[374] EFAs also reduce the growth retardation and dermal lesions in zinc-deficient rats.[138,346,799]

Lysozyme has also been shown to decrease the onset of dermal lesions in zinc-deficient rats by decreasing bacterial colonization.[1026] Diodoquin added to the diet at 1% was shown to reduce the dermal lesions in zinc-deficient rats without affecting growth retardation or altering skin, plasma, or liver zinc levels.[136] Neidner et al.[1184] have shown that diodoquin increases linoleic acid absorption in acrodermatitis enteropathica (AE). A beneficial effect of diodoquin on linoleic acid absorption would explain the lack of effect of diodoquin on zinc status of the zinc-deficient rat, as well as the beneficial effect of supplemental EFAs in zinc deficiency.

III. OTHER SPECIES

A. Ruminant

Zinc deficiency in ruminants is characterized by parakeratosis, increased salivation, defective hoof formation, and bacterial infiltration of the mouth.[1051] In many countries, ruminants grazing on natural forage are susceptible to zinc deficiency.[1025,1128] Ewes fed a zinc-deficient diet during pregnancy have disrupted parturition and high fetal and neonatal losses,[77] as do those fed an excess of zinc — 750 mg/kg.[221]

One of the genetic models of zinc deficiency is the "lethal trait A-46" in calves. This condition is characterized by hereditary thymic hypoplasia, which is totally responsive to zinc supplementation (500 mg/day).[201,202] Since thymic hypoplasia and decreased production of T lymphocytes is characteristic of zinc depletion associated with protein-energy malnutrition in children,[612,614] this model of zinc deficiency may have direct clinical relevance.

A defect in sperm morphology has been reported in Jersey bulls and ascribed to "toxic" amounts of zinc in the sperm.[152] This abnormality in the sperm tails causes coiling, folding, or splitting of the fibers. Zinc toxicity in the horse (caused by zinc excess in the pasture) has been documented to cause periarticular enlargement of the long bones resulting in lameness.[437]

B. Pig

Studies of zinc deficiency in the pig were initially concerned with the condition, parakeratosis, which is characterized by erythema, seborrhea and hyperkeratinization of the skin, and growth retardation.[691,1289] These studies demonstrated two important points: (1) that the zinc requirement of the pig fed on soy-based diets is considerably higher (about 50 mg/kg) than would be anticipated from studies with soy-based diets fed to other species (15 to 20 mg/kg) and (2) that the effects of zinc deficiency could be partly ameliorated by EFAs. Parakeratosis was induced in 80% of pigs fed suboptimal zinc, but addition of corn oil to the diet completely prevented the effect.[691,1289] The interactions between zinc, copper, calcium, and EFAs in the pig have been recently reviewed.[342]

Pathological and biochemical changes consistent with the effects of zinc deficiency in other species also occur in the pig, including thymic atrophy,[1125] testicular degeneration in boars,[734] impaired parturition in sows,[873,1688] and reduced food intake,[1125] but birthweight and weight gain have been reported to be unaffected by zinc deficiency of the sow.[873]

C. Poultry

Chicks fed a zinc-deficient diet develop a leg disorder characterized by an arthritis-like swelling of the hock joint.[1194-1196,1710] Activity of alkaline phosphatase and collagenase is decreased, as is collagen synthesis.[1547] Although joint swelling also develops in zinc-deficient rats, this condition appears to be species-specific with respect to the degree of incapacitation that develops. It can be largely alleviated by feeding nonsteroidal antiinflammatory drugs or histidine.[1194-1196]

D. Cat

Zinc deficiency has not been widely studied in the cat. It has been used to evaluate retinal function in zinc deficiency. Jacobson et al.[847] reported that the electroretinogram threshold of the rods but not cones was increased in cats that were fed for 4 months on a diet containing about 7 mg/kg zinc.

E. Dog

Dogs have been shown to have an unusually high requirement for zinc; at 20 to 35 mg/kg zinc in the diet for 6 weeks, severe deficiency symptoms were observed which were only prevented at 120 to 130 mg/kg.[1410] In beagles, infection causes acute zinc depletion as part of the characteristic immune response-induced mobilization of zinc to the liver.[525] Decreased zinc absorption has been demonstrated in Alaskan malamutes with chondrodysplasia.[199]

F. Monkey

Hurley and colleagues have conducted a detailed study of the effects of zinc deficiency in the rhesus monkey. Zinc was fed at 4 mg/kg. Plasma zinc varied inversely with weight gain. Lymphocyte response to mitogen stimulation was impaired. Fetal and neonatal losses were increased in both pair-fed and zinc-deficient monkeys. Infant monkeys showed delayed development, lethargy, and hypoactivity after being weaned from the mothers and fed the zinc-deficient diet.[97,617-620,813,984] Hallas[664] has shown that the behavior of the zinc-deficient monkey is characterized by reduced activity, greater susceptibility to stress, increased aggressive behavior, and loss of long- and short-term memory.

G. Hamster

Disrupted estrus has been reported in the zinc-deficient hamster.[1438] The Chinese hamster has been shown to be prone to diabetes; it has defective glucose tolerance[161] and when made zinc deficient, rapidly develops diabetes mellitus.[162] Although there is no hyperglycemia or glucosuria, the insulin response to glucose injection is defective.

H. Rabbit

Experimental zinc deficiency has been reported for the rabbit.[1457] Rabbits have been shown to be susceptible to zinc-induced epilepsy; intracerebral injection of 500 to 600 μg zinc per kg is effective within 5 to 6 hr.[1255]

I. Mouse

Mice, particularly the A/J strain, have been used extensively to study immune dysfunction in zinc deficiency. Thymic atrophy, reduced circulating levels of thymic hormone, and impaired cell-mediated and humeral immunity are found in the zinc-deficient A/J mouse.[109,110,392,509,557,559,655,836] In spite of the immune deficiency, both Ehrlich's ascites tumors[1137] and plastocytoma-derived tumors[507] have retarded growth in zinc-deficient mice.

A number of strains of mice have also been described in which zinc deficiency develops spontaneously, e.g., lethal milk (lm/lm)[464,465] and "super mouse".[1353] The "lethal milk" condition is one in which the milk is deficient in various nutrients, including zinc. As a result, the weanlings do not survive without nutrient supplementation, including zinc.

In view of low serum and femur zinc levels and inability to incorporate supplemental zinc into serum or tissues, the genetically diabetic mouse (db/db) has been suggested to be zinc deficient.[997] Nevertheless, db/db mice fed zinc-deficient diets had no further decrease in the already depressed immune response.[405]

In the presence of supplemental zinc, the genetically obese mouse (ob/ob) demonstrates increased pancreatic insulin and reduction of the exaggerated insulin response to oral glucose.[117,119] This effect of zinc is enhanced in the presence of oxytetracycline.[118] Recent data suggests that in spite of increased plasma zinc, ob/ob mice have significantly lower tissue zinc and may, in fact, be zinc deficient.[896]

Issacson and Sandow[833] reported that a strain of dystrophic mice had markedly elevated zinc levels in the skeletal muscles, specifically in the muscle fibers themselves. This, they suggested, made the "fast" fibers more like "slow" fibers, which normally have more zinc and might therefore be of etiological significance to the muscular dystrophy. Horrobin and Morgan[777] have reasoned along similar lines and hypothesized that myotonic dystrophy may be in part attributable to abnormal utilization of zinc by skeletal and cardiac muscle.

In spite of the obvious similarities between the effects of zinc deficiency in mice and rats, Dreosti et al.[413] recently reported that two distinct differences exist: (1) cyclical feeding was not observed in the zinc-deficient mice and (2) zinc deficiency was teratogenic at 5 mg/kg in the mouse diet, considerably above the degree of depletion required in the rat (<2 mg/kg).

J. Guinea Pig

Zinc deficiency has been produced in the guinea pig, although this species is notorious for starving in preference to consuming a diet of low palatability, e.g., zinc deficient.[35,627,652,1329] With the notable exception of no anorexia,[651] symptoms of dietary zinc deficiency typically observed in other species, e.g., skin lesions, alopecia,[651] and impaired cell-mediated immunity[225] are also noted in the guinea pig.

IV. LIMITATIONS

One major limitation prevents the animal models of zinc deficiency from being widely applicable to human zinc deficiency; the majority of studies have utilized diets in which (1) only zinc is deficient and (2) the zinc is almost totally absent. This creates two conditions which, I believe, do not exist in human zinc deficiency, except under experimental conditions: namely (1) zinc deficiency does not exist without deficiency of other nutrients and (2) human do not consume ''zinc-free'' diets. Rare exceptions to both these conditions do exist, e.g., AE and zinc-free total parenteral nutrition. Since reduced food consumption is one of the early signs and complications of ''zinc-free'' diets, protein-energy malnutrition needs to be controlled for pair feeding.

Two alterations to the methodology of current zinc deficiency research might be helpful: (1) feeding diets not totally devoid of zinc (for the rat, 4 to 5 mg/kg works very effectively) and (2) attempts to mimic human zinc deficiency or depletion more closely. Since alcoholism is probably a major contributor to chronic zinc depletion, the use of marginal zinc deficiency in animal models of alcoholism ought to yield promising results.

Another problem is that, although the rat is the most commonly used laboratory animal model and more is known about zinc deficiency in the rat than in any other species, we must accept that, in many instances, the rat is only a model for itself. Since research on zinc deficiency in animals is ultimately aimed at resolving human zinc deficiency, animal models need to be carefully evaluated for their applicability to human zinc metabolism. In view of my particular interest in the role of zinc in lipid and fatty acid metabolism, it is particularly unfortunate that the rat is so widely used because, in relation to EFAs, the rat is probably the worst model for humans.[778]

On balance, we have probably learned as much about zinc metabolism from human studies as from animals. There is a lot more that humans can still tell us about what goes wrong with zinc metabolism. Therefore, it is essential to keep applying what we find out about zinc metabolism in animal models to the human situation and maintain a feedback between the two in order to maximize the long-term gains made using animal nutritional experimentation.

Chapter 12

PROTEINS, NUCLEIC ACIDS, AND CELL REPLICATION

I. INTRODUCTION

The biological role of zinc is invariably associated with protein synthesis and metabolism (see Table 23). While this is unquestionably a dominant role for zinc, it should be borne in mind that zinc has significant interactions with other major and minor nutrient classes as well, particularly lipids. Furthermore, it has as yet been difficult to definitively relate the effects of experimental zinc deficiency to specific alterations in protein synthesis. Zinc is also a structural and catalytically active component of the enzymes involved in nucleoprotein synthesis. Whereas a functional deficiency in protein synthesis caused by zinc deficiency has not been demonstrated, a failure to adequately synthesize nucleoproteins and to complete the processes of cell replication is a recognized effect of zinc deficiency. Hence, zinc deficiency more significantly affects cell division, which is a function of nucleoprotein synthesis than cell growth and enlargement, which is a function of protein synthesis.

II. PROTEIN METABOLISM

A. Amino Acids

Zinc deficiency in rats increases the rate at which amino acids are oxidized — an effect reversed by zinc supplementation. This has been reported for lysine, leucine and glutamine,[1607] and for methionine.[790] Since protein incorporation of a variety of amino acids in several tissues has been shown to be normal in zinc deficiency, enhanced oxidation of these amino acids cannot be equated with reduced incorporation into tissue proteins.[790] Nevertheless, increased oxidation of amino acids in zinc-deficient rats is undoubtedly associated with the increase in protein catabolism observed in zinc-deficient humans and animals (see Chapter 5).

Cysteine incorporation into skin proteins has clearly been shown to be decreased in zinc deficiency,[789] but its incorporation into proteins in other tissues, such as liver and testes, was not affected. Urinary excretion of cysteine is also increased in zinc deficiency.[789] The incorporation of various other amino acids into skin protein has also been shown to be impaired in zinc deficiency.[790] In view of the rapid onset of dermal lesions in zinc-deficient rats, it would be encouraging to obtain further evidence that these two events are related. Taurine is a sulfur-containing amino acid synthesized from cysteine, and its excretion is increased in zinc deficiency.[793]

Arginine supplementation increases the severity of zinc deficiency in the chick, an effect prevented by zinc supplementation.[295] Since soybean protein increases the zinc requirement of chicks and contains arginine, it is possible that soy protein increases the zinc requirement not only through its content of the zinc chelator, phytic acid, but also because of its content of arginine.

Histidine given acutely by i.v. injection or chronically by gastric intubation significantly enhances zinc excretion.[719] Histidine chelates tissue zinc through its imidazole group and can prevent the effect of zinc reducing lactate production by muscle.[826] Both of these effects are suggestive of a pharmacological interaction between excess histidine and zinc. Physiologically, histidine forms important complexes with zinc, particularly in skin.[1339] Histidine also prevents the effects of zinc deficiency in the chick.[1194] Nonsteroidal antiinflammatory drugs such as aspirin also have this effect and Suso and Edwards[1585] established that both histidine and aspirin form complexes with zinc that can be absorbed intact.

Table 23
INTERACTION OF ZINC WITH PROTEINS

- Direct effects of zinc
  - Chelation by sulfhydryl-containing amino acids (cysteine)
  - Chelation by nitrogen-containing amino acids (histidine)
  - Induces metallothionein
  - Increases hemoglobin affinity for oxygen
  - Stabilizes and binds tubulin
  - Facilitates DNA denaturation/renaturation
  - Stimulates protein phosphorylation
- Zinc-deficiency causes
  - Increased
    - Amino acid oxidation
    - Amino acid excretion
    - 5′ AMP amino hydrolase activity
    - Adenosuccinate lyase activity
    - Ribonuclease activity
  - Decreased
    - Incorporation of cysteine and methionine into proteins
    - Collagen cross-linking
    - Total collagen (tissue-specific)
    - DNA and RNA polymerase (tissue-specific)
    - Thymidine kinase
    - Methionine and thymidine incorporation into DNA

B. Protein Synthesis

Although zinc deficiency in the rat increases amino acid oxidation and excretion, until recently,[646] evidence has not consistently demonstrated that protein synthesis per se is inhibited by zinc deficiency. Thus, the demonstration that total protein in various tissues is lower in zinc-deficient rats and that nonprotein nitrogen is increased[910] could not be directly attributed to decreased protein synthesis. Sandstead et al.[1402] have observed decreased protein synthesis in the brains of neonatal zinc-deficient rats. Wallwork and Duerre[167] have demonstrated impaired methionine uptake by the perfused liver from zinc-deficient rats. This was associated with decreased methylation of DNA.

C. Protein Depletion

In humans, zinc deficiency does not usually occur in the absence of some degree of protein depletion, e.g., either reduced intake or increased excretion of protein (urinary or fecal). It is therefore important to consider whether there is an interaction between depletion of zinc and protein. Severe zinc deficiency in the rat does result in net protein loss due to a combination of reduced protein synthesis and enhanced protein degradation. Reduced circulating insulin and increased circulating corticosteroids may contribute to this effect.[646] Zinc deficiency may also intensify protein depletion by increasing oxidation and urinary excretion of amino acids.[763,796] Enzymes associated with protein catabolism, e.g., 5′ adenosine monophosphate (AMP) aminohydrolase, adenylosuccinate synthetase, and adenosuccinate lyase have been reported to be increased in zinc-deficient weanling rats.[194] Nevertheless, total muscle protein was unchanged in the zinc-deficient rats in this study.

Low protein (normal zinc) intake in the rat is associated with lower zinc levels in intestine and liver, an effect suggested to induce secondary zinc deficiency.[1643] Zinc deficiency has been shown not to affect protein uptake by the mesenteric lymphatic system.[846] In zinc-deficient pregnant rats, nitrogen retention has been shown to become negative toward term as a consequence, not of increased nitrogen excretion, but of decreased intake.[638] This situation might equally apply in humans.

III. METALLOTHIONEIN

Metallothionein is a protein of molecular weight 6300 to 6600 daltons, which is composed of 20 cysteine residues and contains 7 g of atoms of bound zinc per mole. It is inducible in liver, kidney, intestinal mucosa, thymus, and malignant cell lines by divalent metals such as zinc, copper, and cadmium.[173,1226,1687] Metallothionein synthesis in the intestine appears to be a function of zinc status, and it may assist in zinc absorption.[316]

Metallothionein induced in liver is generally reported to be dependent on zinc status; when zinc status is low, metallothionein is not synthesized, but following zinc administration, metallothionein-bound zinc is immediately detectable.[169,315-317,642,1415] Zinc deficiency is associated with lower plasma metallothionein[1413] and in zinc-deficient pregnant rats, fetal liver metallothionein levels are also reduced.[577]

Metallothionein catabolism is associated with the release of zinc.[172] Ferritin has been shown to donate zinc to metallothionein following zinc administration to rats, suggesting that it may "detoxify" high levels of zinc prior to metallothionein synthesis,[1323] a process dependent on the production of new protein.[316,741]

The physiological relevance of the induction of metallothionein by high doses of zinc has been questioned by Chen et al.,[260] who found that metallothionein was not induced in the liver until dietary zinc reached a level 40 times normal. In conditions favoring synthesis of metallothionein, zinc excreted in the bile was not found in association with metallothionein. Since zinc loading at such levels is normally unlikely, direct induction of metallothionein by increasing dietary zinc may not be physiological. Rather, such a mechanism may function to cope with toxic amounts of zinc and other metals, such as copper and cadmium, which also induce metallothionein.

Metallothionein is also synthesized by the liver in conditions of acute stress, e.g., acute infection, an effect due partly to stimulation by glucocorticoids.[316,317,472,1411] The increase in liver metallothionein following infection is considered to be steroid-dependent and to be the principal reason for the rapid decline in plasma zinc.[402] However, adrenalectomy in the rat causes an increase of ten times in liver metallothionein.[167]

Mediators of acute stress reactions are associated with metallothionein induction. Interleukin I from immunologically challenged monocytes also stimulates metallothionein synthesis.[912] As well, catecholamines have been shown to have a quantitatively greater effect on liver metallothionein synthesis than steroids.[168,320] Polypeptides, including glucagon and angiotensin II but not arginine vasopressin, induce a twofold increase in rat liver metallothionein.[705] Catecholamines and not steroids may therefore be the primary messenger for stress-induced metallothionein synthesis. The mobilization of zinc to the liver and the synthesis of zinc-metallothionein as part of the reaction to acute stress are not understood in terms of a defense mechanism. Is this to facilitate (1) stimulation of the immune system or (2) new protein synthesis? Recent evidence suggests that one of the physiological benefits of zinc-metallothionein is as an effective antioxidant; in erythrocyte ghosts, lipid peroxidation induced by xanthine oxidase and/or iron was prevented by zinc-metallothionein.[1610]

IV. COLLAGEN

A number of enzymes involved in collagen synthesis are zinc metalloenzymes, including alkaline phosphatase, collagenase, and DNA and RNA polymerase.[798] Fernandez-Madrid et al.[513] have reviewed the evidence relating the effects of zinc deficiency in rats to collagen metabolism and have concluded that total collagen is reduced in zinc deficiency. The effect is partly due to a generalized impairment of protein synthesis and partly to a specific effect on collagen cross-linking. A more fundamental role of zinc in DNA metabolism may also be involved. However, others have reported that the total content of collagen in skin, aorta, and cartilage is unaffected by zinc deficiency.[1278] Therefore, it appears to be collagen cross-linking per se that is defective in zinc-deficient rats. Defective collagen cross-linking in the skin of zinc-deficient rats[1303] is probably due, at least in part, to the relationship of zinc to lysyl oxidase. Interestingly, in vitro, the addition of 5 to 500 μM zinc inhibits proline hydroxylation,[70] suggesting the interaction of zinc with collagen metabolism may be biphasic.

Alkaline phosphatase in epiphysial plates is not as readily stained in zinc deficient as control chicks, particularly in areas remote from the blood supply.[1709] In zinc-deficient chicks, it was also found that chondrocytes remote from the blood supply did not mature and degenerate normally.[1709] Although collagen and mucopolysaccaride secretion have been shown to be defective in zinc deficiency, formation of the calcified matrix is apparently normal in zinc deficiency.

Westmorland[1709] has emphasized that the effect of zinc deficiency on collagen metabolism appears to be strongest in tissues and/or cell layers to which blood supply is low or minimal, e.g., skin, some areas of cartilage, and the epithelium of the esophagus. He has indicated that blood supply and hence the supply of an essential nutrient (not necessarily zinc, but a nutrient whose synthesis is zinc-dependent) is a factor correlated with the degree to which zinc deficiency affects that tissue. To my knowledge, this hypothesis has not been further investigated. It may be simply that zinc supply to the tissue is dependent on the blood supply and hence cells furthest away from the nutrient (zinc) supply will be most affected. Alternatively, in view of the link between zinc and cholesterol metabolism (Chapter 13) and the fact that it is the less vascular tissues (collagenous) which normally accumulate cholesterol, the relationship between zinc and collagen metabolism may be linked to cholesterol.

The fundamental issue of whether the effect of zinc deficiency in animals can be related to humans is applicable in discussing the relationship of zinc to collagen metabolism. From the data reviewed here, it would appear reasonable to say that zinc deficiency in humans would be a cause of impaired wound healing and that zinc supplementation would shorten the time to heal a wound. In reality, zinc seems only to be beneficial if the individual was zinc depleted for other reasons; if zinc depletion prior to wounding was not present, zinc supplementation is of no benefit to the healing of various types of wounds (Chapter 4). The fact that pure zinc deficiency rarely if ever exists in humans must be the cause of this discrepancy between the effects of zinc demonstrated in rats and humans in relation to collagen metabolism.

V. HEMOGLOBIN

The interaction of zinc with hemoglobin involves both its synthesis and oxygen affinity. Amino-levulinic acid dehydratase is a zinc-metalloenzyme and catalyzes the condensation of two molecules of δ-amino-levulinic acid to form porphobilinogen, a precursor in the formation of heme. The rate of hemoglobin synthesis has not been reported in conditions of zinc deficiency; in fact, the hematocrit is elevated in zinc-deficient rats.[1248] This is more likely due to hemoconcentration than increased hemoglobin synthesis. Impaired heme synthesis in uremic patients has been suggested to potentially benefit from zinc supplementation.[1750]

Zinc increases the affinity of hemoglobin for oxygen and favors the formation of oxyhemoglobin.[871,1217] The interaction of zinc with hemoglobin, which increases the affinity of hemoglobin for oxygen, involves the binding of zinc directly to heme; the saturation of zinc (zinc to heme, 1:2) at this site increases its affinity for oxygen by 3.7 times.[1360] The effect of zinc is reduced in the presence of calcium[380] and diphosphoglycerate.[1218,1360] The high permeability of the erythrocyte membrane to zinc[951] favors zinc interaction with hemoglobin.

VI. MICROTUBULES AND TUBULIN

Zinc stabilizes microtubule proteins and prevents their depolymerization when homogenates of microtubule-rich tissues are prepared, e.g., brain.[1190] Drugs such as colchicine readily bind to microtubule proteins, an effect prevented by zinc. Since the properties of the zinc-stabilized microtubules stabilized in vitro by zinc are similar to those in vivo, the zinc effect has been considered physiological. Cells in which the microtubules are thought to be stabilized by zinc include leukocytes, spermatogenic epithelial cells,[1190] and brain.[736]

Zinc has been shown to have high-affinity binding sites on tubulin, which are thought to participate in its assembly.[249,436,733,735,736] When the ratio of zinc to tubulin in low, microtubules are formed, but when the ratio is high, protofilaments are formed.[701] In in vitro preparations of brain from zinc-deficient pigs, tubulin assembly has been shown to be disorganized.[732,733]

VII. IMMUNOLOGICAL PROTEINS

The essential role of zinc in optimizing the cellular immune system may so far be linked with both interferon and thymus-derived peptide hormones. Interferon-β synthesis by *Escherichia coli* is unstable in the absence of additional zinc; 0.1 to 0.3 m*M* of zinc increases the yield of interferon-β by inhibiting the proteases which would otherwise degrade the interferon.[643] Thymulin (serum thymic factor) is the best known of the thymic hormones. It is a polypeptide of molecular weight 2000 to 3000 daltons. Zinc is essential for its activity and structural conformation.[975]

VIII. NUCLEIC ACIDS

Zinc has a central role in the metabolism of RNA and DNA. Both RNA and DNA polymerases contain two intrinsic zinc ions; in RNA polymerase, one zinc ion is structural, whereas the other is catalytic.[597]

Zinc deficiency impairs the synthesis of both RNA and DNA and also stimulates the activity of the enzyme, ribonuclease, which catalyzes their degradation. However, it has been pointed out that the ''side effects'' of experimental zinc deficiency in animals, including anorexia and cyclical food intake, also have influences on the activity of thymidine kinase.[1766] Hence, results need to be interpreted in light of the types of controls used and the length of time that zinc-deficient diets were fed. Furthermore, many of the effects of zinc on nucleoprotein synthesis and degradation are tissue-specific; in the liver, kidney, spleen, testes, thymus, and pancreas of zinc-deficient rats, nucleoprotein synthesis is inhibited (reviewed by Kirchgessner et al.[910]), but, in both esophagus and buccal mucosa, hyperkeratinization occurs during zinc deficiency and, in both tissues, enhanced DNA synthesis has been demonstrated.[43,397] In spite of marked thymic atrophy in zinc-deficient animals of all species studied, Stephan and Hsu[1557] showed that thymic incorporation of thymidine into DNA was *increased*.

Although reports have been published describing a reduction in total tissue content of both DNA and RNA in zinc deficiency,[1031,1646] these effects are not consistently observed. Recently, however, it has been clearly demonstrated that a specific reduction in methionine incorporation into DNA occurs in zinc-deficient rats.[1671] Therefore, in spite of a possible effect of zinc deficiency on *tissue content* of nucleoprotein polymerases, including DNA polymerase, RNA polymerase, and thymidine kinase, the most clear-cut effect of zinc deficiency still seems to be on their *activity*.[414,910,1312,1379,1402,1406,1515,1595]

The other important aspect of the interaction of zinc with nucleoproteins is in relation to their *synthesis*. It has been shown that within a few days of having initiated the zinc-deficient diet, thymidine incorporation into DNA is inhibited.[1726,1727] The temporal relationship between growth retardation and inhibition of DNA synthesis caused by zinc deficiency is therefore close and probably *not* a consequence of impaired food intake and generalized protein-energy malnutrition, both of which are complications of longer-term studies. These results are supported by in vitro data showing impaired thymidine uptake by melanoma cells raised in zinc-deficient media.[1166]

The rapid onset of either the inhibitory effect of zinc deficiency or the stimulatory effect of zinc supplementation on DNA and RNA synthesis implicates a tissue pool of zinc that can be very rapidly depleted, e.g., one with a high rate of turnover.[267,1735] The likely importance of such a zinc pool has been alluded to earlier.[910] Identification of such a pool will be a significant boost to the understanding of conditions controlling zinc metabolism during zinc deficiency. Since the effect of zinc deficiency on DNA synthesis has been so clearly demonstrated to occur within a short time after inducing zinc deficiency,[1726,1727] it would seem that effects of zinc deficiency that take weeks to develop are less likely to be specific for zinc deficiency, e.g., those related to zinc metalloenzymes and tissue zinc levels (Chapters 10 and 11).

Zinc supplementation in vitro has been shown to have effects opposite to zinc deficiency on the activity of DNA and RNA polymerase,[1707] ribonuclease,[1221] and RNA transcription.[1735] Hence, the effects of zinc depletion, which have often been indirectly demonstrated, e.g., using EDTA to chelate zinc thereby reducing its concentration and availability, have been shown to be reversible by zinc addition. This provides strong evidence of a specific role of zinc in synthesis of nucleoproteins.

RNA and DNA polymerase from bacteriophage T7 contain no intrinsic zinc, and exogenous supplemented zinc inhibits the DNA polymerase,[1478] but does not affect the RNA polymerase.[905] This may be a significant means by which bacteriophage can synthesize protein without depending on the availability of host zinc.

IX. CELL REPLICATION

Chesters[267] has reviewed the relationship between zinc and cell replication. He has pointed out that DNA synthesis is more sensitive to the effects of zinc deficiency than RNA synthesis and has proposed that cell replication (a function of DNA synthesis) is more susceptible to the effects of zinc depletion than cell growth (a function of RNA synthesis).

The inhibition of DNA synthesis in cells in culture by zinc depletion of the medium appears to be related primarily to impaired synthesis of proteins directly involved in the cell cycle and secondarily to reduced activity of nucleic acid polymerases. The arrest of replication of cells grown in zinc-deficient media[495] would therefore appear to be due to impaired *induction* of DNA synthesis, ultimately a function of genetic expression.[497]

For the purposes of inducing DNA synthesis, a particular zinc metalloenzyme may not be as important as the reversible *binding* of zinc to DNA,[1126] which uniquely permits DNA denaturation and renaturation.[452] This may be the critical role for zinc in DNA synthesis.

Alternatively, stimulation of protein phosphorylation, which is exquisitely sensitive to zinc,[38,875] may also be a significant function for zinc in regulating cell replication. Either function would involve a pool of zinc that was freely exchangeable.[267,910]

Chapter 13

FATTY ACIDS, LIPIDS, AND MEMBRANES

I. INTRODUCTION

No previous review on zinc metabolism has adequately covered the important interactions of zinc and lipids. This is not for lack of research, because approximately 140 articles have been published on the subject since 1958. Of these, nearly half have been published prior to 1980, so the subject is not a new one. In view of the lack of a previous review on the subject of zinc interactions with lipids (other than essential fatty acids (EFAs)[341,342,776] and membranes [137,276]), a fairly detailed review is given here.

II. EFAs

The physiologically important long-chain fatty acids are those of 16 to 24 carbons in length. These fatty acids belong to different families, depending on the position of the first double bond from the methyl end of the molecule. Only two of these families of fatty acids comprise the EFAs, those with the n-6 configuration (first double bond 6 carbons from the methyl terminal), or those with the n-3 configuration (first double bond 3 carbons from the methyl terminal). Their metabolism is outlined in Figure 3. The parent fatty acids of these two families (linoleic acid, 18:2n-6 and α-linolenic acid, 18:3n-3) cannot be formed by animals or humans, hence their *essentiality*. Their products are formed by the stepwise desaturation and elongation reactions characteristic of metabolism of the long-chain fatty acids.

Zinc has been shown to affect two main aspects of EFA metabolism: (1) the desaturation-elongation pathway and (2) lipid incorporation of EFA (Figure 4). Most of the interactions have been demonstrated through the effects of zinc deficiency and this, it will be appreciated, is complicated by the effects of reduced food intake.[940] Nevertheless, the effects of zinc deficiency on EFA metabolism are relatively consistent in various experimental systems, whether controls are fed *ad libitum* or pair fed.[348]

The symptoms of zinc deficiency in rats are superficially similar to those of EFA deficiency (see Table 24). The majority of these symptoms of deficiencies of both these nutrients were recognized in the 1930s, but the possibility of an interaction of these nutrients was not described until 1958.[691] The exacerbation of EFA deficiency by zinc deficiency or high calcium intake has been reported.[757]

A. Tissue Levels

The single largest area of research on the interaction between zinc and EFA has focused on the effects of zinc deficiency on tissue levels of EFAs. The fatty acid analysis is done initially by extraction of tissue total lipids.

Sometimes, the total lipid fatty acid composition is analyzed without separating the lipid classes. Changes in the fatty acid composition of the various lipid classes, particularly phospholipids and triglycerides, in response to zinc deficiency,[360] can be opposite to each other and thereby cancel the effect observed if only the total fatty acid pattern is analyzed.[543] It is therefore preferable to subdivide the lipids into their constituent classes, e.g., triglyceride, phospholipid, cholesterol esters, and free-fatty acids, prior to fatty acid analysis.

One other problem with the analysis of fatty acids is that currently, only the *proportional* composition is determined, e.g., differences in relative *concentration* can be assessed. The concentration of a fatty acid relative to other fatty acids indicates its accessibility to enzymes

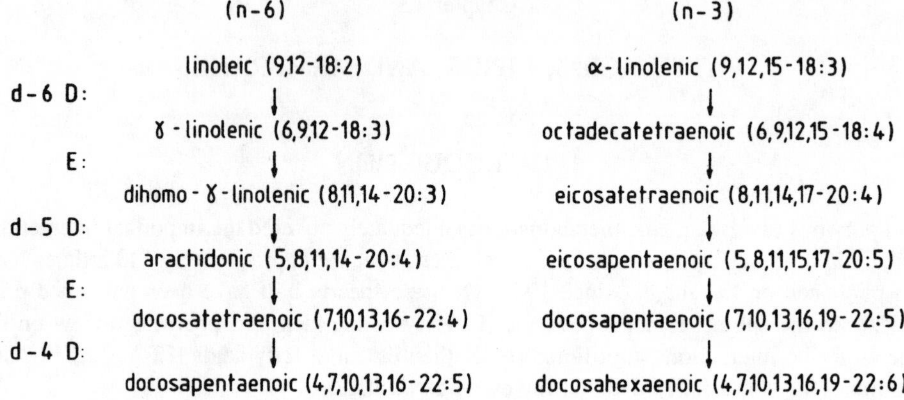

FIGURE 3. Metabolism of the EFAs. The two families of EFAs are distinguished by the positions of the double bonds in the fatty acid molecules. The linoleic acid family comprises those fatty acids sequentially synthesized from linoleic acid, all of which have the first double bond six carbons from the methyl terminal of the fatty acid. The α-linolenic acid family has fatty acids with the double bonds initially positioned at the third carbon from the methyl terminal. Both families are metabolized alternately by the desaturases and elongases (d-6 D — Δ-6 desaturase, d-5-D — Δ-5 desaturase, and d-4 D — Δ-4 desaturase, respectively; E — elongase).

for which other fatty acids may also compete. Most laboratories do not measure the quantitative amount of the parent lipids, so quantitative fatty acid composition has not so far been described for zinc-deficient conditions. In spite of these limitations, a lot of significant progress has been made concerning the interactions of zinc with EFA.

1. Humans

Clinical conditions associated with altered metabolism of both zinc and EFAs are shown in Figure 3 and Table 25.

Since the paper by Cash and Berger[236] suggesting that EFA metabolism might be defective in acrodermatitis enteropathica (AE), a number of reports of fatty acid levels in AE have been published.[357,869,881,1184,1719] With the exception of the study of Kayden and Cox,[881] who found no difference in EFA in AE, these reports clearly demonstrated that EFA metabolism was impaired in AE. Julius et al.[869] noted that *free* arachidonic acid was *increased* in serum of a patient with AE, an effect consistent with the known effects of zinc deficiency on EFA incorporation into lipids (see later). Neldner et al.[1184] reported low arachidonic acid levels in AE and suggested that there was a defect in both EFA and zinc metabolism. These reports appeared at the time of the demonstration of impaired zinc absorption in AE,[103] but have never been acknowledged by researchers reporting the role of zinc in AE.

Before zinc was used for treating AE, diodoquin was the only therapy. Although it had been suggested that the main effect of diodoquin in AE was to increase zinc absorption by zinc chelation, Neldner et al.[1184] thought it might also increase EFA absorption. This has received some support recently in studies of diodoquin effects in zinc-deficient rats in which the symptoms were corrected but zinc status was unchanged.[136] Hambidge et al.[682] alluded to fatty acid changes in AE being corrected by zinc supplementation, but did not specify further.

Holman[758] presented fatty acid data on a patient with AE, which also suggested that EFA metabolism is interrupted in AE, not at the level of linoleic acid desaturation, but at the next step, elongation of γ-linoleic acid (18:3n-6, see Figure 3). Cash and Berger[236] made similar observations. Either way, arachidonic acid synthesis would be impaired. Recently, Cunnane and Krieger[357] have reported that AE patients have raised linoleic acid levels and lowered metabolites of linoleic acid in plasma phospholipids, results that are consistent with

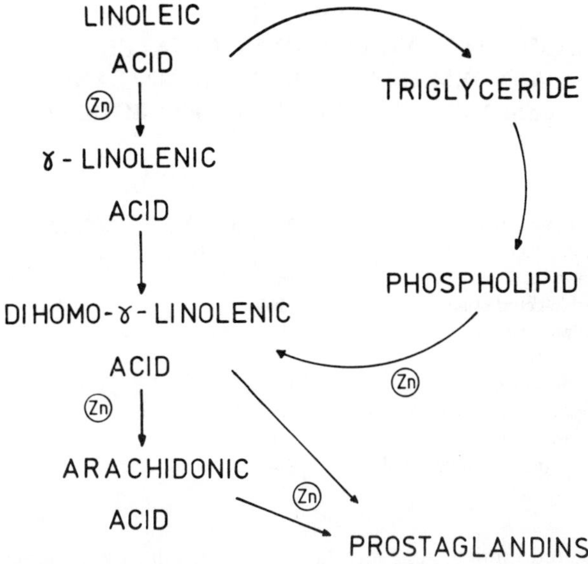

FIGURE 4. Sites at which zinc is known to influence lipid and fatty acid metabolism. Zinc deficiency in both humans and animals increases the level of linoleic acid, increases dihomo-γ-linolenic acid, and decreases arachidonic acid, steps involving the Δ-6 and Δ-5 desaturases. Although the desaturases contain iron as the metal cofactor, microsomal zinc levels directly determine electron transfer from nicotinamide-adenine-dinucleotide hydride (NADH) or nicotinamide-adenine dinucleotide phosphate hydride (NADPH) through the cytochromes to the desaturase protein, which is the terminal electron acceptor. The effects of zinc deficiency on this electron transfer pathway are opposite to those of zinc supplementation, suggesting a direct role of zinc in this pathway, rather than an indirect effect of zinc deficiency through, for example, food intake reduction. Zinc also has complex interactions in the synthesis of prostaglandins (PGs), inhibiting some of the enzymes involved, including the phospholipases and thromboxane synthetase. In zinc deficiency, the overwhelming effect is to increase the tissue and serum levels of "2 series" PGs (those derived from arachidonic acid), whereas zinc supplementation decreases PG production. Levels of free (nonesterified) EFAs tend to increase in both clinical and experimental zinc deficiency, an effect possibly related to the phospholipases.

Table 24
SIMILARITIES BETWEEN DEFICIENCIES OF ZINC AND ESSENTIAL FATTY ACIDS (EFAs)

Growth retardation
Dermal lesions
Immunodeficiency
Alopecia
Male and female infertility
Impaired parturition
High perinatal losses
Increased capillary permeability
Increased epidermal water loss
Exacerbation by calcium and copper

Table 25
CLINICAL CONDITIONS ASSOCIATED WITH ABNORMALITIES OF BOTH ZINC AND ESSENTIAL FATTY ACID METABOLISM

Condition	Ref.
Acrodermatitis enteropathica	236, 357, 690, 758, 869, 922, 1157, 1184, 1363, 1674, 1719
Anorexia nervosa	16, 1500
Sickle-cell disease	1169
Atopic eczema	382, 1049
Cystic fibrosis	758, 1509
Crohn's disease	153, 345
Protein-energy malnutrition	608, 923, 1736
Multiple sclerosis	410, 761
Transient neonatal zinc deficiency	944

the concept of impaired linoleic acid metabolism as a result of zinc depletion. Furthermore, zinc supplementation of the AE patient was shown to increase arachidonic acid levels to control values in serum phospholipids.

Walldius et al.[1669] have recently described two adolescents with AE, in one of whom EFA and zinc treatments were alternated. Lower linoleic acid levels were noted when serum zinc was low and vice versa. A child manifesting symptoms of both AE and cystic fibrosis was found to have low zinc and EFA status, but raised serum prostaglandins (PGs).[690] Zinc treatment raised EFA and lowered PG levels. Zinc treatment has also been shown to significantly raise linoleic acid and arachidonic acid in serum triglycerides and cholesteryl esters, but not phospholipids in a female child with AE.[922]

In sickle-cell disease, erythrocyte levels of linoleic acid have been shown to be decreased and levels of dihomo-γ-linolenic acid (20:3n-6) to be increased. In the same patients, plasma zinc was decreased, but erythrocyte zinc was unchanged from controls.[1169]

In a report of the possible beneficial effects of zinc in tropical skin ulcers, Watkinson et al.[1683] noted that the levels of EFA (linoleic acid and arachidonic acid) were unchanged in plasma *total* lipid samples following zinc supplementation. Of interest was the decrease in oleic acid (18:1n-9) after zinc supplementation, an effect also demonstrated in animals[343] and predicted from the competitive nature of the metabolism of n-6 and n-9 fatty acids.[341]

Plasma zinc levels in cystic fibrosis have been shown to correlate positively with the levels of dihomo-γ-linolenic acid (20:3n-6) and arachidonic acid, but not with linoleic acid.[687] The authors suggested that this was evidence in favor of the role of zinc in linoleic acid desaturation. Parallel observations were made by Fogerty et al.,[543] who have shown that, in infants and young children, liver levels of arachidonic acid are significantly positively correlated with liver zinc levels.

2. *Animals*

In animal studies of zinc deficiency, effects on tissue EFA levels have been inconsistent. Some reports indicate that the *ratio* of linoleic acid to longer-chain fatty acids, e.g., dihomo-γ-linolenic acid and arachidonic acid, is increased.[144,254,289,360] Others have reported that arachidonic acid is *increased* in some tissues such as skin, liver, and mammary tissue of zinc-deficient rats.[138,139,352,355,366,543,799,1214] Two reasons for this discrepancy are possible: (1) *total* lipid rather than individual lipid fatty acid profiles were determined (particularly in liver) and (2) zinc-deficiency effects are tissue-specific (particularly evident when comparing effects on mammary tissue with other tissues).[366] Equally important is the recent demonstration that skin does not convert linoleic acid to arachidonic acid.[256] The increase in arachidonic acid in the skin of zinc-deficient rats and chicks therefore indicates that it is transported there in greater amounts, not that it is being synthesized in greater amounts. The transport of arachidonic acid to the skin in zinc deficiency may be to help correct the dermal lesions.

It should not be overlooked that most of the studies demonstrating an effect of zinc deficiency on EFA levels have been conducted over a period of 3 to 6 weeks, during which reduced food intake would be present. Although it has been claimed that reduced food intake can account for all of the effects of zinc deficiency in the rat,[861,940] conclusive evidence has been presented showing that comparison of zinc-deficient rats to rigorously pair fed controls still presents a fatty acid profile consistent with impaired linoleic acid metabolism.[343,348,360]

B. Desaturation

The metabolic steps in the EFA pathway that appear most susceptible to the effects of zinc deficiency are the conversion of linoleic acid to longer-chain metabolites, a reaction involving metabolism of linoleic acid (Δ-6 desaturase), and dihomo-γ-linoleic acid (Δ-5 desaturase). A further desaturation step (Δ-4 desaturase) is also present, but the effect of zinc on this step has not been studied.

Studies of the microsomal desaturation of linoleic acid and dihomo-γ-linolenic acid have shown that the effect of zinc deficiency is tissue-dependent and also sensitive to the degree of zinc deprivation. Pregnant rats fed 5 mg/kg zinc had linoleic acid desaturation values that were lower than controls (uterus), higher than controls (mammary gland), and not different than controls (liver).[365,366] Δ-9 desaturation has been shown to be increased in zinc-deficient rat testes.[290] Subsequently, in rats fed minimal zinc (1 to 2 mg/kg), linoleic and dihomo-γ-linolenic acid desaturation has been unequivocally shown to be decreased in comparison with both *ad libitum* and pair-fed controls.[87,289,518,1619]

The increase in skin levels of arachidonic acid in zinc-deficient rats[138,799] and chicks[139] are not inconsistent with impaired linoleic acid desaturation, because the skin does not synthesize arachidonic acid from linoleic acid.[256] Hence, its accumulation there is probably a result of a transport phenomenon and is unrelated to linoleic acid desaturation.

The mechanism by which zinc might interact with the desaturases is, at present, unknown. Certain factors, however, increase the likelihood of such an interaction. Zinc is present in relatively high amounts in liver microsomes,[137] the cellular component responsible for fatty acid desaturation. Electrons required for the desaturation of long-chain fatty acids are provided by nicotinamide-adenine dinucleotide hydride (NADH) B_5. Cytochrome B_5 reductase activity is impaired in liver microsomes from zinc-deficient rats[1771] causing interrupted electron transfer from the donor (NADH) to the terminal acceptor (desaturase-acyl CoA complex). Cytochrome P-450 activity is also significantly decreased in zinc-deficient rats,[114] suggesting a second possible site at which zinc deficiency would inhibit the terminal desaturase reaction. Furthermore, purified linoleoyl CoA desaturase has 12 histidine and 4 cysteine residues.[1223] The confirmation of the enzyme might therefore depend on zinc bound to these residues.

One important consequence of an effect of zinc deficiency on the desaturases is that EFA content of the diet can be adequate, but *metabolic* EFA deficiency is nonetheless induced, e.g., impaired synthesis of arachidonic acid. The classical biochemical sign of EFA deficiency, raised eicosatrienoic acid (20:3n-9), does not occur in zinc-deficient animals[341,757,799] or humans,[357,869,944] because its synthesis is also dependent on the Δ-6 desaturase; if the desaturase activity is decreased, 20:3n-9 will not be synthesized.

C. EFA Supplementation

1. Humans

Cash and Berger[236] showed that cottonseed oil (54% linoleic acid) given i.v. to three patients with AE reduced the dermal lesions; arachidonic acid was not effective.

2. Animals

In zinc-deficient pigs with parakeratosis, Hansen et al.[691] and Pond et al.[1289] have shown that supplementation with corn oil (45 to 65% linoleic acid), with or without zinc, markedly reduced the dermal lesions. It has been widely demonstrated that growth retardation, dermal lesions, and altered weights of organs, such as thymus, in zinc-deficient rats can be partly corrected by EFA supplementation.[138,334,340,350,351,353,355,799]

D. Fatty Acid Synthesis and Lipid Incorporation

Pregnant zinc-deficient rats at term have been reported to have significantly lower Δ-9 desaturase and fatty acid synthetase activity in liver microsomal preparations.[398] These findings are in contrast to those made in young male zinc-deficient rats in which both of these parameters were significantly increased.[290] Nevertheless, these inconsistencies are probably related to differences in the physiological condition of the rats (young male vs. pregnant female) and reflect differences also seen in Δ-6 desaturase activity between these two groups.[290,366]

EFAs are mainly incorporated into triglycerides, phospholipids, and cholesterol esters; in the rat, arachidonic acid is favored in cholesterol esters and phospholipids and linoleic acid in triglycerides. EFAs in the diet are mainly present as triglycerides, but are absorbed as free-fatty acids and monoglycerides and are then incorporated into the appropriate lipid classes. This step is influenced by zinc deficiency (Figure 4).

Free dihomo-γ-linolenic acid has been shown to accumulate in triglyceride and as the free acid in zinc-deficient rat pups.[334,354] Arachidonic acid also is increased in triglycerides of leukocytes of zinc-deficient pregnant rats.[356] In both Crohn's disease[345] and AE,[869] free arachidonic acid is increased. This also occurs in leukocytes during pregnancy,[362] a condition in which peripheral leukocytes contain lower zinc.[1100]

E. Physiological Interactions

The physiological actions of zinc and dihomo-γ-linolenic acid and PG E_1 in mesenteric vessels in vitro are similar (see Chapter 18) and may reflect an effect of zinc on dihomo-γ-linolenic acid release from endothelial phospholipids.[352,1048,1160]

F. Zinc Absorption

Possible mechanisms controlling zinc absorption and ligands that might be involved have been discussed in detail in Chapter 9. However, the possible function of EFA and/or PGs in zinc absorption is worth reviewing briefly. Roles for both EFA and PGs in zinc absorption have been suggested largely on the basis of rat studies and are, as yet, inconclusive. PG effects are more controversial because of the inconsistency of their effects. Depending on the type of PG and dose studied, they have been shown to (1) increase,[339,1520-1522] (2) have no effect on,[339,1524] or (3) decrease[1492] zinc absorption. Nevertheless, PG E_1 and zinc levels are correlated in the gut mucosa.[1117] Whether PGs bind zinc directly in the gut is controversial.[482,1521] In one clinical study of therapeutic levels of a PG synthetase inhibitor, indomethacin, given for 3 days prior to a zinc-tolerance test, zinc absorption was not affected over the 4-hr test period.[1568]

Low concentrations (10 to 1 ng μg/mℓ) of linoleic acid, γ-linolenic acid, and dihomo-γ-linolenic acid,[339] as well as higher concentrations of arachidonic acid,[1524] have been shown to increase zinc absorption. Zinc deficiency causes increased zinc absorption and is associated with higher EFA and PG levels in the gut.[339,344,1523] Since about 30% of the total zinc in human milk is bound to fat,[562,1016] and human milk is richer in EFA than cow's milk or artificial formula,[857] it is reasonable to consider a role of EFA and/or PGs in stimulating zinc absorption. The role is not necessarily as a ligand, but perhaps as a facilitator of mucosal uptake of zinc-ligand complexes.

III. PROSTIGLANDINS — LEVELS AND SYNTHESIS

Concurrent with the start of studies in zinc interaction with EFA, zinc was also shown to have physiological and biochemical interactions with PGs. In general, zinc deficiency increases the measurable amounts of PGs and, in physiological to pharmacological doses, zinc inhibits PG synthesis, but many inconsistencies have been reported, even by the same authors.

Indirect evidence from (1) in vitro vascular preparations[775,779,1048,1050] and (2) the similarity of zinc deficiency and aspirin toxicity to the pregnant rat[1211] initially suggested that PG synthesis would be directly affected by zinc status. Direct assays have since confirmed that PG E_1, at least in gut contents, varies, as does the zinc concentration.[1117] These data are consistent with the in vitro data suggesting a relationship between zinc, dihomo-γ-linolenic acid, and PG E_1.[334,341,352,1048] Release of PGs from ionophore-stimulated human neutrophils has been shown to be increased by 0.1 m*M* zinc.[626] The route of zinc administration (p.o. or i.p.), the PG being measured, and the assay site (intestine vs. plasma) are also variables affecting the impact of zinc on PG levels.[1524]

PG levels in the serum of a patient with cystic fibrosis complicated by AE-like dermal lesions were shown to be above control values for thromboxane B_2 and PG I_2 (prostacyclin).[690] Treatment with zinc brought the PG levels down within 10 days. The ratio of PG E_2/PG $F_{2\alpha}$ in monocytes of pregnant women also varies directly with the zinc status of the individual.[1469]

Increased levels of "2 series" PGs in vivo were not expected to be found in zinc deficiency but, with few exceptions,[253,254,485] this appears to be the predominant effect.[59,96,200,255,486,582,821,1207,1209] Conversely, zinc supplementation generally appears to decrease PG synthesis/levels.[363] In NZB/W mice, increased PG synthesis in liver and kidney associated with autoimmune disease was shown to be completely inhibited by a 160 mg zinc per kg diet.[1552]

Increased conversion of labeled arachidonic acid to "2 series" PGs in placentas of zinc-deficient pregnant rats has also been demonstrated,[337] although uterine PG synthesis was decreased. The presence of excess progesterone can account for these apparently opposite effects of zinc deficiency on uterine and placental PG synthesis.[208,358] Zinc deficiency has also been shown to increase the number of binding sites, but not the affinity for PG $F_{2\alpha}$ in the ovaries of pregnant rats.[1001] Hence, it would not appear as though PG synthesis or actions are impaired in zinc-deficient animals. In addition to their effects on PG synthesis, aspirin and other nonsteroidal antiinflammatory drugs have recently been shown to impair linoleic acid metabolism to arachidonic acid in rats.[800] The similarity between zinc deficiency and aspirin toxicity[1211] may therefore be related to impaired EFA metabolism (as suggested by the desaturase studies) rather than to decreased synthesis or action of PGs.

Zinc inhibits the activity of enzymes related to PG synthesis, including platelet thromboxane synthetase,[752] phospholipase A_2,[1038,1626,1705] and phospholipase C.[1007,1230] Zinc inhibits arachidonic acid release from leukocytes,[1053] platelets,[1650] and endo/myometrium.[890] In platelets, zinc does not affect synthesis of thromboxane from arachidonic acid, even though it inhibits platelet aggregation by 50%.[1272] Inhibition of PG synthesis with indomethacin or aspirin has been shown to have no effect on tissue zinc levels.[1118]

IV. CHOLESTEROL

Klevay[915-918] has presented evidence that elevated levels of zinc in the diet of rats raises serum total cholesterol. The effect of zinc was suggested to be related to copper, since high zinc intake reduces serum copper, and copper deficiency is associated with elevated serum cholesterol. Klevay has therefore advocated increased copper intake and reduced zinc intake to decrease the proatherosclerotic effects of high zinc intake in relation to cholesterol metabolism.[918]

A number of researchers have tried to assess Klevay's hypothesis by determining the degree of correlation between zinc and cholesterol in serum. A significant positive correlation between serum zinc and total cholesterol in animals has been demonstrated by some researchers,[217,854,1265,1277] and between serum zinc and aortic cholesterol;[453,878,930,931,934] others have found no correlation.[240,331,522,523,564,1168,1267,1474,1740,1756] Most of these studies have not differentiated between cholesterol in different lipoprotein fractions, a significant variable in relation to atherosclerosis.

Clinical evidence on the subject of zinc, cholesterol, and atherogenesis is no more conclusive than the studies cited above, most of which were done in healthy volunteers. The study by Bustamante et al.[217] gives the strongest support for a direct relationship between zinc and cholesterol, since the relationship of raised serum zinc/copper and cholesterol was seen in atherosclerotic patients. Okuyama et al.[1225] have reported evidence to the contrary; they noted that the higher than normal incidence of atherosclerosis in hemodialysis patients was associated with low serum zinc or zinc/copper and a decrease in high-density lipoprotein cholesterol (HDL).

At least five factors seem to interplay in the zinc-cholesterol relationship: (1) zinc, (2) copper, (3) cholesterol, (4) lipoproteins, and (5) species. If the dietary zinc intake of rats is raised sufficiently, particularly in relation to copper, serum total cholesterol will increase. Koo and Ramlet[930,931] and Koo and Williams[934] have also added 1% cholesterol to the diet in the studies in which they observed the positive relationship between zinc and cholesterol in rats. Supplementation with both zinc (40 mg/kg diet) and cholesterol (choleate) is associated with a decrease in HDL cholesterol.[273] The effect of zinc appears to be specific for HDL cholesterol, elevation of which is associated with a significantly lower risk of atherosclerosis (see Chapter 7).

The question of physiological significance of the zinc-cholesterol relationship in rats, therefore, becomes pertinent. Since none of the studies showing a zinc-induced increase in serum cholesterol involved physiological intakes of zinc (<100 mg/kg) under normal dietary conditions, there does not seem to be reason to associate zinc with raised serum total cholesterol in the rat. Nevertheless, the data of Bustamante et al.[217] for humans suggest that further work is still required to establish the clinical importance of this relationship. Klevay[917] feels that a lack of correlation between serum zinc and cholesterol does not negate his hypothesis that there is a causal relationship between zinc *intake* and plasma cholesterol. His reasoning is based on the frequent lack of correlation between zinc intake and zinc levels in plasma (see Chapter 2). Further details of the effect of zinc on plasma cholesterol in humans are given in Chapter 8.

Zinc deficiency is associated with lower adrenal cholesterol in parturient rats.[76] Zinc-deficient male rats, however, have been shown to have higher adrenal cholesterol.[996,1326,1378] Lower serum total cholesterol has been shown in zinc-deficient pigs,[211] but not in zinc-deficient rats.[1206] Although the intestinal mucosal synthesis of cholesterol has been reported to be increased in male zinc-deficient rats,[583] incorporation of ^{14}C-cholesterol into mesenteric lymph is 40% decreased, as is hepatic uptake of ^{14}C-cholesterol.[926,929] In both cases, the abnormal cholesterol metabolism was attributed to impaired chylomicron synthesis due to low apolipoproteins C and E.

V. PHOSPHOLIPIDS

Much less has been published about interactions of zinc with lipids other than cholesterol. Petering et al.[1267] reported that serum total phospholipids in rats were largely unaffected by increasing dietary zinc from 2.5 to 40 mg/kg. Sandstead et al.[1402] demonstrated that in zinc-deficient neonatal rats, the brain had increased phosphorus in relation to total lipid suggesting that phospholipid represented a greater proportion of total lipids in zinc deficiency. This has recently been confirmed and the increased phospholipid phosphorus confined to phosphatidylcholine.[1334] Sullivan et al.[1579] reported that, in zinc-deficient rats, serum zinc was inversely proportional to liver total phospholipid content, consistent with the data of Sandstead et al.[1402] It has recently been reported that zinc deficiency is not only associated with increased phosphatidylcholine levels, but also *synthesis* by the choline phosphotransferase pathway in liver.[290,305] This effect is associated with decreased phosphatidylethanolamine methylation to phosphatidylcholine in the brain.[305]

The uptake of labeled EFA into phospholipid has been shown to be diminished in zinc-deficient rats.[354,356] Since zinc inhibits phospholipase A_2,[1705] this enzyme may be more active in zinc deficiency, hence decreasing net EFA incorporation into phospholipid. Zinc also inhibits bacterial lipase, thereby decreasing skin-surface free-fatty acids in acne vulgaris.[1340]

Zinc has been shown to form salts with phospholipids in in vitro membrane preparations[1584,1660] and to cause fusion of phospholipid vesicles.[102] The physiological significance of these observations is presently unclear. However, the ability of zinc to increase the resistance of phospholipid monolayers to temperature-induced phase transition[1022] suggests an enhanced stability of membranes, specifically membrane phospholipids in the presence of zinc.

Zinc levels in total lipid extracts of erythrocytes from patients with multiple sclerosis are elevated three times.[753,754] These membranes contain large amounts of phospholipid, so altered phospholipid content or composition may be associated with the increase in zinc.

VI. TRIGLYCERIDES

Young zinc-deficient animals contain very little body fat (primarily triglyceride). However, few reports of an interaction between zinc and triglyceride have been published. Rana and Tayal[1337] have shown that the increase in liver triglycerides caused by carbon tetrachloride can be prevented by zinc. Halevy and Sklan[666] have recently isolated a protein from chick liver which stimulates triglyceride lipolysis. This protein contains zinc and copper (4:1) and has a molecular weight of 6000, but is not metallothionein.

Intestinal transport of absorbed triglyceride has been shown to be markedly diminished in zinc-deficient rats.[933] The defect was related to chylomicron formation and may have been due to decreased synthesis or availability of phospholipid or transport proteins. Liver TG (which is a function of both synthesis and secretion) has been reported to be 50% decreased in zinc-deficient rats.[667]

VII. FREE FATTY ACIDS

Zinc-deficient rats have been reported to have increased plasma free-fatty acids.[1325,1328,1330] This would more likely be due to increased triglyceride lipolysis rather than to increased phospholipase activity (zinc inhibits phospholipase A_2, see Chapter 10). Zinc (100 to 500 μM) in vitro directly stimulates lipogenesis by rat adipocytes, an effect consistent with zinc deficiency stimulating lipolysis.[314] Direct evidence for inhibition of lipase by zinc has been presented;[1340] in acne vulgaris, skin-surface bacterial lipase was inhibited by oral skin resulting in lower sebum and skin-surface free-fatty acids.

VIII. LIPOPROTEINS

As described under "Cholesterol", increased dietary zinc is generally associated with increased cholesterol in plasma HDL. These findings have recently been challenged by Lefevre et al.;[985] they found that zinc *deficiency* increased the HDL content of cholesterol. Roth and Kirchgessner[1375] have reported that zinc deficiency in the rat does not alter serum concentrations of β-lipoproteins.

Prasad and Oberleas[1310] have shown that zinc has a high affinity for serum lipoproteins. Apart from this, the relationship between zinc, HDL, and cholesterol is quite confused. Synthesis of the apoprotein component of HDL has been shown to be decreased by zinc fed to rats (100 to 500 mg/kg).[1741] Conversely, the content of apolipoproteins C and E in lymph is decreased, whereas apolipoprotein A-I is increased in zinc deficiency.[926,928,929] Contributing to the triglyceride, cholesterol, and protein changes in lipoproteins of zinc-deficient rats is the factor of reduced food intake.[1424]

IX. LIPID PEROXIDATION

Chvapil[276] has been a major proponent of the role of zinc as a lipid antioxidant in biological membranes. In membranes, zinc is associated to a large extent with the lipid component.[137,276,281] Its role there has not been elucidated, but is consistent with that of an antioxidant; reducing lipid peroxidation and stabilizing membranes by a mechanism suggested to involve decreasing oxidation of nicotinamide-adenine dinucleotide phosphate hydride (NADPH).[279,280] Such membrane stabilization by zinc has been shown in platelets,[278,882,884,885,1059] leukocytes,[276] liver lysosomes,[283,285] erythrocytes,[135,281,1701] lymphoblastoid cells,[1744] and in the retina.[1244]

Zinc protects against malonaldehyde generation (indirect measure of lipid peroxidation).[282] Zinc deficiency increases malonaldehyde formation by three to four times[1412,1579] and is associated with increased in vitro peroxidation in microsomal and mitochondrial membranes from tumors[214] and lung but not liver.[171] Zinc can also reversibly bind directly to unsaturated fatty acids such as arachidonic acid, an effect that protects arachidonic acid from iron-catalyzed oxidation.[1272]

Reduced glutathione is an electron donor and free radical scavenger, thereby protecting lipid membranes from peroxidation. Its levels are reduced in plasma of zinc-deficient rats,[510] an observation consistent with enhanced lipid peroxidation in zinc deficiency. Zinc-metallothionein is a very effective antioxidant against xanthine oxidase and iron-induced lipid peroxidation in erythrocyte ghosts.[1610]

X. MEMBRANES

Chvapil[276,1022] and Bettger and O'Dell[137] have been major proponents of the role of zinc in membranes. Within membranes, zinc binds to both proteins and phospholipids. Zinc binds to the sulfhydryl groups of proteins forming mercaptides and to the phosphate groups of phospholipids. The binding of zinc to membranes stabilizes them with the following effects: (1) resistance to temperature-induced phase transition,[1022] (2) inhibition of macrophage activation and platelet aggregation (see Chapter 17), (3) inhibition of phospholipases (Chapter 10), (4) inhibition of osmotic and toxic lysis of erythrocytes,[870] and (5) inhibition of carbon tetrachloride-induced lipid peroxidation in liver and lysosomes. The destabilizing (activating) effects of calcium on inflammatory cells and platelets are prevented by zinc, possibly by inhibition of calmodulin.[178] The free radical scavenging enzyme, superoxide dismutase, is partially a zinc metalloenzyme.[586] The membrane-stabilizing and antioxidant properties of zinc are listed in Table 26.

Zinc is also present in high concentrations in the membranes of microsomes[137,1545] and erythrocytes.[753,754] Zinc concentration in erythrocyte membranes is decreased in zinc-deficient rats,[135] a possible reason for their increased fragility in conditions of osmotic stress. Aspects of membrane disruption in zinc deficiency include reduced extracellular fluid (function of membrane-bound carrier proteins), increased microsomal lipid peroxidation, and altered membrane morphology. Membrane components such as EFAs and vitamin E are protective against zinc deficiency in animals and humans. Zinc chelating agents, including EDTA and diodoquin, are also membrane protective by themselves and more so in the presence of zinc.[283]

XI. RECEPTORS

Norepinephrine-binding to hypothalamic receptors has been suggested to be impaired in young zinc-deficient rats. This has been proposed to account for the increased norepinephrine in the hypothalamus and the cyclic food intake in young male zinc-deficient rats.[877]

Insulin-induced stimulation of glucose uptake by adipocytes is enhanced by zinc.[314] Zinc also stimulates insulin binding to various cell types.[727] Combined with the fact that zinc deficiency appears to be associated with peripheral insulin resistance,[1239] it would appear that the insulin receptor is in some way modulated by zinc.

XII. SUMMARY

Evidence is beginning to accumulate that zinc has a major role in the regulation of membrane stability and long-chain fatty acid metabolism. It is not yet clear to what extent these effects are relevant to the pathology of zinc deficiency in humans or animals. Since at least ten enzymes involved in (1) synthesis of long-chain fatty acids from their dietary precursors (desaturases) and (2) metabolism of lipid classes (lipases) and synthesis of various PGs are activated or inhibited by zinc, it is evident that we cannot speak of the independent roles of zinc in lipid and protein metabolism. Considering, too, that the interactions of zinc with the metabolism of hormones, particularly insulin (see Chapter 15), now appear to involve the insulin receptors on numerous organs, it becomes evident that all these aspects need to be integrated before we will fully understand the role of zinc in mammalian biology.

Chapter 14

CARBOHYDRATES

I. INTRODUCTION

The relationship between zinc and the metabolism of carbohydrates has generally been linked to lipids and insulin. Recently, however, a direct link has been demonstrated; zinc-deficient rats have been shown to have abnormal absorption of simple sugars. The effects of zinc deficiency on hexose absorption and interactions of zinc with insulin in relation to glucose tolerance is discussed in this chapter.

II. HEXOSE ABSORPTION

A recent series of papers from Southon and colleagues[1529,1531-1533] proposes an effect of zinc deficiency on absorption of simple sugars. The initial report indicated that the elevated absorption of galactose in zinc deficient rats was reduced following zinc supplementation and recovery from zinc depletion.[1529]

The studies that followed confirmed this effect and showed that hexose absorption in zinc-deficient rats was markedly increased.[1530-1534]

In the previous chapter, it was suggested that the increase in hexose absorption in zinc deficiency might adversely affect the metabolism of essential fatty acids (EFAs) and that some of the effects of zinc deficiency on the composition of EFAs might be due to increased levels of simple sugars, which among many other effects, inhibit the desaturation of linoleic acid.

III. MUCOPOLYSACCHARIDES

Zinc has been shown to bind to heparin, but not to other mucopolysaccharides, including chondroitin, dermatin, and hyaluronic acid.[1242] Increased hyaluronic acid has been reported in the skin of zinc-deficient pigs.[1612] Decreased mucopolysaccharide secretion has been demonstrated in the bone of zinc-deficient chicks.[1709]

IV. GLUCOSE TOLERANCE

Zinc-deficient rats have been shown to have impaired glucose tolerance.[783,1239,1330] In fasted zinc-deficient rats, however, plasma glucose and insulin were essentially normal. The impaired glucose tolerance was later suggested to be related to insulin resistance in the presence of elevated plasma levels of free fatty acids.[1239,1325,1328] Impaired glucose tolerance in zinc-deficient rats was also demonstrated to be dependent on the dietary carbohydrate source, starch, causing much greater impairment than sucrose.[1325]

V. INSULIN

Zinc-insulin interactions is discussed in greater depth in Chapter 16, but it is worth noting here that, in vitro, zinc has insulin-like effects on glucose uptake by isolated adipocytes.[314] In view of the possible zinc depletion in noninsulin-dependent diabetic mice,[997] a physiologically important interaction of zinc with insulin, perhaps at the insulin receptor, may exist, which controls glucose uptake by adipocytes. EFAs and prostaglandin (PG) E_1 also enhance the stimulatory effect of insulin on glucose uptake by adipocytes.[1013] The interaction between zinc and EFAs (Chapter 13) may therefore not be limited to EFA metabolism per se, but may also involve the peripheral actions of EFAs on, for example, insulin.

Chapter 15

VITAMINS, MACROELEMENTS, AND TRACE METALS

I. INTRODUCTION

In the search to define the biological role of zinc, the interaction of zinc with vitamins, minerals, and trace metals has sometimes been overlooked. Nevertheless, it is quite clear that zinc depletion in both humans and animals profoundly influences the biological activity of other essential nutrients. Some of these interactions are discussed in this chapter.

II. VITAMINS

A. Vitamin A

The relationship between zinc and vitamin A has been reviewed in detail.[63,1484,1488] In human plasma, zinc has been reported to be positively correlated with retinol-binding protein.[1484,1514] In zinc-depleted patients, the effectiveness of zinc in restoring plasma vitamin A to normal seems to depend on whether the patients were also protein-energy malnourished[1461,1484] (see Chapter 4).

Zinc-deficient animals have generally been reported to have low serum levels of vitamin A and retinol-binding protein, and low liver retinol-binding protein, but normal liver vitamin A.[1487] Vitamin A secretion from the liver may therefore be decreased in zinc deficiency.[424,1171] That zinc supplementation helps mobilize vitamin A from the liver to the plasma does suggest that the interaction is specific.[471] The role of depressed food intake in the interaction between zinc deficiency and vitamin A metabolism should not be overlooked in view of the similarity between these parameters in zinc-deficient and zinc-adequate, pair-fed rats.[1486] Vitamin A does not prevent teratogenic effects of zinc deficiency in the cat.[1268]

B. Vitamin B_6

Two interactions have been documented between zinc and vitamin B_6: (1) zinc effects on pyridoxal phosphate kinase and (2) tissue zinc levels in relation to vitamin B_6 status. The enzyme-catalyzing conversion of pyridoxine, pyridoxal, and pyridoxamine (collectively — vitamin B_6) to their active phosphate forms is pyridoxal phosphate kinase, which has been shown to be activated more or less specifically by zinc.[391,1183,1629] Its activity has been shown to be decreased in zinc deficiency.[1593] Pyridoxamine has also been reported to be capable of complexing with zinc.[1611]

Zinc levels in chick and rat liver have been reported to vary directly with the dietary vitamin B_6 intake.[7,1516] In vitamin B_6-deficient rats, tissue zinc levels have been reported to be unchanged, or generally decreased, [788] except in the kidneys.[825] Zinc absorption has been shown to be increased by both vitamin B_6 deficiency[788,1322] and elevated vitamin B_6 intake (40 mg/kg diet).[477]

The gross pathologies of vitamin B_6 and zinc deficiency are superficially similar; both cause hypophagia, growth retardation, dermal lesions, alopecia, and immunodeficiency.[1443] Deficiencies of both have been shown to be at least partially corrected by essential fatty acid (EFA) supplementation.[346,349] Deficiencies of both vitamin B_6 and zinc are associated with decreased protein utilization,[1516] with impaired metabolism of linoleic acid, and with an increased ratio of linoleic acid to arachidonic acid in tissue phospholipids.[348,349,360] The essentiality of both zinc and vitamin B_6 for the adequate utilization of both protein and EFAs may be responsible in part for the similar pathology of their deficiencies. Similar effects of zinc deficiency and vitamin B_6 deficiency are listed in Table 27.

Table 27
SIMILAR EFFECTS OF DEFICIENCY OF ZINC OR VITAMIN B_6

Growth retardation
Alopecia
Dermal lesions
Immunodeficiency
Infertility
Increased sodium-to-potassium ratio in muscle
Increased linoleic acid-to-arachidonic acid ratio in serum and tissue phospholipids

C. Vitamin C

At concentrations normally consumed by humans, vitamin C has been shown to have no effect on zinc absorption.[1507]

D. Vitamin D

The interaction between zinc and vitamin D also involves calcium; the increase in zinc excretion caused by calcium has been shown to be blocked by vitamin D_3.[533] Vitamin D_3 supplementation in uremic patients (concentration not given) had no effect on zinc absorption.[12] Vitamin D-induced DNA synthesis in femoral diaphyses has been shown to be stimulated by zinc.[1752] Vitamin D_3 increases zinc concentration in the livers of rats following subtotal nephrectomy.[751]

E. Vitamin E

Vitamin E and zinc are frequently implicated in similar biological phenomena, but their interaction has rarely been studied directly. They are both considered to have antioxidant and membrane-stabilizing properties in the face of free-radical excess, such as occurs following administration of carbon tetrachloride (CCl_4).[137] Experimentally, an interaction between zinc and vitamin E has been demonstrated in zinc-deficient chicks; the dermal pathology and malonaldehyde release from the skin of the feet was significantly reduced by vitamin E.[140]

F. Folic Acid

Liver content of folic acid has been shown to be decreased in zinc-deficient rats.[1729] Folic acid absorption[1596] and plasma levels[1135] have been shown to be decreased in young men fed zinc-deficient diets. These and related studies[53] suggest that folic acid absorption may be a direct function of zinc status.

More recent data suggest the inverse: fecal zinc excretion in men is increased after folate supplementation (400 μg/2 days)[1134] and folic acid supplementation (500 μg/kg for 14 days in vivo or 200 μg added in vitro) significantly decreased zinc absorption in male rats.[592] This study may also simply indicate that biotin deficiency was inadvertently present along with the zinc deficiency.

G. Biotin

Symptoms of zinc deficiency in rats, including growth retardation, alopecia, and dermatitis are also seen in biotin-deficient rats and, in zinc-deficient rats, can be partially alleviated by biotin.[34]

III. MACROELEMENTS

A. Calcium

At the dietary level, zinc and calcium have an antagonistic relationship such that increasing the intake of one increases the excretion of the other and vice versa.[508,1287,1432,1751,1753] The relationship between parakeratosis and zinc depletion in pigs was shown to be partly due to high levels of dietary calcium in the presence of low zinc intake.[691] The exacerbation of EFA deficiency by zinc deficiency was shown to be dependent on calcium; high calcium enhanced the effect of zinc deficiency and vice versa.[757] Fetal malformations in rats induced by zinc deficiency are also dependent on calcium intake; with coexisting calcium deficiency the malformations do not occur, whereas with increased calcium intake they are more severe.[819]

At the cellular level, calcium prevents the zinc-induced inhibition of histamine release from human neutrophils; this effect of calcium is, in turn, prevented by additional zinc.[1058] Calcium also inhibits zinc uptake by erythrocytes from parakeratotic (zinc-deficient) pigs.[131] One of the mechanisms by which zinc has been proposed to interact with calcium is through suppression of the calcium-regulating protein, calmodulin.[108,177,178,181] In humans, calcium has not been shown to affect zinc status in the absence of an effect of phytate (see Chapter 4).

B. Magnesium

Many of the enzyme reactions catalyzed by magnesium can also be catalyzed by zinc, e.g., pyridoxal phosphokinase.[1090] Mild magnesium deficiency in the rat is associated with lower femur and whole-carcass zinc.[954]

C. Sodium

Zinc (0.1 to 0.9 m*M*) infused into the jejunum decreases sodium absorption in humans.[1551] Low dietary sodium intake is associated with increased zinc excretion in sickle-cell disease,[1070] possibly indicating that a sodium-dependent mechanism controls zinc reabsorption in the kidney. Zinc deficiency in the rat is associated with increased sodium/potassium in muscle.[142] Zinc deficiency also decreases the adrenal-hormonal response to sodium depletion, e.g., there is no increase in the secretion of aldosterone in sodium-depleted rats.[662]

D. Sulfur

The sulfhydryl groups (–SH) of amino acids such as cysteine can be linked through zinc to form disulfide bridges. Such bonds are a principal means by which zinc stabilizes polypeptide chains.

E. Nitrogen

The other major bond partner of zinc is nitrogen, frequently in such structures as the imidazole ring of histidine. As such, it is at the active site of molecules such as insulin and glucagon.[631]

IV. TRACE METALS

A. Copper

The negative interaction between zinc and copper absorption has primarily been observed in animal studies (see Table 28). Humans do not normally encounter ratios of dietary copper to zinc on the order of 25:1, nor of zinc to copper on the order of 100 to 1000:1, which are required in order to demonstrate the inhibitory effects of copper on zinc absorption and metabolism and vice versa.[341] Hence, the physiological relevance of the zinc-copper inter-

Table 28
INVERSE EFFECTS OR INTERACTIONS OF ZINC AND COPPER

Zinc and copper have opposing effects on:
- Zinc and copper absorption
- Proteins
  - Metallothionein
  - Ceruloplasmin
  - Lysyl oxidase
- Membrane peroxidation
  - Erythrocytes
    - Sickle-cell disease
    - Experimental hemolytic stress
  - Essential fatty acids (EFAs)

Blood levels of zinc and copper affected in opposite directions by:
- Increased steroid levels
  - Pregnancy
  - Oral contraceptives
- Acute infection
- Malignancy
- Cardiovascular disease
- Renal disease
- Iron- or copper-dependent anemia
- Schizophrenia
- Endocrine disease (acromegaly, Addison's disease)

action is debatable.[524,1219,1600] Nevertheless, Festa et al.[515] have recently shown that an increase of 25% above the recommended zinc intake in humans (from 15 to 20 mg/day for 9 weeks) is sufficient to increase fecal copper excretion.

A few pathological conditions increase the relevance of this interaction, including sickle-cell anemia, Wilson's disease (copper overload), Menkes' disease (genetic copper deficiency), and acrodermatitis enterpathica (AE) (genetic zinc deficiency). Among these diseases, the interaction of zinc and copper has only been studied in Wilson's disease; zinc is effective at reducing copper absorption and inducing copper excretion (see Chapter 7, Section IV). The imbalance in plasma levels of zinc and copper caused by the use of oral contraceptives may also have physiological relevance. Where the zinc-copper interaction may also be of importance in humans is the use of excess amounts of zinc during supplementation; ten times the normal zinc intake (about 100 mg/day) is capable of interfering with copper metabolism and decreasing serum copper.[1398]

In animals, the zinc-copper interaction is well documented[341,342] with respect to (1) diet,[174,599,634,743,746,858,1210,1527] (2) absorption,[523,1644] (3) transport and storage proteins,[169,888,982,1458,1717] (4) metallothionein binding,[483] (5) tissue levels,[1167,1672] lysosome stability,[283,285] and (6) erythrocyte zinc levels[143] (see Table 15, Chapter 9). Interestingly, the enhancement of copper excretion by zinc appears to be a phenomenon limited to oral zinc; 10 mg/kg zinc given s.c. had no effect on copper balance.[744]

Recently, the negative interaction of zinc and copper and the inverse correlation of their levels in plasma in various physiological and pathological conditions have been suggested to be correlated with opposing effects of zinc and copper on the metabolism of EFAs.[338,341-343] This hypothesis was based on the fact that copper stimulates the metabolism of stearic acid to oleic acid via the Δ-9 desaturase, while zinc stimulates the metabolism of linoleic acid to arachidonic acid via the Δ-6 and Δ-5 desaturases. Deficiency of zinc in rats leads to reduced levels of arachidonic acid and increased oleic, whereas deficiency of copper has the opposite effect. Cunnane[343] reported that in the same series of rats, varying the zinc to copper ratio from the normal of 7:1 to 70:1 increased arachidonic acid and decreased oleic

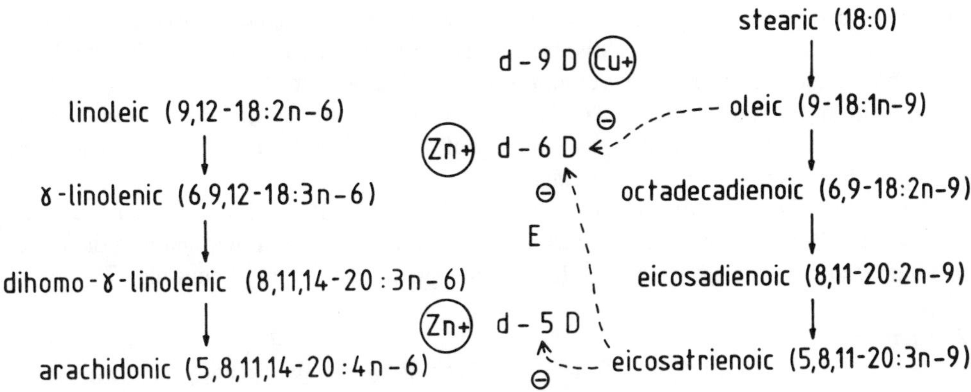

FIGURE 5. Interactions of zinc and copper in the metabolism of the n-6 and n-9 families of long-chain fatty acids. As outlined in Chapter 13, zinc is closely but indirectly associated with the rates of desaturation of the EFAs (d-6 D — Δ-6 desaturase, E — elongase, and d-5 D — Δ-5 desaturase), but not with the Δ-9 desaturation (d-9 D - Δ-9 desaturase) of stearic acid to oleic acid. This is opposite to the effects of copper, which stimulates the synthesis of oleic acid and, as a consequence, eicosatrienoic acid (20:3n-9). Both oleic and eicosatrienoic competitively inhibit the EFA desaturases (Δ-6 and Δ-5). This creates a competitive antagonism between zinc and copper in the control of the metabolism of the essential and nonessential long-chain fatty acids (the former stimulated by zinc and the latter stimulated by copper). In the presence of sufficient zinc and linoleic acid, eicosatrienoic acid is not synthesized, whereas in the presence of excess copper, oleic and eicosatrienoic acids are synthesized in excess, and they competitively inhibit the synthesis of arachidonic acid.

acid, whereas decreasing the ratio to 1:6 had the opposite effect (Figure 5). These results are consistent with the hypothesis that zinc and copper interact physiologically and pathologically, in part, through differential regulation of EFA metabolism.[341,343]

B. Cadmium

Similar to its antagonistic interaction with other divalent cations, zinc interacts negatively with cadmium. Zinc increases cadmium excretion and protects against its toxicity.[27,438,1021,1431,1562] High renal levels of cadmium to zinc have been reported in humans and rats with hypertension. In rats, zinc displaces cadmium from the kidney and decreases blood pressure and vascular responsiveness to various vasoconstrictors.[1431,1432] Cadmium also exacerbates the decrease in rectal temperature in zinc-deficient rats.[1266]

C. Iron

Zinc and iron have, under experimental conditions, been shown to interact negatively in both humans and animals. With the possible exception of iron supplementation in pregnancy, which has been reported to decrease zinc absorption,[680,1100] the interaction of zinc and iron only occurs under extreme conditions of overload or deficiency of either element[911,1409] (see Chapter 4).

D. Selenium

Although zinc and selenium both have antioxidant properties and in selected conditions have antitumor properties, a direct interaction of these two elements has not, to my knowledge, been studied.

E. Other

1. Aluminum

In hemodialyzed uremic patients being tested for zinc absorption, a solution of aluminum hydroxide (concentration not stated) was shown to decrease the plasma increment in zinc by >75%; and a 60% decrease in zinc absorption in controls was also observed.[13] In view of the association of Alzheimer's disease (a form of senility) with aluminum accumulation in the brain, and the generally lower zinc status of elderly people (Chapter 3), it would be worthwhile to determine whether zinc supplementation would reduce the aluminum accumulation in the brain and whether, as the study of Abu-Hamdah et al.[13] suggests, aluminum may exacerbate zinc deficiency in humans.

Marginally suboptimal dietary zinc (10 mg/kg) and 0.1 mg/kg aluminum fed to rats for 120 days has been shown to be associated with the accumulation of aluminum in the cortex and hippocampus, but not the cerebellum, in amounts greater than in controls.[1706]

2. *Manganese*

Manganese (3 mg/kg i.p. for 30 days) has been shown to significantly decrease zinc in the amygdala and hypothalamus of the rat brain.[1422]

3. *Nickel*

Nickel has been demonstrated to have a sparing effect on zinc utilization in zinc-deficient rats; it reduces the increase in urinary zinc, hematocrit, erythrocyte count, and hemoglobin count.[1535]

4. *Lead*

Marginal zinc deficiency (6 mg/kg diet) in the rat leads to greater lead accumulation in rat pups whose mothers have been administered lead during lactation.[80]

V. SUMMARY

Zinc has important effects on the metabolism of vitamin A in relation to retinol-binding protein. With vitamins B_6 and E, zinc seems to have similar, possibly synergistic effects, especially involving EFAs and antioxidant effects/membrane stability, respectively. The most significant interactions of zinc with the macroelements are with calcium (antagonistic), nitrogen, and sulfur (bonding). With two of the essential trace elements, copper and iron, zinc has a largely competitive association. The role of zinc with the toxic trace metals (cadmium, aluminum, and lead) appears to be one of competitive inhibition of their uptake, thereby preventing their toxicity.

Chapter 16

HORMONES

I. INTRODUCTION

Effects of zinc on the biological activity of adrenal and gonadal steroids, as well as pituitary hormones, are well documented. As with insulin, the significance of the interaction of zinc with steroids and steroid-releasing hormones is partly due to its ability to prolong the biological activity of hormones. Studies in the 1940s and 1950s demonstrated that crude extracts of pituitary hormones contained zinc and that zinc prolonged the biological activity of these extracts (Chapter 1). Zinc has two additional roles governing hormones: zinc deficiency appears to interfere with secretion of gonadotropins and zinc may also be an important component or modulator of hormone receptors, e.g., insulin. This chapter addresses the relationship between zinc and steroids and polypeptide hormones and enkephalins.

II. ADRENAL STEROIDS

Research on the interaction between zinc and the adrenal steroids has indicated that, in general, their blood levels are inversely related; blood levels of adrenal steroids are increased in zinc deficiency,[1327] while excess adrenal steroids, e.g., in Cushing's syndrome[709] or with steroid supplementation,[1028] cause plasma zinc levels to be decreased. Conversely, adrenocortical insufficiency or adrenalectomy are associated with increased plasma zinc concentration.[713] Adrenal steroid therapy causes zinc levels to decrease and urinary zinc excretion to increase.[709,843,1628] No doubt part of the hypozincemic effect of adrenal steroids is mediated by increasing zinc uptake by the liver in association with enhanced metallothionein synthesis.[425] In contrast to the general increase in catabolic steroids in zinc-deficient rats, aldosterone does not increase, even in sodium-depleted rats.[662]

The hypozincemic effect of adrenal steroids is particularly relevant to clinical zinc nutrition because so many pathological, as well as physiological, conditions are associated with hypozincemic (see Chapter 4). In many of these conditions, particularly related to infection, surgery, and chronic disease, endogenous steroids will be elevated or steroid therapy will have been instituted. The lowering of plasma zinc by corticosteroids may be an obligatory part of their mode of action, e.g., in infection, postsurgery, and pregnancy. Preventing the decrease in plasma zinc in infected pigs by zinc supplementation was associated with higher mortality than in unsupplemented pigs.[267]

III. GONADAL STEROIDS

Delayed progesterone withdrawal has been implicated in the prolonged and delayed parturition observed in zinc-deficient rats.[208] Elevated serum progesterone levels were attributed to delayed activation of the enzyme, 20 α-hydroxysteroid dehydrogenase, possibly through decreased synthesis of prostaglandin $F_{2\alpha}$.

Hypogonadism in the rat has been related more or less specifically to Leydig cell failure to synthesize testosterone.[1082] A similar effect in the Leydig cells of the zinc-deficient pig was suggested by the fat droplet accumulation and disorganized smooth endoplasmic reticulum seen by electron microscopy.[734]

Urinary zinc excretion is increased in zinc-deficient rats but, following testosterone injection in zinc-deficient rats, zinc retention is increased.[241] Hence, zinc balance may be governed in part by testosterone, which will, in turn, ensure adequate testosterone secretion.

Increased urinary excretion of zinc in males with renal failure (see Chapter 4) could therefore be either the cause or consequence of hypogonadism and infertility.

IV. POLYPEPTIDES

A. Insulin

In 1934, the crystalline structure of insulin was shown to contain zinc.[1437] Conversion of proinsulin to insulin in vitro is decreased in zinc-deficient media.[786] The conversion of proinsulin to insulin may be zinc-dependent because proinsulin binds five times more zinc than does insulin.[632] Zinc also increases proinsulin stability and decreases insulin solubility,[606] which may contribute to increasing the biological activity of insulin in peripheral tissues.[79] The pancreatic islets of Langerhans readily accumulate zinc.[1024]

Circulating insulin has been reported to be either normal[1239] or decreased[646] in zinc-deficient rats. In the study of Park et al.[1239] in which impaired glucose tolerance, but normal plasma insulin, was observed in intragastric force-fed zinc-deficient rats, the impaired glucose tolerance was considered to be a function of peripheral insulin resistance.

Zinc is secreted with insulin and is essential for its release.[976] Although zinc added to islet cells in culture stimulates insulin release, the effect was considered nonphysiological.[520] In spite of the apparently close association between zinc and insulin secretion, islet zinc turnover has been reported to be unrelated to insulin release.[519] Nevertheless, insulin prevents the increase in zinc excretion caused by somatostatin.[1645]

One particularly interesting and relevant observation is that an ''insulin-like'' stimulation of glucose uptake by adipocytes occurs in the presence of 0.1 to 0.3 m*M* zinc.[314,1073] This effect is identical to that demonstrated for prostaglandin (PG) E_1.[774] Although this effect occurs in the absence of added insulin, zinc (250 to 1000 μM) does stimulate insulin binding to adipocytes and, at lower concentrations (25 to 50 μM), stimulates insulin binding to liver, lymphocytes, and placenta.[727] In view of the postulated relationship between zinc and PG E_1 (Chapter 13), it is possible that the insulin-like effect of zinc on glucose uptake by adipocytes is mediated by locally synthesized PG.

There appears to be a better clinical association between hypozincemic and noninsulin-dependent diabetes rather than insulin-dependent diabetes. The latter has been associated with hyper-, normo-, and hypozincemic,[274,1065,1282] whereas the former has been clinically[908] and experimentally[997] associated only with zinc depletion. This may indicate that insulin resistance is a phenomenon associated with zinc depletion and the insulin receptor function is zinc-dependent, either directly or in association with PGs. This possibility is corroborated by the observation that zinc supplementation helps reduce clinical obesity.[299]

Zinc and insulin actions are not entirely complementary; zinc inhibits the insulin-stimulated uptake of uridine into RNA in mouse mammary gland explants.[1361]

B. Prolactin

The initial association between zinc and prolactin was shown in the prostate; zinc uptake by the dorso-lateral prostate was stimulated by prolactin.[649,1141] This has recently been confirmed in the human prostate.[978] the prolactin secretion antagonist, bromocryptine, has been shown to significantly decrease the zinc content of the rat prostate.[692] Zinc supplementation reduces plasma prolactin levels by 30% in men with hyperprolactinemia,[1039] possibly by its inhibitory effect on prolactin secretion from the pituitary.[845,868,1010,1061]

The association between prolactin and zinc may involve PGs; both have prostaglandin E_1-like effects in vascular smooth muscle which are inhibited by PG synthetase inhibitors such as indomethacin and by phospholipase inhibitors such as cortisol.[334,1048] Many of the effects of prolactin are mediated by PGs.[774] Therefore, the stimulation of zinc uptake by the prostate may be one instance of zinc being a messenger between prolactin and PGs.

C. Somatomedin

Reports have recently appeared describing reduced levels of somatomedin-C in zinc-deficient rats.[309-311] Since somatomedin has growth-promoting properties, decreased somatomedin levels may be related to growth retardation associated with zinc deficiency.

D. Somatostatin

Similar to its effect on insulin half-life, zinc prolongs the postprandial increase in plasma glucose, triglyceride, and glucagon caused by somatostatin given to alloxan-diabetic dogs. A zinc-somatostatin complex might therefore have a beneficial effect as an adjunct therapy to insulin in diabetes mellitus.[1060]

E. Other

Immunoreactive cholecystokinin is located in areas of the rat hippocampus very similar to those containing both zinc and enkephalins, and its presence there can be altered by divalent metal chelators.[1556] Its degradation was suggested to possibly be mediated by a (zinc?) metalloenzyme.

Administration of growth hormone to constitutionally short (growth hormone-deficient) children has been reported to increase hair zinc and to decrease urinary zinc excretion.[264] It was suggested that growth hormone effects may be mediated in part by zinc. Growth stimulation by growth hormone might also increase the requirement for zinc (see Chapter 4).

V. ENKEPHALINS

Zinc is highly localized in the mossy fibers of the rat hippocampus.[738] In the hippocampus, the localization of zinc and enkephalins has been shown to be very similar.[1554,1555] Zinc also blocks met-enkephalin binding to opiate receptors in hippocampal synapses.[100,1553] Sufficient endogenous zinc is apparently present for this effect to be physiological.[1553] In vivo, zinc antagonizes the analgesic effect of morphine and, by itself, is hyperalgesic.[100]

VI. BIOGENIC AMINES

Zinc deficiency for 10 days in the rat has been shown to cause an increase in norepinephrine in the whole brain[1670] and in the hypothalamus.[877] Norepinephrine levels in the whole brain were not correlated with food intake changes and were not changed prior to or coincident with cyclic changes in food intake.

In the mouse, pretreatment with zinc increased survival and liver regeneration and prevented the depletion of brain norepinephrine caused by the toxic effects of the mushroom *Amantia phalloides*.[537]

Micromolar concentrations of zinc inhibit the release of histamine from human leukocytes and mast cells in the lung. This effect is blocked by calcium, the effect of which is, in turn, inhibited by zinc.[1058]

Chapter 17

DRUGS

I. INTRODUCTION

Interactions between zinc and drugs are important from two points of view. First, zinc deficiency in rats is associated with slower drug metabolism by the liver.[115] The immediate outcome is a longer half-life of drugs such as anesthetics. The successful outcome of surgery conducted under general anesthetic may therefore depend on the individual's zinc status. Second, many drugs chelate zinc. In some instances this may be desirable, but more often than not this is an unwanted side effect, e.g., for diuretics and anticancer drugs. The examples given are of the commoner drugs known to affect zinc metabolism. The studies are drawn primarily from animal studies, since the human aspects have been covered earlier (Chapter 5).

II. DRUG METABOLISM

To my knowledge, only one paper has been published on the effect of zinc deficiency on drug metabolism (aside from alcohol), that by Becking and Morrison[115] (reviews by Becking[114] and Roe and Campbell[1367]). They noted that various unrelated drugs, including aminopyrine, phenobarbital, and *p*-nitrobenzoic acid were all metabolized more slowly in zinc-deficient rats than in controls, an effect that was attributed in part to reduced activity of liver microsomal cytochrome P-450. Interestingly, zinc supplementation (10 to 20 μM) in vitro inhibits nicotinamide-adenine dinucleotide phosphate hydride (NADPH) oxidation and thereby also reduces the activity of cytochrome P-450. The phosphate group of NADPH combines in a 2:1 ratio with zinc, a factor that may account for decreased oxidation of NADPH by zinc.[279,280] Thus, like zinc deficiency, zinc supplementation causes reduced microsomal drug metabolism.[279,280,855,1023] A biphasic effect would appear to be operative in which both zinc deficiency and zinc excess inhibit microsomal mixed-function oxidases involved in drug metabolism. This is a potentially significant area of research into the metabolic functions of zinc which deserves further research.

III. ALCOHOL

Clinically, there are two important interactions between alcohol and zinc. The first is in relation to pregnancy and fetal outcome, and the second is in relation to the high probability of negative zinc balance in alcoholics due to a combination of increased excretion and, invariably, reduced intake of zinc (recently reviewed by McClain and Su[1085]).

A. Pregnancy

Alcohol consumption during pregnancy constitutes a risk to the normal development of the fetus. If alcohol intake is constant or sporadically high during pregnancy, fetal alcohol syndrome is a possible outcome. The newborn infant is characteristically growth-retarded, mentally deficient, has midfacial hypoplasia, microcephaly, short palpebral fissures, peicanthal folds, cleft palate, and other deformities.[865] These features have also been reported in zinc-deficient neonatal rats.[809]

A number of reports suggest that secondary zinc depletion of the fetus is induced by maternal consumption of ethanol and may therefore be a contributing factor in fetal alcohol syndrome.[897,983,1111,1127,1382,1393,1571,1597,1598] The mechanism may be related to reduced placental zinc transfer to the fetus.[591]

The effects of alcohol consumption during pregnancy on tissue zinc levels seem to be clear-cut. What is not clear-cut is that there is a causal relationship between lower zinc tissue levels caused by alcohol and increased fetal losses and malformations.[58,706] In addition, zinc supplementation to alcohol-fed pregnant rats has been shown not to alter fetal zinc levels[706] or in one study, the degree of fetal teratogenesis.[987]

B. Other Effects

Alcohol dehydrogenase is a zinc metalloenzyme. Its activity in the liver of young zinc-deficient rats has been shown to be either unchanged[412] or decreased.[379,802] Antipyrine half-life (index of rate of drug metabolism) varies inversely as serum zinc in alcoholics.[699] In addition, low serum zinc has been reported to correlate with low liver cytochrome P-450, suggesting that, in alcoholics, drug metabolism may be impaired. In zinc-deficient rats, esophageal parakeratosis is exacerbated by alcohol intake.[1139] In spite of an apparently reduced rate of alcohol clearance, alcohol preference is increased in zinc-deficient rats.[299]

In mice, zinc injection has been reported to reduce the mortality of a normally lethal dose of ethanol.[538,851,1759]

IV. CARBON TETRACHLORIDE (CCl_4)

Administration of CCl_4 to rodents causes liver enlargement and lipid stasis, due primarily to reduced clearance of triglycerides from the liver. The effect of CCl_4 is considered to be associated in part with lipid peroxidation in the liver caused by the CCl_3-radical. One effect of CCl_4 is to reduce serum and liver levels of zinc.[872,1140] CCl_4 was also shown to reduce the uptake and turnover of zinc by the liver.[1747]

The antioxidant properties of zinc have been widely demonstrated in this model; zinc supplementation diminishes the hepatic lipid accumulation and necrosis caused by CCl_4[219,284,1335,1336,1389,1544] and also diminishes the collagen accumulation in the lung.[69] The mechanism of the protective effect of zinc against CCl_4 has been suggested to be due to decreased microsomal metabolism of the free radical-CCl_3 because supplemental zinc reduces NADPH oxidation.[279]

V. CHELATORS

Depending on their effect on zinc absorption, orally administered chelators may induce negative or positive zinc balance (see Chapters 4 and 5). Phytate, for example, reduces zinc absorption, as does ethylenediaminetetraacetic acid (EDTA) in humans.[1505-1507,1539] Diethyldithiocarbamate, on the other hand, increases brain uptake of ^{65}Zn.[4] It may be via reduction of zinc absorption that EDTA is teratogenic in the rat.[1594] Zinc chelators, including dithizone and 8-hydroxyquinoline are both chemical inducers of diabetes mellitus,[462,631] a condition in which zinc metabolism is markedly altered.[326,1202]

Penicillamine appears to increase zinc excretion. Zinc depletion has been reported as a result of penicillamine therapy in Wilson's disease.[919] Autoimmune complications of penicillamine therapy are preventable by nutrient supplementation, including zinc.[1443] Zinc-penicillamine complexes have been shown to be lethal when administered to rats.[1720] Tetracycline also chelates zinc and enhances its excretion.[190]

VI. NONSTEROIDAL ANTIINFLAMMATORY DRUGS

Aspirin toxicity and zinc deficiency during pregnancy have a similar prognosis, including delayed and prolonged parturition, neonatal losses, and prolonged bleeding.[29,265,1211] Aspirin enhances the teratogenic effects of marginal zinc deficiency in rats.[659] Aspirin also delays wound healing, an effect opposite to that of zinc supplementation, but similar to zinc deficiency.[1152] Part of the similarity between aspirin toxicity and zinc deficiency may be related to the zinc-binding capacity of aspirin.[1585]

Observations on the similarity of zinc deficiency and aspirin toxicity, along with the reports demonstrating similar effects of zinc and prostaglandin (PG) E_1 in vascular smooth muscle,[334,352,1048] were instrumental in generating a concerted investigation of zinc-PG interactions. However, zinc deficiency is more often associated with *excess* circulating levels and tissue synthesis of PGs (see Chapter 13). Acetominophen-induced hepatotoxicity (375 mg/kg) is prevented by prior injection of zinc (3 mg/kg, i.p.).[261]

VII. DIURETICS

In humans, diuretics are associated with acute hyperzincuria (see Chapter 5). Similar effects have been reported for volume-expanded dogs; chlorthiazide causes diuresis and thereby hyperzincuria. Chlorthiazide was also shown to reduce zinc reabsorption.[1682] Since the angiotensin-converting enzyme is a zinc metalloenzyme, it has been hypothesized that part of the antihypertensive effect of diuretics is due to reduced activity of the angiotensin-converting enzyme by diuretic-induced hyperzincuria.[1008]

VIII. CENTRAL NERVOUS SYSTEM (CNS) DRUGS

Two reports have indicated that both phenothiazine derivatives and diphenylhydantoin increase ^{65}Zn uptake by the rat brain.[328,1700] Phenothiazine is also associated with decreased erythrocyte zinc levels.[1286]

Two cases of epileptics treated with phenobarbitone followed by valproate have been reported as developing clinical symptoms of zinc deficiency, reversible with zinc supplementation.[1000] Both drugs were shown to increase zinc absorption, but also to increase its excretion. Hurd et al.[808] have maintained that valproate binds zinc and that its side effects (anorexia, hyperammonemia, alopecia, and teratogenicity) could be related to or exacerbated by zinc depletion.

IX. STEROIDS

Intravenous infusion of prednisolone or dexamethasone has a biphasic effect on plasma zinc; an initial short-term increase followed by a decrease that is maximal at 48 hr.[1758] Other interactions of zinc with adrenal steroids are discussed in Chapter 5.

X. TERATOGENIC DRUGS

Ethylene thiourea-induced teratology in rats cannot be prevented by zinc supplementation.[900] A thalidomide analog (EM 12) has been shown to have increased teratogenicity in rats fed a low-zinc diet.[837] Aspirin is more teratogenic in the presence of low-zinc intake,[659] as is valproate.[1661]

XI. ANTICANCER DRUGS

The anticancer drugs, methotrexate and 6-mercaptopurine, have been reported to decrease appetite and cause dermal lesions preventable with supplemental zinc.[370] Both of these drugs, as well as the mercaptopurine analog azothioprine, have sulfhydryl groups in open positions, suggesting the possibility of zinc chelation.

XII. MISCELLANEOUS

An interaction between aspirin, anthralin, and zinc has been reported. Anthralin is used in the treatment of psoriasis. Its activity is decreased in the presence of added zinc, but increased by added aspirin.[804,1331] Complexes of zinc with lidocaine decrease rat mast cell histamine release.[884] Aminonucleoside-induced nephrosis in rats is associated with hypozincemia and hyperzincuria.[566] The prolactin secretion antagonist, bromocryptine, has been shown to significantly decrease prostatic zinc content in the rat.[692]

Chapter 18

PHYSIOLOGY AND PHARMACOLOGY

I. INTRODUCTION

There are three main reasons for describing the physiological and pharmacological actions of ionic zinc. First, zinc is of considerable therapeutic value, both as a topical and as an oral agent, and is rapidly absorbed into the blood from the skin[671] and from the gut. Therapeutic doses in excess of 100 mg elemental zinc per day are not uncommon. The degree to which free, unbound zinc exists in the blood is normally small (<1%), but this could change significantly after large oral doses. Therefore, some of the physiological and pharmacological effects of zinc on vascular smooth muscle could have clinical relevance. Second, the physiological and pharmacological effects of zinc have been widely reported, but no systematic review has been written. Third, some of the direct effects of zinc on tissues, e.g., vascular smooth muscle and the neuromuscular junction, may suggest new approaches to understanding its mechanism of action.

II. CARDIAC MUSCLE

At low concentrations (0.001 to 0.1 m*M*), zinc decreased the mechanical contractility of a variety of heart muscle preparations, including (1) dog, rabbit, and monkey papillary muscle, (2) rat atria, (3) rat hearts, and (4) toad and tortoise heart muscle.[1182] Above 0.5 m*M* zinc, mechanical arrest was induced. Zinc also increases the bidirectional permeability of rat heart mitochondria to potassium.[188] Isoproterenol-induced cardiomyopathy is preventable by zinc (10 mg/kg/day, 7 days).[1473]

In zinc-deficient pregnant rats at term, cardiac output has been shown to be reduced by 50% — 45 vs. 88 mℓ/min.[359] The proportion of cardiac output to the uteroplacental mass was 50 to 65% lower, but to the kidneys was 65% increased in the zinc-deficient rats.

III. VASCULAR SMOOTH MUSCLE

Arterial vascular smooth muscle has been shown to readily take up zinc (1) during perfusion in vitro,[363] (2) after experimental myocardial infarction,[1005,1292] and (3) in aged male rats.[1564] The mechanism of zinc accumulation in damaged vascular smooth muscle has not been explained, but could be related to increased protein synthesis as part of a repair process or could be part of a feedback mechanism attempting to regulate vascular responsiveness to vasoconstrictors and, ultimately, blood pressure.

One of the clinically known effects of high zinc intake is hypotension.[192] Although this effect was toxicological, in vitro studies have demonstrated a possible mechanism through which this might occur. The rat mesenteric vascular bed is a widely used in vitro preparation in which vascular sensitivity to a variety of agents, particularly prostaglandins (PGs) can be tested. In view of the hypothesis that the actions of zinc might be mediated via PGs,[779] the effects of zinc have been studied in the rat mesenteric vascular bed preparation. Zinc has been shown to have a biphasic dose-response curve over a concentration range of 1 pg/mℓ to 1 μg/mℓ, which mimics that of PG E_1 and its precursor, dihomo-γ-linolenic acid.[334,1048,1160] The ability of zinc to depress the constrictor effects of norepinephrine could be inhibited by indomethacin.[352] Like prolactin, which is also thought to stimulate PG E_1 synthesis,[774] the effects of zinc in vascular smooth muscle are seasonally variable.[351,1176]

Zinc antagonizes calcium and calcium-agonist-induced contractility in rat aorta.[308] These effects are consistent with those published elsewhere, suggesting that zinc and PG effects in vascular smooth muscle may be calcium-dependent.[774]

Pinealectomy in the rat is associated with increased blood pressure and premature aging[334] and also causes increased aortic levels of zinc.[350]

IV. UTERINE SMOOTH MUSCLE

The biphasic dose-response curve of the effect of zinc on vascular reactivity[351,1048] has also been demonstrated in uterine smooth muscle.[151,375,376] Although zinc may be affecting membrane permeability to cations such as potassium at higher concentrations,[188] at low concentrations (1 to 100 μ*M*), its effects are independent of calcium and potassium. Uterine contractility in pregnant rats at term is dependent on the zinc status of the animals; if zinc status is low, the rhythmic, high-amplitude, infrequent contractions are replaced by continuous low-amplitude contractions.[352,359]

V. OTHER SMOOTH MUSCLE

At 1 m*M*, zinc suppresses electrically induced contractions in guinea pig *Taenia coli*, an effect only blocked by calcium if the calcium is present prior to addition of zinc.[960] At truly pharmacological doses (10^{-4} to 10^{-3} *M*), zinc increases contraction of *Mitilus* smooth muscle stimulated by cholinergic drugs, caffeine, and electrical stimulus.[1162] As in guinea pig *T. coli*, these effects of zinc are thought to be related to competitive interaction with calcium.

VI. SKELETAL MUSCLE

Slow-contracting skeletal muscle has 3 to 7 times the amount of zinc contained in fast-contracting muscle.[204] The difference occurs postnatally and is primarily associated with an increase in zinc in myofibrils and nucleoli.[239] The addition of zinc to in vitro skeletal muscle preparations has been shown to prolong twitch time and the duration of the action potential in frog skeletal muscle[832,833,1062,1203] and to lengthen the tetanic period of rat diaphragm.[1354] In each of these cases, a competitive interaction with calcium binding to sarcoplasmic reticulum and an effect on membrane flux of potassium have been suggested.[230]

That the effects of zinc in skeletal muscle might be clinically relevant is suggested by the observations of Isaccson and Sandow[833] that skeletal muscle in genetically dystrophic mice contains more than twice as much zinc as do the controls. They suggested that excess zinc might be responsible for the normally fast-contracting gastroenemius behaving as a slow-contracting muscle in the dystrophic animals.

VII. CENTRAL NERVOUS SYSTEM

Intracerebral injection of zinc induces seizures in rats and rabbits and has been suggested to be a model for epilepsy[159,835,1255] (see also Chapter 11).

The effects of zinc in vascular, uterine, and skeletal muscle may be mediated by its effects on impulse transmission at the neuromuscular junction. Zinc (50 μ*M*) reversibly blocks end-plate potentials.[1394] At higher concentrations (3.3 m*M*), it inhibits both depolarization and hyperpolarization of squid[1116] and snail[879] giant neurons.

Recently, the turnover of zinc present in the hippocampus has been shown to be linked to the transmission of neuronal electrical impulses.[83,785] The preferential uptake of zinc by the mossy fiber synaptic boutons in the hippocampus is suggestive of a specific role for zinc in the hippocampus, possibly related to opiate binding.[1553]

VIII. PLATELETS

Zinc (10 to 15 μ*M*) inhibits adenosine diphosphate (ADP) and collagen-induced platelet aggregation.[272,287,517,1272] Since PG E_1 has an identical effect to that of zinc over a similar concentration range,[774] and some of the physiological effects of zinc have been shown to be dependent on "1 series" PGs,[334,352] its inhibitory effect on platelet aggregation may be mediated by PG E_1. The inhibitory effect of zinc on platelet aggregation is not mediated by inhibition of thromboxane synthesis from arachidonic acid.[1272] At 0.1 to 0.3 m*M* in vitro, zinc *induces* platelet aggregation.[742] The effect is inhibited by prostacyclin and does not appear to involve increased thromboxane generation.

CONCLUSION

This book was written with the intention of providing a comprehensive and up-to-date review of the clinical and biochemical significance of zinc. Within that framework, the two objectives were (1) to emphasize the common etiological aspects of clinical abnormalities of zinc metabolism and (2) to constructively examine the interactions of zinc with essential nutrients. Some of the major reviews on the clinical aspects of zinc metabolism have dealt very well with the etiological aspects of zinc depletion, but the clinical and biochemical implications of the interactions of zinc with nutrients other than proteins have not previously been adequately reviewed.

From the clinical point of view, the biggest problem remains one of assessing zinc nutriture. As a corollary, there is the problem of not knowing whether biochemical parameters suggestive of zinc depletion are accurate enough to diagnose a requirement for zinc therapy. In other words, when does low plasma zinc indicate low zinc nutriture? The answer should be clear from the chapters on secondary and acute zinc depletion. It very much depends on the cause of the low plasma zinc level — whether pathological or physiological. Ultimately, where a disease entity is suspected, the answer often cannot be definitively established until zinc supplementation is carried out.

I feel that stepping outside the confines of zinc assessment by zinc analysis per se, e.g., of plasma, erythrocytes, or even the zinc tolerance test, may prove rewarding in the search for a sensitive indicator of zinc nutriture. It is for this reason that some of the functional and metabolic tests are described, not because they are proven, but because they have potential. It is now also apparent, from having reviewed the literature fairly extensively, that closer attention needs to be paid to zinc analysis of erythrocytes, particularly erythrocyte ghosts. A number of conditions, ranging from multiple sclerosis to uremia and bone metastases are characterized by *increased* erythrocyte zinc levels. If the increase in zinc can be localized and its cause determined, this might contribute significantly to understanding the role of zinc in these diseases.

In Part II (Biochemistry), the main difference with other reviews of the biochemical role of zinc is the discussion of its interactions with lipids and long-chain fatty acid metabolism. It is a mystery to me why, with the exception of the membrane effects of zinc, this subject has received so little attention previously. Although zinc may stabilize membranes by directly binding to the lipid (and protein) components, there are also many enzyme-dependent steps in lipid and long-chain fatty acid metabolism which preliminary reports suggest are affected by zinc status or zinc levels in the assay system. These observations require the same scrutiny and sophisticated techniques that have characterized the recent research on nucleic acid and metallothionein metabolism to solidify the initial studies. Even without a full understanding of the interaction between zinc and lipids, there is considerable clinically useful data being generated in this field. For example, it is through the interaction of zinc with cholesterol and essential fatty acid (EFAs) that we can rationalize *some* of the interactions of zinc with copper and some of its similarities with vitamin B_6 and EFA deficiency. The interaction between zinc and EFAs may also have a particularly important role in the superiority of human vs. cow's milk for the absorption of zinc by neonates. In fact, the role of zinc in EFA metabolism may turn out to be one of its clinically more important. Interpreting the pathological effects of zinc depletion in terms of decreased zinc metalloenzyme activity or altered protein or DNA synthesis has not so far been rewarding. Perhaps a better understanding of the importance of zinc in lipid metabolism and membrane function will lead to a closer link between zinc biochemistry and the pathology of zinc depletion.

Zinc deficiency studies using laboratory animals have been plagued by the effects on appetite and food intake. However, this is primarily a problem experienced in young animals. Rather than devising elaborate nutrient energy control groups, two alternative methods would perhaps yield useful information. First, since humans rarely experience the extreme dietary zinc deficiency that is used routinely with rodents (a <1 mg zinc per kg diet), working with diets containing 3 to 5 mg zinc per kg might be more realistic. This level of zinc intake has been successfully used to induce the symptoms of zinc deficiency that are uncomplicated by reduced food intake. Second, older animals can also be used in which there is a lower appetite sensitivity to low zinc intake. These alternatives need to be considered more seriously in order to sustain the usefulness of the rodent as a model animal for dietary zinc deficiency studies. It is perhaps equally important to realize that expecting whole-tissue zinc values to reflect zinc status is a little fanciful. This is particularly true when one realizes that extracellular fluid volume appears to be dependent on zinc nutriture. Some researchers have investigated the subcellular localization of zinc, and more research in this field would undoubtedly demonstrate subcellular fractions or organelles sensitive to zinc nutriture. Hence, a refinement of our approach may be all that is necessary to forge the elusive bond between the established, but almost independent roles, of zinc in clinical medicine, nutrition, and biochemistry.

Clinical zinc deficiency/depletion masquerades in many forms, with no overriding feature or diagnostic criterion predominating. This is perhaps the greatest difficulty in identifying zinc as a frequent denominator for such conditions as growth retardation, dermal lesions, susceptibility to infection, anorexia, or dysgeusia, none of which need be present simultaneously with the others. Neither are these symptoms specifically linked to zinc depletion or, for that matter, necessarily responsive to zinc supplementation. A good example is the disease epidermolysis bullosa, which is characterized in the recessive dystrophic form by growth retardation, alopecia, anemia, and severe bullous, edematous skin lesions induced by friction or pressure. The symptoms would suggest that zinc depletion might be present or, alternatively, that a therapeutic response to zinc supplementation could be achieved. In one case in which zinc supplementation was attempted, it was without effect.[1693] This reinforces the current maxim that zinc treatment is the only reliable means of establishing preexisting zinc deficiency/depletion. It should not discourage the search for improved means of diagnosing zinc depletion, either by more discriminating zinc analysis, e.g., of a particular cell type or subcellular organelle, or by detection of a change in a metabolite directly linked to zinc nutriture, e.g., serum ammonia, EFAs, or perhaps a zinc metalloenzyme.

I realize with some despair that my initial concept of creating a comprehensive and up-to-date monograph on zinc is already slipping from grasp. It is painfully evident that in many of the areas of research on zinc that I have reviewed here, I have either done an inadequate job through an incomplete understanding of that field or the papers that are currently appearing in the zinc literature should have appeared 2 months ago so I could have included them. It is obvious, therefore, that this book is just a start and that the material presented here needs to be continually updated if it is to retain its usefulness. It is nevertheless satisfying to realize that this book may make it a little easier for those who want a "beginners guide to research on zinc".

References

REFERENCES

1. **Aamodt, R. L., Rumble, W. F., Babcock, A. K., Foster, D. M., and Henkin, R. I.,** Effects of oral zinc loading on zinc metabolism in humans. I. Experimental studies, *Metabolism,* 31, 326, 1982.
2. **Aamodt, R. L., Rumble, W. F., Johnson, G. S., and Henkin, R. I.,** Malabsorption of zinc and hyposmia, *Clin. Res.,* 27, 224A, 1979.
3. **Aamodt, R. L., Rumble, W. F., O'Reilly, S., Johnson, G., and Henkin, R. I.,** Studies on metabolism of zinc-65 in man, *Fed. Proc. Fed. Am. Soc. Exp. Biol.,* 34, 922, 1975.
4. **Aaseth, J., Soli, N. E., and Forre, O.,** Increased brain uptake of copper and zinc caused by diethyldithiocarbamate, *Acta Paham Toxicol.,* 45, 41, 1979.
5. **Abbassi, A. A., Prasad, A. S., and Rabbini, P.,** Experimental zinc deficiency in man: effect on testicular function, *J. Lab. Clin. Med.,* 96, 544, 1980.
6. **Abbassi, A. A., Prasad, A. S., and Rabbini, P.,** Experimental zinc deficiency in man: effect on spermatogenesis, *Clin. Res.,* 27, 503A, 1979.
7. **Aboaysha, A. M., Kratzer, F. H., and Sifri, M.,** Vitamin B_6, plasma amino acids and liver zinc relationships, *Poult. Sci.,* 55, 2005, 1976.
8. **Abdulla, M.,** Copper levels after oral zinc, *Lancet,* i, 616, 1979.
9. **Abdulla, M., Andersson, B., Evander, A., Lilja, P., Lundquist, I., Svensson, S., and Ihse, I.,** Zinc and copper concentrations in serum, blood and liver in moderate experimental pancreatic insufficiency, *Digestion,* 18, 86, 1978.
10. **Abou-Mourad, N. N., Farah, F. S., and Steel, D.,** Dermatopathic changes in hypozincemia, *Arch. Dermatol.,* 115, 956, 1979.
11. **Abu-Hamdan, D. K., Mahajan, S. K., Migdal, S. D., Prasad, A. S., and McDonald, F. D.,** Zinc absorption in uremia: effects of phosphate binders and iron supplements, *J. Am. Coll. Nutr.,* 3, 283, 1984.
12. **Abu-Hamdan, D. K., Mahajan, S. K., Migdal, S. D., Prasad, A. S., and McDonald, F. D.,** Effect of $1,25(OH)_2$ vitamin D_3 on zinc absorption in uremia, *J. Am. Coll. Nutr.,* 4, 362, 1985.
13. **Abu-Hamdan, D. K. Mahajan, S. K., Migdal, S. D., Prasad, A. S., and McDonald, F. D.,** Zinc tolerance test in uremia. Effect of ferrous sulfate and aluminum hydroxide, *Ann. Intern. Med.,* 104, 50, 1986.
14. **Acosta, P. B., Fernhoff, P. M., Warshaw, H. S., Elas, L. J., Hambidge, K. M., Ernest, A., and McCabe, E. R. B.,** Zinc status and growth of children undergoing treatment for phenylketonuria, *J. Inherit. Metab. Dis.,* 5, 107, 1982.
15. **Adeloye, A. and Warkany, J.,** Experimental congenital hydrocephalus: a review with special consideration of hydrocephalus produced by zinc deficiency, *Child's Brain,* 2, 325, 1976.
16. **Adams, C. E., Holman, R. T., Erdman, J. W., Nelson, R. A., Jaskiewicz, J. A., Johnson, S. B., and Grater, S. J. E.,** Plasma fatty acid profiles from lipid classes in anorexia nervosa, *Fed. Proc. Fed. Am. Soc. Exp. Biol.,* 44, 936, 1985.
17. **Adham, N. F. and Song, M. K.,** Effect of calcium and copper on zinc absorption in the rat, *Nutr. Metab.,* 24, 281, 1980.
18. **Agarwal, B. N. and Agarwal, P.,** Zinc and copper in nephrology, in *Zinc and Copper in Medicine,* Karcioglu, Z. A. and Sarper, R. M., Eds., Charles C. Thomas, Springfield, Ill., 1980, 383.
19. **Agarwal, R. P. and Henkin, R. I.,** Zinc and copper in human cerebrospinal fluid, *Biol. Trace Elem. Res.,* 4, 117, 1982.
20. **Aggett, P. J.,** Zinc metabolism in chronic renal insufficiency with or without dialysis therapy, *Contrib. Nephrol.,* 38, 95, 1984.
21. **Aggett, P. J., Atherton, D. L., More, J., Davey, J., Delves, H. T., and Harries, J. T.,** Symptomatic zinc deficiency in a breast-fed pre-term infant, *Arch. Dis. Child.,* 55, 547, 1980.
22. **Aggett, P. J., Delves, H. T., and Harries, J. T.,** The possible role of diodoquin as a zinc ionophore in the treatment of acrodermatitis enteropathica, *Biochem. Biophys. Res. Commun.,* 87, 513, 1979.
23. **Aggett, P. J. and Harries, J. T.,** Current status of zinc in health and disease states, *Arch. Dis. Child.,* 54, 909, 1979.
24. **Aggett, P. J., Thorn, J. M., Delves, H. T., Harries, J. T., and Clayton, B. E.,** Trace element malabsorption in exocrine pancreatic insufficiency, *Monogr. Paediatr.,* 10, 8, 1979.
25. **Ahmed, S. and Blair, A. W.,** Symptomatic zinc deficiency in a breast-fed infant, *Arch. Dis. Child.,* 56, 315, 1981.
26. **Ahmed, S. B. and Russell, R. M.,** The effect of ethanol on zinc balance and tissue zinc levels in rats maintained on zinc deficient diets, *J. Lab. Clin. Med.,* 100, 211, 1982.
27. **Ahokas, R. A., Dilts, P. V., and Lahaye, E. B.,** Cadmium-induced fetal growth retardation: protective effect of excess dietary zinc, *Am. J. Obstet. Gynecol.,* 136, 216, 1980.
28. **Aihara, K., Nishi, Y., Hatano, S., Kihara, M., Yoshimutsu, K., Takeichi, N., Ito, T., Ezaki, H., and Usui, T.,** Zinc, copper, manganese and selenium metabolism in thyroid disease, *Am. J. Clin. Nutr.,* 40, 26, 1984.

29. **Aiken, J. W.,** Aspirin and indomethacin prolong parturition in rats: evidence that prostaglandins contribute to expulsion of the fetus, *Nature (London),* 240, 21, 1972.
30. **Aitken, J. M.,** Factors affecting the distribution of zinc in the human skeleton, *Calcif. Tissue Res.,* 20, 23, 1976.
31. **Aitken, J. M., Lindsay, R., and McKay-Hart, D.,** Plasma zinc in pre- and post-menopausal women: its relationship to estrogen therapy, *Clin. Sci.,* 44, 91, 1973.
32. **Ainscough, E. W., Brodie, A. M., and Plowman, J. E.,** Zinc transport by lactoferrin in human milk, *Am. J. Clin. Nutr.,* 33, 1314, 1980.
33. **Akar, N.,** Anorexia and zinc, *Lancet,* 2, 874, 1984.
34. **Alaoui, L., McClain, C. J., and Essatara, M. B.,** Some aspects of biotin and zinc interactions; effects on growth and feed efficiency in the rat, *Nutr. Res.,* Suppl. 1, 203, 1985.
35. **Alberts, J. C., Lang, J. A., Reyes, P. S., and Briggs, G. M.,** Zinc requirement of the young guinea pig, *Fed. Proc. Fed. Am. Soc. Exp. Biol.,* 34, 906, 1975.
36. **Alcala-Santaella, R., Castellanos, D., Velo, J. L., and Gonzalez Lara, V.,** Zinc acexamate in treatment of duodenal ulcer, *Lancet,* 2, 157, 1985.
37. **Alegre, C., Baro, J., and Obach, J.,** Zinc and rheumatic disease, *Arthritis Rheum.,* 27, 1073, 1984.
38. **Alitalo, K., Keski-oja, J., and Bornstein, P.,** Effects of zinc ions on protein phosphorylation in epithelial cell membranes, *J. Cell. Physiol.,* 115, 305, 1983.
39. **Allara, E.,** Modificazioni rell'organo del gusto di Mus rattus albinus in sequito a castrazioni, *Monit. Zool. Ital. Suppl.,* 58, 46, 1950.
40. **Allen, J. I., Bell, E., Boosalis, M. G., Oken, M. M., McClain, C. J., Levine, A. S., and Morley, J. E.,** Association between urinary zinc excretion and lymphocyte dysfunction in patients with lung cancer, *Am. J. Med.,* 79, 209, 1985.
41. **Allen, J. I., Kay, N. E., and McClain, C. J.,** Severe zinc deficiency in humans. Association with a reversible T-lymphocyte dysfunction, *Ann. Intern. Med.,* 95, 154, 1981.
42. **Allen, J. I., Perri, R. T., McClain, C. J., and Kay, N. E.,** Alterations in human natural killer cell activity and monocyte cytotoxicity induced by zinc deficiency, *J. Lab. Clin. Med.,* 102, 577, 1983.
43. **Alvares, O. F. and Meyer, J.,** Regional differences in parakeratotic response to mild zinc deficiency, *Arch. Dermatol.,* 98, 191, 1968.
44. **Amador, M., Pena, M., Garcia-Miranda, A., Gonzalez, A., and Hermelo, M.,** Low hair zinc in acrodermatitis enteropathica, *Lancet,* 1, 1379, 1975.
45. **Amon, R. B., Swenson, K. H., Hanifan, J. M., and Hambidge, K. M.,** The glucagonoma syndrome (necrolytic migratory erythema) and zinc, *N. Engl. J. Med.,* 295, 962, 1976.
46. **Anderson, B. M., Gibson, R. S., and Sabry, J. H.,** The iron and zinc status of long-term vegetarian women, *Am. J. Clin. Nutr.,* 34, 1042, 1981.
47. **Andersson, K.-E., Bratt, L., Dencker, H., and Lanner, E.,** Some aspects of intestinal absorption of zinc in man, *Eur. J. Clin. Pharmacol.,* 9, 423, 1976.
48. **Andrews, G. S.,** Studies of plasma zinc, copper, ceruloplasmin and growth hormone, *J. Clin. Pathol.,* 32, 325, 1979.
49. **Anke, M. and Schneider, H.-J.,** Zinc, cadmium and copper metabolism in man, *Arch. Exp. Veterinaermed.,* 25, 805, 1971.
50. **Anon.,** Liver vitamin A mobilization during zinc deficiency and restricted food intake, *Nutr. Rev.,* 35, 213, 1977.
51. **Anon.,** Zinc, *Med. Lett.,* 20, 57, 1978.
52. **Anon.,** Zinc deficiency and bone metabolism in rats, *Nutr. Rev.,* 36, 152, 1978.
53. **Anon.,** Experimental zinc deficiency in humans, *Nutr. Rev.,* 37, 76, 1979.
54. **Anon.,** Zinc and intestinal absorption of folates, *Nutr. Rev.,* 37, 221, 1979.
55. **Anon.,** Mobilization of hepatic vitamin A by supplementation in zinc deficiency associated with protein-energy malnutrition, *Nutr. Rev.,* 38, 275, 1980.
56. **Anon.,** Clinical application of a zinc tolerance test, *Nutr. Rev.,* 39, 129, 1981.
57. **Anon.,** On the entero-pancreatic circulation of endogenous zinc, *Nutr. Rev.,* 39, 162, 1981.
58. **Anon.,** The role of zinc deficiency in fetal alcohol syndrome — suggestive but not conclusive, *Nutr. Rev.,* 40, 43, 1982.
59. **Anon.,** Prostaglandin metabolism as related to vitamin E and zinc status, *Nutr. Rev.,* 40, 338, 1982.
60. **Anon.,** Oral zinc and immunoregulation: a nutritional or pharmacological effect of zinc supplementation?, *Nutr. Rev.,* 40, 72, 1982.
61. **Anon.,** Plasma levels of zinc in protein-calorie malnutrition and after nutritional rehabilitation, *Nutr. Rev.,* 41, 209, 1983.
62. **Anon.,** Zinc and fetal alcohol syndrome: another dimension, *Nutr. Rev.,* 44, 359, 1986.
63. **Anon.,** The interaction of alcohol, vitamin A and zinc in rats, *Nutr. Rev.,* 45, 62, 1987.
64. **Antoniou, L. D. and Shalhoub, R. J.,** Zinc-induced enhancement of lymphocyte function and viability in chronic uremia, *Nephron,* 40, 13, 1985.

65. **Antoniou, L. D., Shalhoub, R. J., and Elliot, S.,** Zinc tolerance tests in chronic uremia, *Clin. Nephrol.*, 16, 181, 1981.
66. **Antoniou, L. D., Sudhakar, T., Shalhoub, R. J., and Smith, J. C., Jr.,** Reversal of uremic impotence by zinc, *Lancet,* ii, 895, 1977.
67. **Antonson, D. L., Barak, A. J., and Vanderhoff, J. A.,** Determination of the site of zinc absorption in rat small intestine, *J. Nutr.*, 109, 142, 1979.
68. **Antonson, D. L. and Vanderhoff, A.,** Effect of chronic ethanol ingestion on zinc absorption in rat small intestine, *Dig. Dis. Sci.*, 28, 604, 1983.
69. **Anttinen, H., Oikarinen, A., Puistola, U., Paakko, P., and Ryhanen, L.,** Prevention by zinc of rat lung collagen accumulation in carbon tetrachloride injury, *Am. Rev. Respir. Dis.*, 132, 536, 1985.
70. **Anttinen, H., Puistola, U., Pihlajaniemi, T., and Kivirikko, K. I.,** Differences between proline and lysine hydroxylation and their inhibition by zinc or by ascorbate deficiency during collagen synthesis in various cell types, *Biochim. Biophys. Acta,* 674, 336, 1981.
71. **Anttinen, H., Ryhanen, L., Puistola, U., Arranto, A., and Oikarinen, A.,** Decrease in liver collagen accumulation in carbon tetrachloride-injured and normal growing rats upon administration of zinc, *Gastroenterology,* 86, 532, 1984.
72. **Apgar, J.,** Effect of zinc deficiency on parturition in the rat, *Am. J. Physiol.*, 215, 160, 1968.
73. **Apgar, J.,** Comparison of the effect of copper, manganese and zinc deficiencies on parturition in the rat, *Am. J. Physiol.*, 215, 1478, 1968.
74. **Apgar, J.,** Effect of zinc deprivation from day 12, 15 or 18 of gestation on parturition in the rat, *J. Nutr.*, 102, 343, 1972.
75. **Apgar, J.,** Use of EDTA to produce zinc deficiency in the pregnant rat, *J. Nutr.*, 107, 539, 1977.
76. **Apgar, J.,** Effects of zinc repletion for limited times on parturition in rats, in *Trace Element Metabolism in Man and Animals,* Vol. 3, Kirchgessner, M., Ed., Arbeitskreis fur Tierernahrungsfirschung, Weihenstephan, F.R.G., 1978, 436.
77. **Apgar, J. and Travis, H. F.,** Effect of a low zinc diet on the ewe during pregnancy and lactation, *J. Anim. Sci.*, 48, 1234, 1979.
78. **Arakawa, T., Tamura, T., Igarashi, Y., Suzuki, H., and Sandstead, H. H.,** Zinc deficiency in two infants during parenteral nutrition, *Am. J. Clin. Nutr.*, 29, 197, 1976.
79. **Arquilla, E. R., Packer, S., Tarmas, W., and Miyamoto, S.,** The effect of zinc on insulin metabolism, *Endocrinology,* 103, 1440, 1978.
80. **Ashrafi, M. H. and Fosmire, G. J.,** Effects of marginal zinc deficiency on subclinical lead toxicity in the rat neonate, *J. Nutr.*, 115, 334, 1985.
81. **Ashrafi, S. H., Meyer, J., and Squier, C. A.,** Effects of zinc deficiency on the distribution of membrane-coating granules in rat buccal epithelium, *J. Invest. Dermatol.*, 74, 425, 1980.
82. **Assadi, F. K. and Ziai, M.,** Zinc status of infants with fetal alcohol syndrome, *Pediatr. Res.*, 20, 551, 1986.
83. **Assaf, S. Y. and Chung, S.-H.,** Release of endogenous zinc from brain tissue during activity, *Nature (London),* 308, 734, 1984.
84. **Atherton, D. J., Muller, D. P. R., Aggett, P. J., and Harries, J. T.,** A defect in zinc uptake by jejunal biopsies in acrodermatitis enteropathica, *Clin. Sci.*, 56, 505, 1979.
85. **Atsumi, T. and Numano, F.,** Blood zinc levels in patients with atherosclerosis obliterans, thromboangiitis obliterans and Takahashu's disease, *Jpn. Heart J.*, 16, 664, 1975.
86. **Avigad, L. S. and Bernheimer, A. W.,** Inhibition of hemolysis by l-histidine, *Infect. Immun.*, 19, 1101, 1978.
87. **Ayala, S. and Brenner, R. R.,** Essential fatty acid status in zinc deficiency. Effect on lipid and fatty acid composition desaturation activity and structure of microsomal membranes of rat liver and testes, *Acta Physiol. Lat. Am.*, 33, 193, 1983.
88. **Babcock, A. K., Henkin, R. I., Aamodt, R. I., Foster, D. M., and Berman, M.,** Effects of oral zinc loading on zinc metabolism in humans. II. In vivo kinetics, *Metabolism,* 31, 335, 1982.
89. **Baer, M. T. and King, J. C.,** Tissue levels and zinc excretion during experimental zinc depletion in young men, *Am. J. Clin. Nutr.*, 9, 556, 1984.
90. **Baer, M. T., King, J. C., Tamura, T., and Margen, S.,** Acne in zinc deficiency, *Arch. Dermatol.*, 114, 1093, 1978.
91. **Baer, M. T., King, J. C., Tamura, T., Margen, S., Bradfield, R. B., Weston, W. L., and Daugherty, N. A.,** Nitrogen utilization, enzyme activity, glucose intolerance and leucocyte chemotaxis in human experimental zinc depletion, *Am. J. Clin. Nutr.*, 41, 1220, 1985.
92. **Balogh, Z., El-Ghobarey, A. F., Fell, G. S., Brown, D. N., Dunlop, J., and Dick, W. C.,** Plasma zinc and its relationship to clinical symptoms and drug treatment in rheumatoid arthritis, *Ann. Rheum. Dis.*, 39, 329, 1980.
93. **Bakan, R.,** The role of zinc in anorexia nervosa: etiology and treatment, *Med. Hypoth.*, 5, 731, 1979.
94. **Bakan, R.,** Anorexia and zinc, *Lancet,* ii, 874, 1984.

95. **Bales, C. W., Steinman, L. C., Freeland-Graves, J. H., Stone, J. M., and Young, R. K.,** The effect of age on plasma zinc uptake and taste acuity, *Am. J. Clin. Nutr.*, 44, 664, 1986.
96. **Bales, C. W., Wang, M. C., Freeland-Graves, J. H., and Pobocik, R. S.,** The effect of zinc deficiency and food restriction on prostaglandin E_2 and thromboxane B_2 in saliva and plasma of rats, *Prostaglandins*, 31, 859, 1986.
97. **Baly, D. L., Golub, M. S., Gershwin, M. E., and Hurley, L. S.,** Studies of marginal zinc deprivation in Rhesus monkeys. III. Effects on vitamin A metabolism, *Am. J. Clin. Nutr.*, 40, 199, 1984.
98. **Banaszak, C. J., Watson, H. C., and Kendrew, J. C.,** The binding of cupric and zinc ions to crystalline sperm whale myoglobin, *J. Mol. Biol.*, 12, 130, 1965.
99. **Banford, J. C., Brown, D. H., Hazelton, R. A., McNeil, C. J., Sturrock, R. D., and Smith, W. E.,** Serum copper and erythrocyte superoxide dismutase in rheumatoid arthritis, *Ann. Rheum. Dis.*, 41, 458, 1982.
100. **Baraldi, M., Caselgrandi, E., and Santi, M.,** Reduction of withdrawal symptoms in morphine-dependent rats by zinc: behavioural and biochemical studies, *Neurosci. Lett.*, Suppl. 18, S371, 1984.
101. **Barbeau, A. and Donaldson, J.,** Zinc, taurine and epilepsy, *Arch. Neurol.*, 30, 52, 1974.
102. **Barfield, K. D. and Bevan, D. R.,** Fusion of phospholipid vesicles induced by zinc, cadmium and mercury, *Biochem. Biophys. Res. Commun.*, 128, 389, 1985.
103. **Barnes, P. M. and Moynahan, E. J.,** Zinc deficiency in acrodermatitis enteropathica: multiple dietary intolerance treated with synthetic diet, *Proc. R. Soc. Med.*, 66, 327, 1973.
104. **Barney, G. H., Orgebin-Crist, M. C., and Macapinlac, M. P.,** Genesis of esophageal parakeratosis and histologic changes in the testes of the zinc deficient rat and then reversal by zinc repletion, *J. Nutr.*, 95, 526, 1968.
105. **Baster, J., Bogden, J., Cinotti, A., Tenhove, W., Stephens, G., Markopoulos, M., and Charles, J.,** Trace metals in a family with sex-linked retinitis pigmentosa, *Adv. Exp. Biol. Med.*, 77, 43, 1977.
106. **Bates, J. and McClain, C. J.,** The effect of severe zinc deficiency on serum levels of albumin, transferrin and pre-albumin in man, *Am. J. Clin. Nutr.*, 34, 1655, 1981.
107. **Batstone, G. F., Helliwell, M., Coombes, E. J., Moody, B. J., and Robertson, J. C.,** Nutritional status in rheumatoid arthritis, *Proc. Nutr. Soc.*, in press.
108. **Baudier, J., Haglid, K., Haiech, J., and Gerard, D.,** Zinc ion binding to human brain calcium-binding proteins, calmodulin and S100b protein, *Biochem. Biophys. Res. Commun.*, 114, 1138, 1983.
109. **Beach, R., Gershwin, M. E., and Hurley, L. S.,** Gestational zinc deprivation in mice: persistence of immunodeficiency for three generations, *Science*, 218, 469, 1982.
110. **Beach, R. S., Gershwin, M. E., and Hurley, L. S.,** Persistent immunological consequences of gestational zinc deprivation, *Am. J. Clin. Nutr.*, 38, 579, 1983.
111. **Beauchamp, C. J., Connors, M. H., Sheikholislam, B. M., Clegg, M. S., and Hurley, L. S.,** Alterations of urinary, plasma and hair zinc levels associated with growth hormone therapy of hypopituitary dwarfs, *Clin. Res.*, 27, 98A, 1979.
112. **Beck, J. E.,** Zinc pyrithione and peripheral neuritis, *Lancet*, ii, 444, 1978.
113. **Becker, W. M. and Hoekstra, W. G.,** The intestinal absorption of zinc, in *Intestinal Absorption of Metal Ions, Trace Elements and Radionuclides*, Skoryna, S. C. and Waldron-Edwards, D., Eds., Pergamon Press, Elmsford, N.Y., 1971, 229.
114. **Becking, G. C.,** Trace elements and drug metabolism, *Med. Clin. N. Am.*, 60, 813, 1976.
115. **Becking, G. C. and Morrison, A. B.,** Hepatic drug metabolism in zinc deficient rats, *Biochem. Pharmacol.*, 19, 895, 1970.
116. **Beerbower, K. S. and Raess, B. U.,** Erythrocyte, plasma, urinary and dialysate zinc levels in patients on continuous ambulatory peritoneal dialysis, *Am. J. Clin. Nutr.*, 41, 697, 1985.
117. **Bégin-Heick, N., Dalpe-Scott, M., Rowe, J., and Heick, H. M. C.,** Zinc supplementation attenuates insulin secretory activity in pancreatic islets of the ob/ob mouse, *Diabetes*, 34, 179, 1984.
118. **Bégin-Heick, N., Heick, H. M. C., and Norman, M. G.,** Regranulation and normalization of in vivo insulin secretion in ob/ob mice treated with tetracycline, *Diabetes*, 28, 65, 1979.
119. **Bégin-Heick, N., Valpe-Scott, M., Rowe, J., and Heick, H. M. C.,** Zinc supplementation improves the insulin secretory response in the ob/ob mouse, *Fed. Proc. Fed. Am. Soc. Exp. Biol.*, 41, 1088, 1982.
120. **Beisel, W. R.,** Trace elements in infectious processes, *Med. Clin. N. Am.*, 60, 831, 1976.
121. **Beisel, W. R.,** Zinc metabolism in infection, in *Zinc Metabolism*, Prasad, A. S. and Brewer, G. J., Eds., Alan R. Liss, New York, 1977, 155.
122. **Beisel, W. R., Pekarek, R. S., and Wannemacher, R. W., Jr.,** Homeostatic mechanisms affecting plasma zinc levels in acute stress, in *Trace Elements in Human Health and Disease*, Prasad, A. S., Ed., Academic Press, New York, 1976, 87.
123. **Bell, L. T., Branstrator, M., Roux, C., and Hurley, L. S.,** Chromosomal abnormalities in maternal and fetal tissue in magnesium or zinc deficient rats, *Teratology*, 12, 221, 1975.
124. **Beng, B. O., Kit, Y. K., Greaves, M. W., and Plummer, V. M.,** Trophic skin ulceration of leprosy: skin and serum zinc concentrations, *Br. Med. J.*, ii, 531, 1974.

125. **Benkovic, P. A.,** Binding and kinetic data for rabbit liver fructose 1,6biphosphate with zinc as a cofactor, *Proc. Natl. Acad. Sci. U.S.A.,* 75, 2185, 1978.
126. **Berfanstam, R.,** Studies on blood zinc. A clinical and experimental investigation into the zinc content of plasma and blood corpuscles with special reference to infancy, *Acta Paediatr.,* 41(Suppl. 87), 1, 1952.
127. **Bergmann, K. E., Marosch, G., and Tews, K. H.,** Abnormalities of hair zinc concentration in mothers of newborn infants with spina bifida, *Am. J. Clin. Nutr.,* 33, 2145, 1980.
128. **Berkelhammer, C. H., Baker, J. P., Jeejeebhoy, K. N., Whittall, R., Slater, A., Leiter, L. A., Uldall, P. R., and Wolman, S. L.,** Whole body protein turnover in adult hemodialysis patients as measured by stable isotope techniques, *Am. J. Clin. Nutr.,* 41, 340, 1985.
129. **Berman, M. B. and Manabe, R.,** Corneal collagenases: evidence for zinc metalloenzymes, *Ann. Ophthalmol.,* 5, 1193, 1973.
130. **Berman, W. F., Keathley, P. S., and Chan, W. M-Y.,** Demonstration of active zinc absorption by rat small intestine, *Gastroenterology,* 80, 1109, 1981.
131. **Berry, R. K., Bell, M. D., and Wright, P. L.,** Influence of dietary calcium, zinc and oil upon the in vitro uptake of zinc-65 by porcine blood cells, *J. Nutr.,* 88, 284, 1966.
132. **Berthon, G.,** Histamine as a ligand in blood plasma. V. Computer simulated distribution of metal histamine complexes in normal blood plasma and discussion of a possible role of zinc and copper in histamine catabolism, *Agents Actions,* 12, 398, 1982.
133. **Bertrand, G. and Bhattcherjee, R. C.,** L'action combinée du zinc et des vitamines dans l'alimentation des animeaux, *C. R. Acad. Sci.,* 198, 1823, 1934.
134. **Bertrand, G. and Vladesco, R.,** Zinc in male reproduction, *C. R. Acad. Sci.,* 173, 176, 1921.
135. **Bettger, W. J., Fernandez, M. F., and O'Dell, B. L.,** Effect of zinc deficiency on the zinc content of rat red cell membranes, *Fed. Proc. Fed. Am. Soc. Exp. Biol.,* 39, 896, 1980.
136. **Bettger, W. J. and O'Dell, B. L.,** Diodoquin therapy of zinc deficient rats, *Am. J. Clin. Nutr.,* 33, 2223, 1980.
137. **Bettger, W. J. and O'Dell, B. L.,** A critical physiological role of zinc in the structure and function of biomembranes, *Life Sci.,* 28, 1425, 1981.
138. **Bettger, W. J., Reeves, P. G., Moscatelli, E. A., Reynolds, G., and O'Dell, B. L.,** Interaction of zinc and essential fatty acids in the rat, *J. Nutr.,* 109, 480, 1979.
139. **Bettger, W. J., Reeves, P. G., Moscatelli, E. A., Savage, J. E., and O'Dell, B. L.,** Interaction of zinc and polyunsaturated fatty acids in the chick, *J. Nutr.,* 110, 50, 1980.
140. **Bettger, W. J., Reeves, P. G., Savage, J. E., and O'Dell, B. L.,** Interaction of zinc and vitamin E in the chick, *Proc. Soc. Exp. Biol. Med.,* 163, 432, 1980.
141. **Bettger, W. J., Reeves, P. G., and O'Dell, B. L.,** Effect of copper and zinc status of rats on erythrocyte stability and superoxide dismutase activity, *Proc. Soc. Exp. Biol. Med.,* 158, 279, 1978.
142. **Bettger, W. J., Savage, J. E., and O'Dell, B. L.,** Extracellular zinc concentration and water metabolism in chicks, *J. Nutr.,* 111, 1013, 1981.
143. **Bettger, W. J. and Taylor, C. G.,** Effect of copper and zinc status of rats on the concentration of copper and zinc in the erythrocyte membrane, *Nutr. Res.,* 6, 451, 1986.
144. **Bieri, J. and Prival, E.,** Effect of deficiencies of alpha-tocopherol, retinol and zinc on the lipid composition of rat testes, *J. Nutr.,* 89, 55, 1966.
145. **Birckner, V.,** The zinc content of some food products, *J. Biol. Chem.,* 38, 191, 1919.
146. **Bischoff, F.,** Factors influencing the augmentation effects produced by zinc or copper when mixed with gonadotrophic extracts, *Am. J. Physiol.,* 121, 765, 1938.
147. **Bjorksten, B., Back, O., Gustavson, K. H., Hallmans, G., Hagglof, B., and Tarnvik, A.,** Zinc and immune function in Down's syndrome, *Acta Paediatr. Scand.,* 69, 183, 1980.
148. **Blakeborough, P. and Salter, D. N.,** the intestinal transport of zinc using brush border membrane vesicles from the piglet, *Br. J. Nutr.,* 57, 45, 1987.
149. **Blakeborough, P., Salter, D. N., and Gurr, M. I.,** Zinc binding in cow's milk and human milk, *Biochem. J.,* 209, 505, 1983.
150. **Blamberg, D. L., Blackwood, U. B., Supplee, W. C., and Combs, G. F.,** Effect of zinc deficiency in hens on hatchability and embryonic development, *Proc. Soc. Exp. Biol. Med.,* 104, 217, 1960.
151. **Blekta, M., Kobilkova, J., Andrasova, V., Koleilatova, A., Trnka, V., Hlavaty, V., Sychra, V., and Zvrova, J.,** The role of trace elements in the excitability of uterine muscle, *Sb. Lek.,* 82, 146, 1980.
152. **Blom, E. and Wolstrup, C.,** Zinc as a possible causal factor in the sterilizing sperm tail defect, the "Dag defect", in Jersey bulls, *Nord. Veterinaermed.,* 28, 515, 1976.
153. **Bloomfield, F. J., Maxwell, W. J., Walsh, J. P., Hogan, F. P., Kelleher, D., Love, W. C., and Keeling, P. W. N.,** Essential fatty acid composition and prostaglandin E_2 production by peripheral blood cells from patients with Crohn's disease, *Gut,* 25, 1157, 1984.
154. **Bloxam, D. L., Tan, J. C. Y., and Parkinson, C. E.,** Non-protein bound zinc concentration in human plasma and amniotic fluid measured by ultracentrifugation, *Clin. Chim. Acta,* 144, 81, 1984.

155. **Blum, J. J.,** Observations on the role of sulphydryl groups on the enzymatic activity of myosin, *Arch. Biochem.*, 97, 309, 1962.
156. **Boeckner, L. S. and Kies, C.,** Zinc content of selected tissues and taste perception in zinc deficient and zinc adequate rats, *Nutr. Rep. Int.*, 34, 921, 1986.
157. **Bogden, J. D., Lintz, D. I., Joselow, M. M., Charles, J., and Salaki, J. S.,** Effect of pulmonary tuberculosis on blood concentrations of copper and zinc, *Am. J. Clin. Pathol.*, 67, 251, 1977.
158. **Bonewitz, R. F., Voner, C., and Foulkes, E. C.,** Uptake and absorption of zinc in perfused rat jejunum: the role of endogenous factors in the lumen, *Nutr. Res.*, 2, 301, 1982.
159. **Bonta, I. L., Van Der Berg, W. J., and Greaven, H. M.,** Tremor-inducing effect of intracerebral administration of zinc, *Acta Physiol. Pharmacol. Neerl.*, 13, 81, 1964.
160. **Boosalis, M. A., Evans, G. W., and McClain, C. J.,** Impaired handling of orally administered zinc in pancreatic insufficiency, *Am. J. Clin. Nutr.*, 37, 268, 1983.
161. **Boquist, L.,** Impaired glucose tolerance in Chinese hamsters fed a zinc deficient diet, Abstr. 250, *6th Congr. Int. Diabetic Federation,* Ostman, J., Hales, C. N., Miles, L. E., and Milner, R. D. G., Eds., Excerpta Medica, Amsterdam, 1967.
162. **Boquist, L. and Lernmark, A.,** Effects on the endocrine pancreas in Chinese hamsters fed zinc deficient diets, *Acta Pathol. Microbiol. Scand.*, 76, 215, 1969.
163. **Borisova, M. A.,** The indices of ceruloplasmin activity. The blood content of copper and zinc in patients with thyphoid and dysentary on levomycetin therapy, *Sov. Med.*, 29, 59, 1966; **Borovansky, T., Horcicko, J., and Duchon, G.**, The hair melanosome: another tissue reservoir of zinc, *Physiol. Bohemoslov.*, 25, 87, 1976.
164. **Boyett, J. D. and Sullivan, J. F.,** Zinc and collagen content of cirrhotic liver, *Am. J. Dig. Dis.*, 15, 797, 1970.
165. **Boyette, D. M.,** Zinc requirements in trauma and inflammation, *Laryngoscope,* 92, 648, 1982.
166. **Bradfield, R. B. and Hambidge, K. M.,** Problems with hair zinc as an indicator of body zinc status, *Lancet,* 1, 363, 1980.
167. **Brady, F. O. and Bunger, P. C.,** The effect of adrenalectomy on zinc thionein levels in rat liver, *Biochem. Biophys. Res. Commun.*, 91, 911, 1979.
168. **Brady, F. O. and Helvig, B.,** Effects of epinephrine and norepinephrine on zinc thionein levels and induction in rat liver, *Am. J. Physiol.*, 247, E318, 1984.
169. **Brady, F. O. and Webb, M.,** Metabolism of zinc and copper in the neonate. (Zinc, copper) thionein in the developing rat kidney and testes, *J. Biol. Chem.*, 256, 3931, 1981.
170. **Brandes, J. M., Lightman, A., Itskovitz, J., and Zinder, O.,** Zinc concentration in gravida's serum and amniotic fluid during normal pregnancy, *Biol. Neonate,* 38, 66, 1980.
171. **Bray, T. M., Kubow, S., and Bettger, W. J.,** Effect of dietary zinc on endogenous free radical production in rat lung microsomes, *J. Nutr.*, 116, 1054, 1986.
172. **Bremner, I., Hoekstra, W. G., Davies, N. T., and Young, B. W.,** Effect of zinc status of rats on the synthesis and degradation of copper-induced metallothionein, *Biochem. J.*, 174, 883, 1978.
173. **Bremner, I. and Young, B. W.,** Isolation of (copper-zinc) thionein from the liver of copper-injected rats, *Biochem. J.*, 157, 517, 1976.
174. **Bremner, I., Young, B. W., and Mills, C. F.,** Protective effect of zinc supplementation against copper toxicosis in sheep, *Br. J. Nutr.*, 36, 551, 1976.
175. **Bremner, W. F. and Fell, G. S.,** Zinc metabolism and thyroid status, *Postgrad. Med. J.*, 53, 143, 1977.
176. **Brenner, R. R.,** Regulatory function of delta-6 desaturase. Key enzyme of polyunsaturated fatty acid synthesis, *Adv. Exp. Biol. Med.*, 83, 85, 1977.
177. **Brewer, G. J.,** Calmodulin, zinc and calcium in cellular membrane regulation, *Am. J. Hematol.*, 8, 231, 1980.
178. **Brewer, G. J.,** Molecular mechanisms of zinc action on cells, in *Trace Elements in the Pathogenesis and Treatment of Inflammation,* Rainsford, K. D., Brune, K., and Whitehouse, M. W., Eds., Birkhauser Verlag, Basel, 1981, 37.
179. **Brewer, G. J.,** Oral zinc therapy for Wilson's disease, *Ann. Intern. Med.*, 99, 314, 1983.
180. **Brewer, G. J.,** The treatment of sickle cell anemia and Wilson's disease with zinc, *Prog. Clin. Biol. Res.*, 127, 97, 1983.
181. **Brewer, G. J., Aster, J. C., Knutsen, C. A., and Kruckeberg, W. C.,** Zinc inhibition of calmodulin: a proposed molecular mechanism of zinc action on cellular function, *Am. J. Hematol.*, 7, 53, 1979.
182. **Brewer, G. J., Brewer, L. F., and Prasad, A. S.,** Suppression of irreversibly sickled erythrocytes by zinc therapy in sickle cell anemia, *J. Lab. Clin. Med.*, 90, 519, 1977.
183. **Brewer, G. J., Hill, G. M., and Prasad, A. S.,** Simplified approaches to controlling Wilson's disease with zinc therapy, *Clin. Res.*, 32, 740A, 1984.
184. **Brewer, G. J., Hill, G., Prasad, A. S., and Dick, R.,** The treatment of Wilson's disease with zinc. IV. Efficacy of monitoring using urine and plasma copper, *Proc. Soc. Exp. Biol. Med.*, 184, 446, 1987.

185. **Brewer, G. J. and Kruckeberg, W. C.,** Anti-calcium and erythrocyte membrane effects of zinc and their potential value in the treatment of sickle cell anemia, in *Development of Therapeutic Agents for Sickle Cell Anemia,* Rosa, J., Beuzard, Y., and Hercules, J., Eds., Elsevier/North-Holland, New York, 1979, 195.
186. **Brewer, G. J. and Oelslegel, F. J., Jr.,** Anti-sickling effects of zinc, *Biochem. Biophys. Res. Commun.,* 58, 854, 1974.
187. **Brewer, G. J., Prasad, A. S., Oelshlegel, F. J., Jr., Schoomacker, E. B., Ortega, J., and Oberleas, D.,** Zinc and sickle cell anemia, in *Trace Elements in Human Health and Disease,* Prasad, A. S., Ed., Academic Press, New York, 1976, 283.
188. **Brierley, G. P.,** The effect of zinc on the permeability of isolated heart mitochondria, *Ann. N.Y. Acad. Sci.,* 147, 842, 1969.
189. **Briggs, M. H., Briggs, M., and Austin, J.,** Effects of steroid pharmaceuticals on plasma zinc, *Nature (London),* 232, 480, 1971.
190. **Brion, M., Lambs, L., and Berthon, G.,** Metal ion-tetracycline interactions in biological fluids. V. Formation of zinc complexes with tetracycline and some of its derivatives and assessment of their biological significance, *Agents Actions,* 17, 229, 1985.
191. **Brissot, P., Le Treut, A., Dien, G., Cottencin, M., Simon, M., and Bourel, M.,** Hypervitaminemia A in idiopathic hemochromatosis and hepatic cirrhosis. Role of retinol-binding protein and zinc, *Digestion,* 17, 469, 1978.
192. **Brocks, A., Reid, H., and Glazer, G.,** Acute intravenous zinc poisoning, *Br. Med. J.,* 1, 1390, 1977.
193. **Brody, I.,** Treatment of recurrent furunculosis with oral zinc, *Lancet,* ii, 1358, 1977.
194. **Brody, M. S., Steinberg, J. R., Svingen, B. A., and Luecke, R. W.,** Increased purine nucleotide cycle activity associated with dietary zinc deficiency, *Biochem. Biophys. Res. Commun.,* 78, 144, 1977.
195. **Brooks, K. P., Kim, B. D., and Sawder, E. G.,** Dihydropurimidine Aminohydrolase is a zinc metalloenzyme, *Biochim. Biophys. Acta,* 570, 213, 1979.
196. **Brophy, M. H., Harris, N. F., and Crawford, I. L.,** Elevated copper and lowered zinc in the placentae of pre-eclamptics, *Clin. Chim. Acta,* 145, 107, 1985.
197. **Brown, E. D., Chan, W., and Smith, J. C., Jr.,** Vitamin A metabolism during the repletion of zinc deficient rats, *J. Nutr.,* 106, 563, 1976.
198. **Brown, E. D., Chan, W., and Smith, J. C., Jr.,** Bone mineralization during a developing zinc deficiency, *Proc. Soc. Exp. Biol. Med.,* 157, 211, 1978.
199. **Brown, R. G.,** Alaskan malamute chondrodysplasia. V. Decreased gut zinc absorption, *Growth,* 42, 1, 1978.
200. **Browning, J. D., Reeves, P. G., and O'Dell, B. L.,** Effect of zinc deficiency and food restriction on the plasma levels of prostaglandin metabolites in male rats, *J. Nutr.,* 113, 755, 1983.
201. **Brummerstedt, E., Basse, A., Flagstad, T., and Andresen, E.,** Animal model of human disease: acrodermatitis enteropathica, zinc malabsorption: lethal trait A46 in Friesian cattle, *Am. J. Pathol.,* 87, 725, 1977.
202. **Brummerstedt, E., Flagstad, T., Basse, A., and Andresen, E.,** The effect of zinc on calves with hereditary thymus hypoplasia (lethal trait A46), *Acta Pathol. Microbiol. Scand. Sect. A,* 79, 686, 1971.
203. **Brun, A., Sandberg, S., Hovding, G., Bjordal, M., and Romslo, I.,** Zinc as an oral photoprotective agent in erythropoeitic protoporphyria, *Int. J. Biochem.,* 12, 931, 1980.
204. **Bryan, G. W.,** Zinc concentration of fast and slow contracting muscle of the lobster, *Nature (London),* 213, 1043, 1967.
205. **Bryce-Smith, D. and Simpson, R. I. D.,** Anorexia, depression and zinc deficiency, *Lancet,* ii, 1162, 1984.
206. **Buamah, P. K., Russell, M., Bates, G., Milford-Ward, A., and Skillen, A. W.,** Maternal zinc status: a determination of central nervous system malformations, *Br. J. Obstet. Gynecol.,* 91, 788, 1984.
207. **Buerk, C. A., Chandy, M. G., Pearson, E., MacAuly, A., and Soroff, H. S.,** Zinc deficiency: effect on healing and metabolism in man, *Surg. Forum,* 24, 101, 1973.
208. **Bunce, G. E., Wilson, G. E., Mills, C. F., and Klopper, A.,** Studies on the role of zinc in parturition in the rat, *Biochem. J.,* 210, 761, 1983.
209. **Bunker, V. W., Hinks, L. J., Lawson, M. S., and Clayton, B. E.,** Assessment of zinc and copper status of healthy elderly people using metabolic balance studies and measurement of leucocyte concentrations, *Am. J. Clin. Nutr.,* 40, 1096, 1984.
210. **Burch, R. E., Jetton, M. M., Hahn, H. K. J., and Sullivan, J. F.,** Trace element composition of ascites fluid, *Arch. Intern. Med.,* 139, 680, 1979.
211. **Burch, R. E., Williams, R. V., Hahn, H., Nayak, R. V., and Sullivan, J. F.,** Trace element content and enzymatic activities in tissues of zinc deficient pigs, in *Trace Element Metabolism in Animals,* Vol. 2, Hoekstra, W. G., Suttie, J. W., Ganther, H. E., and Mertz, W., Eds., University Park Press, Baltimore, 1974, 513.
212. **Bureau of Nutritional Sciences,** *Recommended Nutrient Intakes for Canadians,* Food Directorate, Health Protection Branch, Department of National Health and Welfare, Ottawa, 1983.

213. **Burger, F. J.,** Changes in the trace element concentration in the sera and hair of kwashiorkor patients, in *Trace Element Metabolism in Animals,* Vol. 2, Hoekstra, W. G., Suttie, J. W., Ganther, H. E., and Mertz, W., Eds., University Park Press, Baltimore, 1974, 671.
214. **Burke, J. P. and Fenton, M. R.,** Effect of a zinc deficient diet on lipid peroxidation in liver and tumor subcellular membranes, *Proc. Soc. Exp. Biol. Med.,* 179, 187, 1985.
215. **Burr, R. G.,** Blood zinc in the spinal patient, *J. Clin. Pathol.,* 26, 773, 1973.
216. **Businco, L., Menghi, A. M., Rossi, P., D'Amelio, R., and Galli, E.,** Zinc-dependent chemotactic effect in an infant with acrodermatitis, *Arch. Dis. Child.,* 55, 966, 1980.
217. **Bustamante, J. B., Mateo, M. C. M., Fernandez, J., De Quiros, B., and Manchado, O. O.,** Zinc, copper and ceruloplasmin in atherosclerosis, *Biomedicine,* 25, 244, 1976.
218. **Butte, N. F., Garza, C., Smith, E. O'B., Wills, C., and Nichols, B. L.,** Macro- and trace mineral intakes of exclusively breast-fed infants, *Am. J. Clin. Nutr.,* 45, 42, 1987.
219. **Cagen, S. Z. and Klassen, C. D.,** Carbon tetrachloride-induced hepatotoxicity: studies in developing rats and protection by zinc, *Fed. Proc. Fed. Am. Soc. Exp. Biol.,* 39, 3124, 1980.
220. **Campbell, I. A. and Elmes, P. C.,** Ethabutol and the eye: zinc and copper, *Lancet,* ii, 711, 1975.
221. **Campbell, J. K. and Mills, C. F.,** The toxicity of zinc to the pregnant sheep, *Environ. Res.,* 20, 1, 1979.
222. **Campbell-Brown, M., Ward, R. J., Haines, A. P., North, W. R. S., Abraham, R., McFadyen, I. R., Turnlund, J. R., and King, J. C.,** Zinc and copper in Asian pregnancies. Is there evidence for a nutritional deficiency?, *Br. J. Obstet. Gynecol.,* 92, 875, 1985.
223. **Capel, I. D., Spencer, E. P., Daivies, A. E., and Levitt, H. N.,** The assessment of zinc status by the zinc tolerance test in various groups of patients, *Clin. Biochem.,* 15, 257, 1982.
224. **Carlomagano, M. A. and McMurray, D. N.,** Chronic zinc deficiency in rats: its influence on some parameters of humeral and cell-mediated immunity, *Nutr. Res.,* 3, 69, 1983.
225. **Carlomagano, M. A., Mintzer, C. L., Tetzlaff, C. L., and McMurray, D. N.,** Differential effect of protein and zinc deficiencies on lymphokine activity in BCG-vaccinated guinea pigs, *Nutr. Res.,* 5, 959, 1985.
226. **Carney, S. M., Underwood, B. A., and Loerch, J. D.,** Effects of zinc and vitamin A deficient diets on the hepatic mobilization and urinary excretion of vitamin A in rats, *J. Nutr.,* 106, 1773, 1976.
227. **Carpentieri, U., Daescher, C. W., Smith, L. R., and Haggard, M. E.,** Zinc and low birth weight: relationship questioned, *Pediatrics,* 74, 898, 1984.
228. **Carpentieri, U., Myers, J., Thorpe, L., Daeschner, C. W., and Haggard, M. E.,** Copper, zinc and iron in normal and leukemic lymphocytes from children, *Cancer Res.,* 46, 981, 1986.
229. **Carper, W. R., Mehra, A. S., Campbell, D. P., and Levisky, J. A.,** Gluconolactone: a zinc-containing metalloprotein, *Experientia,* 38, 1046, 1982.
230. **Carvalho, A. P.,** Effects of potentiators of muscular contraction on binding of cations by sarcoplasmic reticulum, *J. Gen. Physiol.,* 51, 427, 1968.
231. **Casey, C. E., Hambidge, K. M., Walravens, P. A., Silverman, A., and Neldner, K. H.,** Zinc binding in human duodenal secretions, *Lancet,* ii, 423, 1978.
232. **Casey, C. E., Hambidge, K. M., and Neville, M. C.,** Studies in human lactation: zinc, copper, manganese and chromium in human milk in the first month of lactation, *Am. J. Clin. Nutr.,* 41, 1193, 1985.
233. **Casey, C. E., Moser, M. C., Hambidge, K. M., and Lum, G. M.,** Zinc, copper and vitamin A in pediatric dialysis, *J. Pediatr.,* 98, 434, 1981.
234. **Casey, C. E., Walravens, P. A., and Hambidge, K. M.,** Availability of zinc in loading tests with human milk, cow's milk and infant formulae, *Pediatrics,* 68, 394, 1981.
235. **Caselli, M. and Biocchi, R.,** Serum zinc levels in patients with acquired immunodeficiency syndrome, *Presse Med.,* 15, 1877, 1986.
236. **Cash, R. and Berger, C. K.,** Acrodermatitis enteropathica: defective metabolism of unsaturated fatty acids, *J. Pediatr.,* 74, 717, 1969.
237. **Casper, R. C., Kirschner, B., and Jacob, R. A.,** Zinc and copper status in anorexia nervosa, *Psychopharmacol. Bull.,* 14, 53, 1978.
238. **Casper, R. C., Kirschner, B., Sandstead, H. H., Jacob, R. A., and Davis, J. M.,** An evaluation of trace metals, vitamins and taste function in anorexia nervosa, *Am. J. Clin. Nutr.,* 33, 1801, 1980.
239. **Cassens, R. G., Hoekstra, W. G., Faltin, E. C., and Briskley, E. J.,** Zinc content and subcellular distribution in red versus white porcine skeletal muscle, *Am. J. Physiol.,* 212, 688, 1967.
240. **Caster, W. O. and Doster, J. M.,** Effect of the dietary zinc:copper ratio on plasma cholesterol, *Nutr. Rep. Int.,* 19, 773, 1979.
241. **Castro-Magana, M., Clejan, S., Chen, S. Y., Maddaiah, V. T., and Collipp, P. J.,** Effect of testosterone on zinc metabolism in rats, *Pediatr. Res.,* 15, 511, 1981.
242. **Castro-Magana, M., Collipp, P. J., Chen, S. Y., Amin, S., and Maddaiah, V. T.,** Zinc levels in one case of fetal alcohol syndrome, *Pediatr. Res.,* 12, 515, 1978.
243. **Catalanotto, F. A.,** The trace metal zinc and taste, *Am. J. Clin. Nutr.,* 31, 1098, 1978.

244. **Catalanotto, F. A. and Nanda, R.,** The effects of feeding a zinc deficient diet on taste acuity and tongue epithelium in rats, *J. Oral Pathol.*, 6, 211, 1977.
245. **Cavdar, A. O.,** Fetal alcohol syndrome, malignancies and zinc deficiency, *J. Pediatr.*, 105, 335, 1984.
246. **Cavdar, A. O., Babacan, E., Arsacoy, A., Erten, J., and Ertem, U.,** Zinc deficiency in Hodgkin's disease, *Eur. J. Cancer.*, 16, 317, 1980.
247. **Cavdar, A. O., Babacan, E., Gozdasoglli, S., Erten, J., Cin, S., Arcasoy, A., and Ertem, U.,** Zinc and anergy in pediatric Hodgkin's disease in Turkey, *Cancer,* 59, 305, 1987.
248. **Cavell, P. A. and Widdowson, E. M.,** Intakes and excretions of iron, copper and zinc in the neonatal period, *Arch. Dis. Child.*, 39, 496, 1964.
249. **Ceska, T. A. and Edelstrin, S. J.,** Three dimensional reconstruction of tubulin in zinc-induced sheets. II. Consequences of removal of microtubule-associated proteins, *J. Mol. Biol.*, 175, 349, 1984.
250. **Chandra, R. K.,** Acrodermatitis enteropathica: zinc levels and cell-mediated immunity, *Pediatrics,* 66, 789, 1980.
251. **Chandra, R. K.,** Excessive intake of zinc impairs immune response, *JAMA,* 252, 1443, 1984.
252. **Chandra, R. K., Heresi, G., and Au, B.,** Serum thymic factor in deficiencies of calories, zinc, vitamin A and pyridoxine, *Clin. Exp. Immunol.*, 42, 332, 1984.
253. **Chanmugan, P., Wheeler, C., and Hwang, D.,** Effects of zinc deficiency on the formation of eicosanoids in rat platelets, *Fed. Proc. Fed. Am. Soc. Exp. Biol.*, 42, 809, 1983.
254. **Chanmugan, P., Wheeler, C., and Hwang, D. H.,** The effect of zinc deficiency on prostaglandin synthesis in rat testes, *J. Nutr.*, 114, 2066, 1984.
255. **Chanmugan, P., Wheeler, C., and Hwang, D. H.,** Fatty acid composition of the testes of zinc deficient rats: the effects of docosapentaenoic acid supplementation, *J. Nutr.*, 114, 2073, 1984.
256. **Chapkin, R. S. and Ziboh, V. A.,** Inability of skin enzyme preparations to biosynthesize arachidonic acid from linoleic acid, *Biochem. Biophys. Res. Commun.*, 124, 784, 1984.
257. **Chaudhry, I. M. and Meyer, J.,** Response of the submandibular gland of the rat to nutritional zinc deficiency, *J. Nutr.*, 109, 316, 1979.
258. **Chausmer, A. B., Ward, G., and Sears, R.,** Influence of cholecalciferol on tissue zinc homeostasis in the rat, *Nutr. Metab.*, 24, 314, 1980.
259. **Cheek, D. B., Smith, R. M., and Spargo, R. M.,** Hair and plasma zinc levels in Aboriginal Australians, in *Clinical Applications of Recent Advances in Zinc Metabolism,* Prasad, A. S., Dreosti, I. E., and Hetzel, B. S., Eds., Alan R. Liss, New York, 1982, 151.
260. **Chen, R. W., Vasey, E. J., and Whanger, P. D.,** Accumulation and depletion of zinc in rat liver and kidney metabolism, *J. Nutr.*, 107, 805, 1977.
261. **Chengelis, C. P., Dodd, D. C., Means, J. R., and Kotsonis, F. N.,** Protection by zinc against acetominophen-induced hepatotoxicity in mice, *Fundam. Appl. Toxicol.*, 6, 278, 1986.
262. **Cherry, F. F., Bennett, E. A., Bazzano, G. S., Johnson, L. K., Fosmire, G. J., and Batson, H. K.,** Plasma zinc in hypertension/toxemia and other reproductive variables in adolescent pregnancy, *Am. J. Clin. Nutr.*, 34, 2367, 1981.
263. **Cherry, F., Fosmire, G., Bennett, E., Batson, H., Trosclair, G., and Bazzano, G.,** The relationship of plasma zinc with toxemia and other outcomes in adolescent pregnancy, *Clin. Res.*, 27, 225A, 1979.
264. **Cheruvanky, T., Castro-Magana, M., and Collipp, P. J.,** Effect of growth hormone administration on hair and urine zinc in 30 growth hormone deficient children, *Am. J. Clin. Nutr.*, 35, 668, 1982.
265. **Chester, R., Dukes, M., Slater, S. R., and Walpole, A. L.,** Delay of parturition in the rat by anti-inflammatory agents which inhibit the biosynthesis of prostaglandins, *Nature (London),* 240, 37, 1977.
266. **Chesters, J. K.,** Biochemical function of zinc with emphasis on nucleic acid metabolism and cell division, in *Trace Elements Metabolism in Animals,* Vol. 2, Hoekstra, W. G., Suttie, J. W., Ganther, H. E., and Mertz, W., Eds., University Park Press, Baltimore, 1974, 39.
267. **Chesters, J. K.,** Biochemical functions of zinc in animals, *World Rev. Nutr. Diet.*, 32, 135, 1978.
268. **Chesters, J. K. and Quarterman, J.,** Effect of zinc deficiency on food intake and feeding patterns of rats, *Br. J. Nutr.*, 24, 1061, 1970.
269. **Chesters, J. K. and Will, M.,** Some factors controlling food intake by zinc deficient rats, *Br. J. Nutr.*, 30, 555, 1973.
270. **Chesters, J. K. and Will, M.,** Erythrocyte zinc-65 uptake in vitro as an aid to diagnosing zinc deficiency, in *Trace Element Metabolism in Man and Animals,* Vol. 3, Kirchgessner, M., Ed., Arbeitskreis fur Tiererhnahrungsforschung, Weihenstephan, F.R.G., 1977, 211.
271. **Chez, R. A., Henkin, R. I., and Fox, R.,** Amniotic fluid copper and zinc concentrations in human pregnancy, *Obstet. Gynecol.*, 52, 125, 1978.
272. **Chiara, J. C., Ince, G., Lin, F. C., Narayanan, S., and Levy, S.,** Effect of zinc ions on coagulation assays, *Clin. Chem.*, 28, 1586A, 1982.
273. **Cho, C. H., Chen, S. M., and Ogle, C. W.,** The effects of zinc sulphate on hypercholesterolemia induced by cholesterol-choleate in rats, *Pharmacol. Res. Commun.*, 17, 433, 1985.

274. **Chooi, M. K., Todd, J. K., and Boyd, N. D.,** Influence of age and sex on plasma zinc levels in normal and diabetic individuals, *Nutr. Metab.,* 20, 135, 1976.
275. **Chung, K. W., Kim, S. Y., Chan, W.-Y., and Rennert, O. M.,** Androgen receptors in ventral prostate glands of zinc deficient rats, *Life Sci.,* 38, 351, 1986.
276. **Chvapil, M.,** New aspects in the biological role of zinc: a stabilizer of macromolecules and biological membranes, *Life Sci.,* 13, 1041, 1973.
277. **Chvapil, M.,** Zinc and wound healing, in *Symposium on Zink,* Zederfeldt, B., Ed., A. B. Tika, Lund, Sweden, 1974, 19.
278. **Chvapil, M.,** Effect of zinc on cells and biomembranes, *Med. Clin. North Am.,* 60, 799, 1976.
279. **Chvapil, M., Ludwig, J. C., Sipes, G., and Halladay, S. C.,** Inhibition of NADPH oxidation and oxidative metabolism of drugs in liver microsomes by zinc, *Biochem. Pharmacol.,* 24, 917, 1975.
280. **Chvapil, M., Ludwig, J. C., Spies, G., and Misiorowski, R. L.,** Inhibition of NADPH oxidation and related drug metabolism by zinc in liver microsomes, *Biochem. Pharmacol.,* 25, 1787, 1976.
281. **Chvapil, M., Montgomery, D., Ludwig, J. C., and Zukoski, C. F.,** Zinc in erythrocyte ghosts, *Proc. Soc. Exp. Biol. Med.,* 162, 480, 1979.
282. **Chvapil, M., Peng, Y. M., Aronson, A. L., and Zukoski, C.,** Effect of zinc on ligand peroxidation and metal content in some tissues of rats, *J. Nutr.,* 104, 434, 1974.
283. **Chvapil, M., Ryan, J. N., and Brada, Z.,** Effects of selected chelating agents and metals on the stability of liver lysosomes, *Biochem. Pharmacol.,* 2, 1097, 1972.
284. **Chvapil, M., Ryan, J. N., Elias, S. L., and Peng, Y. M.,** Protective effect of zinc on carbon tetrachloride-induced liver injury in rats, *Exp. Mol. Pathol.,* 19, 186, 1973.
285. **Chvapil, M., Ryan, J. N., and Zukoski, C. F.,** The effect of zinc and other metals on the stability of lysosomes, *Proc. Soc. Exp. Biol. Med.,* 140, 642, 1972.
286. **Chvapil, M., Stankova, L., Weldy, P., Bernhard, D., Campbell, J., Carlson, E. C., Cox, T., Peacock, J., Bartos, Z., and Zukoski, C.,** The role of zinc in the function of some inflammatory cells, in *Zinc Metabolism: Current Aspects in Health and Disease,* Prasad, A. S. and Brewer, G. J., Eds., Alan R. Liss, New York, 1977, 103.
287. **Chvapil, M., Weldy, P. L., Stankova, L., Clark, D. S., and Zukoski, C. F.,** Inhibitory effects of zinc ions on plasma aggregation and serotonin release reaction, *Life Sci.,* 16, 561, 1975.
288. **Cimmino, M. A., Mazzucotelli, A., Rovetta, G., and Cutozo, M.,** The controversy over zinc sulphate efficacy in rheumatoid arthritis and psoriatic arthritis, *Scand. J. Rheumatol.,* 13, 191, 1984.
289. **Clejan, S., Castro-Magana, M., Collipp, P. J., Jonas, E., and Maddaiah, V. T.,** Effects of zinc deficiency and castration on fatty acid composition and desaturation in rats, *Lipids,* 17, 129, 1982.
290. **Clejan, S., Maddaiah, V. T., Castro-Magana, M., and Collipp, P. J.,** Zinc deficiency-induced changes in the composition of microsomal membranes and in the enzymatic regulation of glycerolipid synthesis, *Lipids,* 16, 454, 1981.
291. **Clemmensen, O. J., Siggar, D., Andersen, J., Worm, A. M., Stahl, D., Frost, F., and Bloch, I.,** Psoriatic arthritis treated with oral zinc sulphate, *Br. J. Dermatol.,* 103, 411, 1980.
292. **Coble, Y. D., Schulert, A. R., and Farid, Z.,** Growth and sexual development of male subjects in an Egyptian oasis, *Am. J. Clin. Nutr.,* 18, 421, 1966.
293. **Cohen, I. K., Schechter, P. J., and Henkin, R. I.,** Hypogeusia, anorexia and altered zinc metabolism following thermal burns, *JAMA,* 223, 914, 1973.
294. **Cohen, N. and Guilmette, R.,** Biological effects of the enhanced excretion of zinc after calcium diethylene-triaminepentaacetate chelation therapy, *Bioinorg. Chem.,* 5, 203, 1976.
295. **Coleman, B. W., Reimann, E. M., Grummer, R. H., Sunde, M. L., and Hoekstra, W. G.,** Antagnostic effect of arginine on zinc metabolism in chicks, *J. Nutr.,* 101, 1695, 1971.
296. **Collipp, P. J.,** New developments in the medical therapy of obesity: thyroid and zinc, *Pediatr. Ann.,* 13, 465, 1984.
297. **Collipp, P. J., Castro-Magana, M., Petrovic, M., Thomas, J., Cheruvanky, T., Chen, S. Y., and Sussman, M.,** Zinc deficiency: improvement in growth and growth hormone levels with oral zinc therapy, *Ann. Nutr. Metab.,* 26, 287, 1982.
298. **Collipp, P. J., Chen, S. Y., Maddaiah, V. T., Amin, S., and Castro-Magana, M.,** Zinc deficiency in achondroplastic children and their parents, *J. Pediatr.,* 94, 609, 1979.
299. **Collipp, P. J., Kris, V. K., Castro-Magana, M., Shih, A., Chen, S. Y., Antoszyk, N., Baltzell, J., Moll, J., and Trusty, C.,** The effects of dietary zinc deficiency on voluntary alcohol drinking in rats, *Alcoholism: Clin. Exp. Res.,* 8, 556, 1984.
300. **Condon, C. J. and Freeman, R. M.,** Zinc metabolism in renal failure, *Ann. Intern. Med.,* 73, 531, 1970.
301. **Considine, M. L.,** Zinc deficiency in Australian Aboriginals, *Ecos,* 40, 14, 1984.
302. **Constantanidis, J., Richard, J., and Tissot, R.,** Pick's disease and zinc metabolism, *Rev. Neurol. (Paris),* 133, 685, 1977.

303. **Coppen, D. E. and Davies, N. T.,** Studies on the effect of dietary zinc dose on zinc-65 absorption *in vivo* and on the effects of zinc status on zinc-65 absorption and body loss in young rats, *Br. J. Nutr.*, 57, 35, 1987.

304. **Corder, C. N. and Lowry, O. H.,** The zinc requirement of dinucleotide pyrophosphatase in mammalian organs, *Biochim. Biophys. Acta,* 191, 579, 1969.

305. **Cornatzer, W. E., Haning, J. A., Wallwork, J. C., and Sandstead, H. H.,** Effect of zinc deficiency on the biosynthesis of phosphatidylcholine in rat microsomes, *Biol. Trace Elem. Res.*, 6, 393, 1984.

306. **Cornelise, C., Van Der Hamer, C. J. A., and Van Der Sluys Veer, J.,** Investigation of the zinc status of surgical patients, *Int. J. Nucl. Med. Biol.*, 11, 143, 1984.

307. **Cornelius, R., Mees, L., Ringoir, S., and Hoste, J.,** Serum and red blood cell zinc, selenium, cesium and rubidium in dialysed patients, *Miner. Electrol. Metab.*, 2, 88, 1979.

308. **Cortijo, J., Esplugues, J. V., Sarria, B., Marti-Cabere, M., and Esplugues, J.,** Zinc as a calcium antagonist: a pharmacological approach in strips of rat aorta, *IRCS Med. Sci.*, 13, 292, 1985.

309. **Cossack, Z. T.,** Somatomedin-C in zinc deficiency, *Experentia,* 40, 498, 1984.

310. **Cossack, Z. T.,** Plasma somatomedin-C and zinc status as affected by interactions between varying levels of dietary protein fed in combinations with varying levels of zinc supplement, in *Trace Element Analytical Chemistry in Medicine and Biology,* Bratter, P. and Schramel, P., Eds., Walter de Gruyter, New York, 1984, 657.

311. **Cossack, Z. T.,** Somatomedin-C and zinc status in rats as affected by zinc, protein and food intake, *Br. J. Nutr.*, 56, 163, 1986.

312. **Cossack, Z. T., Prasad, A. S., and Konuich, D.,** Effect of zinc supplementation on retinal reductase in zinc deficient rats, *Nutr. Rep. Int.*, 26, 841, 1982.

313. **Cotzias, G. C., Borg, D. C., and Selleck, B.,** Specificity of the zinc pathway in the rabbit: zinc-cadmium exchange, *Am. J. Physiol.*, 201, 63, 1961.

314. **Coulston, L. and Dandona, P.,** Insulin-like effect of zinc on adipocytes, *Diabetes,* 29, 665, 1980.

315. **Cousins, R. J.,** Regulation of zinc absorption: role of intracellular ligands, *Am. J. Clin. Nutr.*, 32, 339, 1979.

316. **Cousins, R. J.,** Regulatory aspects of zinc metabolism in liver and intestine, *Nutr. Rev.*, 37, 97, 1979.

317. **Cousins, R. J.,** Synthesis and degradation of metallothionein, in *Metallothionein,* Kagi, J. H. R. and Nordberg, M., Eds., Birkhauser Verlag, Basel, 1979, 293.

318. **Cousins, R. J.,** Mechanism of zinc absorption, in *Clinical, Biochemical and Nutritional Aspects of Trace Elements,* Prasad, A. S., Ed., Alan R. Liss, New York, 1982, 117.

319. **Cousins, R. J.,** Absorption, transport and hepatic metabolism of copper and zinc: special reference to metallothionein and ceruloplasmin, *Physiol. Rev.*, 65, 238, 1985.

320. **Cousins, R. J., Dunn, M. A., Leinart, A. S., Yedinak, K. C., and Disilvestro, R. A.,** Coordinate regulation of zinc metabolism and metallothionein gene expression in rats, *Am. J. Physiol.*, 251, E688, 1986.

321. **Cousins, R. J. and Smith, K. T.,** Zinc-binding properties of bovine and human milk in vitro: influence of changes in zinc content, *Am. J. Clin. Nutr.*, 33, 1083, 1980.

322. **Cousins, R. J., Smith, K. T., Failla, M. L., and Markowitz, L. A.,** Origin of low molecular weight zinc-binding complexes from rat intestine, *Life Sci.*, 23, 1819, 1978.

323. **Cowen, L. A., Bell, D. E., Hoadely, J. E., and Cousins, R. J.,** Influence of dietary zinc deficiency and parenteral zinc on rat liver fructose 1,6-bisphosphatase activity, *Biochem. Biophys. Res. Commun.*, 134, 944, 1986.

324. **Cox, D. H. and Harris, D. L.,** Reduction of liver xanthine oxidase activity and iron storage proteins in rats fed excess zinc, *J. Nutr.*, 78, 415, 1962.

325. **Craelius, W., Jacobs, R. M., and Jones, A. O. L.,** Mineral composition of brains from normal and multiple sclerosis victims, *Proc. Soc. Exp. Biol. Med.*, 165, 327, 1980.

326. **Craft, N. E. and Failla, M. L.,** Zinc, iron and copper absorption in the streptozotocin-diabetic rat, *Am. J. Physiol.*, 244, E122, 1983.

327. **Craig, W. J., Balbach, R., Harris, S., and Vymeister, N.,** Plasma zinc and copper levels of infants fed different milk formulas, *J. Am. Coll. Nutr.*, 3, 183, 1984.

328. **Crerniak, P. and Haim, D. B.,** Phenothiazine derivatives and brain zinc. Radioisotope turnover study, *Arch. Neurol.*, 24, 555, 1971.

329. **Crofton, R. W., Glover, S. C., Ewen, S. W. B., Aggett, P. J., Mowat, N. A. G., and Mills, C. F.,** Zinc absorption in celiac disease and dermatitis herpetiformis. A test of small intestinal function, *Am. J. Clin. Nutr.*, 38, 706, 1983.

330. **Crosby, W. H., Metcoff, J., Costiloe, J. P., Mancesh, M., Sanstead, M. M., Jacob, R. A., McClain, P. E., Jacobson, G., Reid, W., and Burns, G.,** Fetal malnutrition: an appraisal of correlated factors, *Am. J. Obstet. Gynecol.*, 128, 22, 1977.

331. **Crouse, S. F., Hooper, P. L., Atterbom, H. A., and Papenfuss, R. L.,** Zinc ingestion and lipoprotein values in sedentary and endurance-trained men, *JAMA,* 252, 785, 1984.

332. **Cunliffe, W. J.,** Unacceptable side-effects of oral zinc sulphate in the treatment of acne vulgaris, *Br. J. Dermatol.*, 101, 363, 1979.
333. **Cunliffe, W. J., Burke, B., Dodman, B., and Gould, D. T.,** Double blind trial of a zinc sulphate citrate complex and tetracycline in the treatment of acne vulgaris, *Br. J. Dermatol.*, 101, 321, 1979.
334. **Cunnane, S. C.,** Vascular, Nutritional and Systemic Zinc Physiology: Interactions with Prostaglandins, Essential Fatty Acids and the Pineal, Ph.D. thesis, McGill University, Montreal, 1980.
335. **Cunnane, S. C.,** Decreased spontaneous contractility in uteri of zinc deficient parturient rats, *Proc. Nutr. Soc.*, 40, 80A, 1981.
336. **Cunnane, S. C.,** Inhibition of arachidonic acid metabolism in the uteri of zinc deficient parturient rats, *Proc. Nutr. Soc.*, 40, 78A, 1981.
337. **Cunnane, S. C.,** Zinc deficiency increases placental prostaglandin synthesis from arachidonic acid, *Proc. Nutr. Soc.*, 40, 114A, 1981.
338. **Cunnane, S. C.,** zinc and copper interact antagonistically in the regulation of essential fatty acid metabolism, *Prog. Lipid Res.*, 20, 831, 1981.
339. **Cunnane, S. C.,** Maternal essential fatty acid supplementation enhances zinc absorption in neonatal rats: relevance to the defect in zinc absorption in acrodermatitis enteropathica, *Pediatr. Res.*, 16, 599, 1982.
340. **Cunnane, S. C.,** Perinatal mortality in zinc deficiency is strictly related to the process of parturition: effect of maternal essential fatty acid supplementation, *Br. J. Nutr.*, 47, 495, 1982.
341. **Cunnane, S. C.,** Differential regulation of essential fatty acid metabolism to the prostaglandins: possible basis for the interaction of zinc and copper in biological systems, *Prog. Lipid Res.*, 21, 73, 1982.
342. **Cunnane, S. C.,** Essential fatty acid-mineral interactions in the pig, in *Fats in Animal Nutrition,* Wiseman, J., Ed., Butterworths, London, 1984, 169.
343. **Cunnane, S. C.,** Contrasting effects of zinc and copper on tissue composition of long chain fatty acids in the rat, in *Trace Element Metabolism in Man and Animals,* Vol. 5, Mills, C. E., Bremner, I., and Chesters, J. K., Eds., Commonwealth Bureaux of Nutrition, Farnham, Slough, U.K., in press.
344. **Cunnane, S. C.,** Levels of essential fatty acids in the gut mucosa in zinc deficiency: relation to altered zinc absorption, presented at the Symp. on Infant Nutrition and Gastrointestinal Disease, Brussels, 1985.
345. **Cunnane, S. C., Ainley, C. C., Keeling, P. W. N., Thompson, R. P. H., and Crawford, M. A.,** Metabolism of linoleic acid and arachidonic acid by peripheral blood leucocytes from patients with Crohn's disease, *J. Am. Coll. Nutr.*, 5, 451, 1986.
346. **Cunnane, S. C. and Horrobin, D. F.,** Parenteral linoleic and gamma-linolenic acids ameliorate the gross effects of zinc deficiency, *Proc. Soc. Exp. Biol. Med.*, 164, 583, 1980.
347. **Cunnane, S. C. and Horrobin, D. F.,** Probable role of zinc in mobilization of dihomo-gamma-linolenic acid, *Prog. Lipid Res.*, 20, 235, 1981.
348. **Cunnane, S. C. and Horrobin, D. F.,** Zinc deficiency, essential fatty acids and reduced food intake, *J. Nutr.*, 115, 500, 1985.
349. **Cunnane, S. C., Horrobin, D. F., and Manku, M. S.,** Accumulation of linoleic and gamma-linolenic acids in tissue lipids of pyridoxine deficient rats, *J. Nutr.*, 114, 1754, 1984.
350. **Cunnane, S. C., Horrobin, D. F., Manku, M. S., and Oka, M.,** Alteration of tissue zinc distribution and serum biochemical analysis following pinealectomy in the rat, *Endocr. Res. Commun.*, 6, 311, 1980.
351. **Cunnane, S. C., Horrobin, D. F., Manku, M. S., and Oka, M.,** The in vitro vascular response to zinc varies seasonally: effect of pinealectomy and melatonin, *Chronobiologia,* 7, 493, 1980.
352. **Cunnane, S. C., Horrobin, D. F., Manku, M. S., and Oka, M.,** Interactions of zinc with prostaglandins E_1 and E_2 in vascular smooth muscle, *Prog. Lipid Res.*, 20, 261, 1981.
353. **Cunnane, S. C., Horrobin, D. F., and Sella, G. E.,** Effect of essential fatty acid supplementation in rats maintained on dietary zinc deficiency, *Trace Subst. Environ. Health.*, 13, 332, 1979.
354. **Cunnane, S. C. and Huang, Y. S.,** Incorporation of dihomo-gamma-linolenic acid into tissue lipids in zinc deficiency, presented at the 5th Int. Conf. on Prostaglandins, Florence, 1982.
355. **Cunnane, S. C., Huang, Y. S., Horrobin, D. F., and Davignon, J.,** Role of zinc in linoleic acid desaturation and prostaglandin synthesis, *Prog. Lipid Res.*, 20, 157, 1981.
356. **Cunnane, S. C., Keeling, P. W. N., Thompson, R. P. H., and Crawford, M. A.,** Leucocyte essential fatty acid metabolism in zinc deficient pregnant rats, *Proc. Nutr. Soc.*, 42, 72A, 1983.
357. **Cunnane, S. C. and Krieger, I.,** Plasma essential fatty acids in human zinc deficiency, presented at the Symp. on Infant Nutrition and Gastrointestinal Disease, Brussels, 1985.
358. **Cunnane, S. C., Majid, E., Senior, J., and Mills, C. F.,** Perinatal mortality in zinc deficiency is associated with significantly reduced utero-placental blood flow, *Proc. Nutr. Soc.*, 41, 69A, 1982.
359. **Cunnane, S. C., Majid, E., Senior, J., and Mills, C. F.,** Utero-placental dysfunction and prostaglandin metabolism in zinc deficient pregnant rats, *Life Sci.*, 32, 2471, 1983.
360. **Cunnane, S. C., Manku, M. S., and Horrobin, D. F.,** Essential fatty acids in tissue phospholipids and triglycerides of the zinc deficient rat, *Proc. Soc. Exp. Biol. Med.*, 177, 441, 1984.

361. **Cunnane, S. C., Manku, M. S., and Horrobin, D. F.,** Effect of vitamin B_6 deficiency on essential fatty acid metabolism, in *Vitamin B_6: Its Role in Health and Disease,* Reynolds, R. and Leklem, J. E., Eds., Alan R. Liss, New York, 1985, 447.

362. **Cunnane, S. C., Meadows, N. J., Keeling, P. W. N., Thompson, R. P. H., and Crawford, M. A.,** Metabolism of linoleic acid and arachidonic acid in peripheral blood leucocytes in human pregnancy at term, *Nutr. Res.,* 5, 373, 1985.

363. **Cunnane, S. C., Nassar, B. A., McAdoo, K. R., and Horrobin, D. F.,** Zinc reduces the release of prostaglandins and polyunsaturated fatty acids from the rat mesenteric vascular bed perfused *in vitro,* in *Trace Element Metabolism in Man and Animals,* Vol. 6, Hurley, L. S., Ed., Plenum Press, New York, 1988.

364. **Cunnane, S. C., Sella, G. E., and Horrobin, D. F.,** Essential fatty acid supplementation inhibits the effect of dietary zinc deficiency, *Adv. Prostagl. Thrombox. Res.,* 8, 1797, 1980.

365. **Cunnane, S. C. and Wahle, K. W. J.,** Differential effects of zinc deficiency on delta-6 desaturase activity and fatty acid composition of various tissues in lactating rats, presented at the 13th Int. Congr. of Nutrition, San Diego, 1981.

366. **Cunnane, S. C. and Wahle, K. W. J.,** Zinc deficiency increases the rate of delta-6 desaturation of linoleic acid in rat mammary microsomes, *Lipids,* 16, 771, 1981.

367. **Cunningham-Rundles, S.,** Effects of nutritional status on immunological function, *Am. J. Clin. Nutr.,* 35 (Suppl. 5), 1202, 1982.

368. **Cunningham-Rundles, C., Cunningham-Rundles, S., Iwata, T., Incefy, G., Garafalo, J. A., Menendez-Botet, C., Lewis, V., Twomey, J. J., and Good, R. A.,** Zinc deficiency, depressed thymic hormones and T-lymphocyte dysfunction in patients with hypogammaglobulinemia, *Clin. Immunol. Immunopathol.,* 21, 387, 1981.

369. **Cuthbertson, D. P., Fell, G. S., Smith, C. M., and Tolstone, W. J.,** Metabolism after injury. I. Effects of severity, nutrition and environmental temperature on protein, potassium, zinc and creatinine, *Br. J. Surg.,* 59, 925, 1972.

370. **Cutler, E. A., Palmer, J., and Kontras, S. B.,** Chemotherapy and possible zinc deficiency, *N. Engl. J. Med.,* 297, 168, 1977.

371. **Daescher, C. W., Matusik, M. C., Carpentieri, U., and Haggard, M. E.,** Zinc and growth in patients with sickle cell disease, *J. Pediatr.,* 98, 778, 1981.

372. **Dagher, R. K., Ellis, G. D., Ranski, D. T., Chakrabarty, M. R., Hoffman, R. V., and Shoemaker, J. P.,** Comparison of levels of zinc in rat prostatic tumors and in normal prostate glands, *IRCS Med. Sci.,* 5, 415, 1977.

373. **Dagostino, L., Acampore, A., Brizio, N., Caporale, O., and Mazzacca, G.,** Zinc in ascites, *Dig. Dis. Sci.,* 26, 861, 1981.

374. **Dahmer, E. J.,** Alleviation of parakeratosis in zinc deficient swine by high levels of dietary histidine, *J. Anim. Sci.,* 35, 1181, 1972.

375. **Daniel, E. E., Fair, S., Kidwai, A. M., and Polacek, I.,** Zinc and smooth muscle contractility. I. Study of the mechanism of zinc-induced contractility changes in rat uteri, *J. Pharmacol. Exp. Ther.,* 178, 282, 1971.

376. **Daniel, E. E., Fair, S., and Kidwai, A. M.,** Zinc and smooth muscle contractility. II. Zinc content and accumulation in rat uterus and their relation to contractility changes from zinc and oubain, *J. Pharmacol. Exp. Ther.,* 178, 290, 1971.

377. **Danks, D. M.,** Diagnosis of trace metal deficiency with emphasis on copper and zinc, *Am. J. Clin. Nutr.,* 34, 278, 1981.

378. **Darlu, P., Lalouel, J. M., Henrotte, J. G., and Rao, D. C.,** A genetic study of red blood cell zinc concentration in man, *Hum. Hered.,* 33, 311, 1983.

379. **Das, I., Burch, R. E., and Hahn, H. K. J.,** Effect of zinc deficiency on ethanol metabolism and alcohol and aldehyde dehydrogenase activities, *J. Lab. Clin. Med.,* 104, 610, 1984.

380. **Dash, S., Brewer, G. J., and Oelshlegel, F. J.,** Effect of zinc on hemoglobin binding by red cell membranes, *Nature (London),* 250, 251, 1974.

381. **Dauncey, M. J., Shaw, J. C. L., and Urman, J.,** The absorption and retention of magnesium, zinc and copper by low birth weight infants fed pasteurized human breast milk, *Pediatr. Res.,* 11, 991, 1977.

382. **David, T. J., Wells, F. E., Sharpe, T. C., and Gibbs, A. C. C.,** Low serum zinc in children with atopic eczema, *Br. J. Dermatol.,* 111, 597, 1984.

383. **Davies, I. J. T., Musa, M., and Dormandy, T. L.,** Measurements of plasma zinc, *J. Clin. Pathol.,* 21, 359, 1968.

384. **Davies, N. T.,** Studies on the absorption of zinc by rat intestine, *Br. J. Nutr.,* 43, 189, 1980.

385. **Davies, N. T. and Nightingale, R.,** The effects of phytate on intestinal absorption and secretion of zinc, and whole body retention of zinc, copper, iron, and manganese in rats, *Br. J. Nutr.,* 34, 243, 1975.

386. **Davies, N. T. and Williams, R. B.,** The effect of pregnancy and lactation on the absorption of zinc and lysine by the rat duodenum *in situ, Br. J. Nutr.,* 38, 417, 1977.

387. **Davies, S.,** Assessment of zinc status, *Int. Clin. Nutr. Rev.*, 4, 122, 1984.
388. **Davies, S.,** Effects of oral zinc supplementation on serum, hair and sweat zinc levels in seven subjects, *Sci. Tot. Environ.*, 42, 45, 1985.
389. **Davis, J. R.,** A comparison of the stimulatory effects of cadmium and zinc on the normal and lead-inhibited human erythrocyte delta-aminolevulenic acid dehydratase activity *in vitro, Toxicol. Appl. Pharmacol.*, 44, 181, 1978.
390. **De Arquer Blanc, A., Pastor Duran, J., Fos Escriva, E., Rodriguez Hiero, F., and Palomique Rico, A.,** Acrodermatitis enteropathica: disparity between clinics and plasma zinc level, *An. Esp. Pediatr.*, 8, 761, 1984.
391. **De Boer, T., Bruinvels, J., and Bonta, I. L.,** Differential effects of GABA analogues and zinc on glutamate decarboxylase, 4-amono butyric-2-oxyglutamic acid transaminase and succinate semialdehyde dehydrogenase in rat brain tissue, *J. Neurochem.*, 33, 597, 1979.
392. **De Pasquele-Jardieu, P. and Fraker, P. J.,** Further characterization of the role of corticosterone in the loss of humeral immunity in zinc deficient A/J mice as determined by adrenalectomy, *J. Immunol.*, 124, 2650, 1980.
393. **Delves, H. T., Alexander, F. W., and Lay, H.,** Copper and zinc concentrations in the plasma of leukemic children, *Br. J. Haematol.*, 24, 525, 1973.
394. **Demetree, J. W., Safer, L. F., and Artis, W. M.,** The effect of zinc on sebum secretion, *Acta Derm. Venereol.*, 60, 166, 1980.
395. **De Roeth, A.,** Treatment of herpetic keratitis, *Am. J. Ophthalmol.*, 56, 729, 1963.
396. **Diamond, L. and Hurley, L. S.,** Histopathology of zinc deficient fetal rats, *J. Nutr.*, 99, 425, 1970.
397. **Diamond, L., Swenerton, H., and Hurley, L. S.,** Testicular and esophageal lesions in zinc deficient rats and their reversibility, *J. Nutr.*, 101, 77, 1971.
398. **Dib, A. and Carreau, J.-P.,** Effects of gamma-linolenic acid supplementation on lipogenesis regulation in the pregnant zinc deficient rat and fetus, *Int. J. Biochem.*, 18, 1053, 1986.
399. **Dinsdale, D. and Williams, R. B.,** The enhancement by dietary zinc deficiency of the susceptibility of the rat duodenum to colchicine, *Br. J. Nutr.*, 37, 135, 1977.
400. **Dinsdale, D. and Williams, R. B.,** Ultrastructural changes in the sperm-tail of zinc deficient rats, *J. Comp. Pathol.*, 90, 559, 1980.
401. **Dinsmore, W. W., Callender, M. E., McMaster, D., and Love, A. H. G.,** The absorption of zinc from a standardized meal in alcoholics and in normal volunteers, *Am. J. Clin. Nutr.*, 42, 688, 1985.
402. **Disilvestro, R. A. and Cousins, R. J.,** Mediation of endotoxin-induced changes in zinc metabolism in rats, *Am. J. Physiol.*, 247, E436, 1984.
403. **Disilvestro, R. A. and Cousins, R. J.,** Glucocorticoid-independent mediation of interleukin-I-induced changes in serum zinc and liver metallothionein levels, *Life Sci.*, 35, 2113, 1984.
404. **Dodge, J. A. and Yassa, J. G.,** Zinc deficiency syndrome in a British youth with cystic fibrosis, *Br. Med. J.*, i, 411, 1978.
405. **Donaldson, D. L., Kubo, C., Smith, C. C., and Good, R. A.,** Effect of genetic diabetes and zinc nutriture on *in vivo* cell mediated immunity in the mouse, *Am. J. Clin. Nutr.*, 43, 263, 1986.
406. **Donaldson, D. L. and Rennert, O. M.,** Trace elements diabetes, in *Metabolism of Trace Elements in Man,* Vol. 2, Rennert, O. M. and Chan, W.-Y., Eds., CRC Press, Boca Raton, Fla., 1984, 114.
407. **Donaldson, J. T., St. Pierre, J. L., Minnich, L., and Barbeau, A.,** Determination of sodium, potassium, magnesium, copper, zinc and manganese in rat brain regions, *Can. J. Biochem.*, 51, 87, 1973.
408. **Dorea, J. G. and Olson, J. A.,** The rate of rhodopsin regeneration in the bleached eyes of zinc deficient rats in the dark, *J. Nutr.*, 116, 121, 1986.
409. **Dorea, J. G. and Paine, P. A.,** Hair zinc in children: its uses, limitations and relationship to plasma zinc and anthopometry, *Hum. Nutr. Clin. Nutr.*, 39C, 389, 1985.
410. **Dore-Duffy, P., Catalanotto, F., Donaldson, J. O., Ostrom, K. M., and Testa, M. A.,** Zinc in multiple sclerosis, *Ann. Neurol.*, 14, 450, 1983.
411. **Dreno, B., Stadler, J. F., Pecquet, C., Boiteau, H.-L., and Barriere, H.,** Variations in cutaneous zinc concentrations after oral adminstration of zinc gluconate, *Acta Derm. Venerol.*, 64, 341, 1984.
412. **Dreosti, I. E., Belling, G. B., and Record, I. R.,** Zinc status and ethanol toxicity in rats, *Nutr. Rep. Int.*, 19, 821, 1979.
413. **Dreosti, I. E., Buckley, R. A., and Record, I. R.,** The teratogenic effect of zinc deficiency and accompanying feeding patterns in mice, *Nutr. Res.*, 6, 159, 1986.
414. **Dreosti, I. E., Gray, P. C., and Wilkins, P. J.,** DNA synthesis, protein synthesis and teratogenesis in zinc deficient rats, *S. Afr. Med. J.*, 46, 1585, 1972.
415. **Dreosti, I. E. and Hurley, L. S.,** Depressed thymidine kinase activity in zinc deficient rat embryos, *Proc. Soc. Exp. Biol. Med.*, 150, 161, 1975.
416. **Dreosti, I. E., Manuel, S. J., Buckley, R. A., Fraser, F. J., and Record, I. R.,** The effect of late prenatal and/or early post-natal zinc deficiency on the development and some biochemical aspects of the cerebellum and hippocampus in rats, *Life Sci.*, 28, 2133, 1981.

417. **Dreosti, I. E., McMichael, A. J., Gibson, G. T., Buckley, R. A., Hartshorne, J. M., and Colley, D. P.,** Fetal and maternal serum copper and zinc levels in human pregnancy, *Nutr. Res.*, 2, 591, 1982.
418. **Dronfield, M. W., Malone, J. D. G., and Langman, M. J. S.,** Zinc in ulcerative colitis: a therapeutic trial and report on plasma levels, *Gut*, 18, 33, 1977.
419. **Drummond, G. S. and Kappas, A.,** Manganese and zinc blockade of enzyme induction. Studies with microsomal heme oxygenase, *Proc. Natl. Acad. Sci. U.S.A.*, 76, 5331, 1979.
420. **Duchateau, J., Delepesse, G., Vrijens, R., and Collet, H.,** Beneficial effects of oral zinc supplementation on the immune response of old people, *Am. J. Med.*, 70, 1001, 1981.
421. **Duncan, G. D., Gray, L. F., and Daniel, L. T.,** Effect of zinc on cytochrome C oxidase activity, *Proc. Soc. Exp. Biol. Med.*, 83, 625, 1953.
422. **Duncan, J. R. and Dreosti, I. E.,** A proposed site of action for zinc in DNA synthesis, *J. Comp. Pathol.*, 86, 81, 1976.
423. **Duncan, J. R. and Hurley, L. S.,** Intestinal absorption of zinc: a role for zinc-binding ligands in milk, *Am. J. Physiol.*, 235, E556, 1978.
424. **Duncan, J. R. and Hurley, L. S.,** An interaction between zinc and vitamin A in pregnant and fetal rats, *J. Nutr.*, 108, 1431, 1978.
425. **Dunn, M. A., Blalock, T. L., and Cousins, R. J.,** Metallothionein, *Proc. Soc. Exp. Biol. Med.*, 185, 107, 1987.
426. **Dura-Trave, T., Da Cunha Ferriera, R. M. C., Monreal, I., Ezcurdia Gurpegui, M., and Villa-Elizaga, I.,** Zinc concentration of amniotic fluid in the course of pregnancy and its relationship to fetal weight and length, *Gynecol. Obstet. Invest.*, 18, 152, 1984.
427. **Dura-Trave, T., Puig-Abuli, M., Monreal, I., and Villa-Elizaga, I.,** Relation between maternal plasmatic zinc levels and uterine contractility, *Gynecol. Obstet. Invest.*, 17, 247, 1984.
428. **Dura-Trave, T., Puig-Abuli, M., Da Cunha Ferriera, R. M. C., and Villa-Elizaga, I.,** Effect of zinc nutrition o parturition and post-partum in the rat, *Gynecol. Obstet. Invest.*, 18, 275, 1985.
429. **Dura-Trave, T., Da Cunha Ferriera, R. M. C., Puig-Abuli, M., Monreal, I., and Villa-Elizaga, I.,** Zinc concentration in amniotic fluid of zinc deficient rats and its relation to fetal weight, *Biol. Neonate*, 47, 230, 1985.
430. **Dutta, S. K. and Iber, F. L.,** Zinc metabolism in patients with exocrine pancreatic insufficiency, *J. Am. Coll. Nutr.*, 3, 274, 1984.
431. **Dvergsten, C. L., Fosmire, G. J., Ollerichi, D. A., and Sandstead, H. H.,** Alterations in the post-natal development of the cerebellar cortex due to zinc deficiency. I. Impaired acquisition of granule cells, *Brain Res.*, 271, 217, 1983.
432. **Dvergsten, C. L., Fosmire, G. L., Ollerich, D. A., and Sandstead, H. H.,** Alterations on the post-natal development of the cerebellar cortex due to zinc deficiency. II. Impaired maturation of the Purkinje cells, *Dev. Brain Res.*, 16, 11, 1984.
433. **Dvergsten, C. L., Johnson, L. A., and Sandstead, H. H.,** Alterations in post-natal development of the cerebellar cortex due to zinc deficiency. III. Impaired dendritic differentiation of basket and stellate cells, *Dev. Brain Res.*, 16, 21, 1984.
434. **Dvorak, H. F. and Heppel, L. A.,** Metalloenzymes released from *E. coli* by osmotic shock. II. Evidence that 5-nucleotidase and cyclic phosphodiesterase are zinc metalloenzymes, *J. Biol. Chem.*, 243, 2647, 1968.
435. **Ead, R. D.,** Oral zinc sulphate in alopecia areata. A double-blind trial, *Br. J. Dermatol.*, 104, 483, 1981.
436. **Eagle, G. R., Zombola, R. R., and Himes, R. H.,** Tubulin-zinc interactions: binding and polymerisation studies, *Biochemistry*, 22, 221, 1983.
437. **Eamens, G. J., MacAdam, J. F., and Laig, E. A.,** Skeletal abnormalities in young horses associated with zinc toxicity and hypocuprosis, *Aust. Vet. J.*, 61, 205, 1984.
438. **Early, J. L. and Schnell, R. C.,** Zinc-induced protection against cadmium alteration of drug action, *Res. Commun. Chem. Pathol. Pharmacol.*, 19, 369, 1978.
439. **Ebbell, B.,** *The Papyrus Ebers, The Greatest Egyptian Medical Documents*, Munksgaard, Copenhagen, 1937.
440. **Eby, G. A., Davis, D. R., and Halcomb, W. W.,** Reduction in duration of common colds by zinc gluconate lozenges in a double-blind study, *Antimicrob. Agents Chemother.*, 25, 20, 1984.
441. **Eby, G. A. and Halcomb, W. W.,** Use of topical zinc to prevent recurrent herpes simplex infection: review of literature and suggested protocols, *Med. Hypoth.*, 17, 157, 1985.
442. **Ecker, R. I. and Schroeter, A.,** Acrodermatitis and zinc deficiency, *Arch. Dermatol.*, 114, 937, 1978.
443. **Eckhert, C. C.,** Isolation of a protein from human milk that enhances zinc absorption in humans, *Biochem. Biophys. Res. Commun.*, 130, 264, 1985.
444. **Eckhert, C. D. and Hurley, L. S.,** Reduced DNA synthesis in zinc deficiency: regional differences in embryonic rats, *J. Nutr.*, 107, 855, 1977.
445. **Eckhert, C. D. and Hurley, L. S.,** Influence of various levels of hypervitaminosis A and zinc deficiency on teratogenesis and DNA synthesis in the rat, *Teratology*, 19, 279, 1979.

446. **Eckhert, C. D., Sloan, M. V., Duncan, J. R., and Hurley, L. S.,** Zinc binding: a difference between human and bovine milk, *Science,* 195, 789, 1977.
447. **Edman, J., Sobel, J. D., and Taylor, M. L.,** Zinc status in women with recurrent vulvo-vaginal candidiasis, *Am. J. Obstet. Gynecol.,* 155, 1082, 1986.
448. **Edman, K. A. P.,** The effect of zinc and certain other bivalent metal ions on the isometric tension development of glycerol-extracted muscle fibre bundles, *Acta Physiol. Scand.,* 43, 275, 1958.
449. **Edman, K. A. P.,** On the binding of zinc and mersalyl to the contractile element in muscle and its relation to relaxing effect, *Acta Physiol. Scand.,* 49, 82, 1960.
450. **Edman, K. A. P.,** Zinc-induced relaxation of muscle fibres, *Acta Physiol. Scand.,* 49, 330, 1960.
451. **Eggleton, W. G. E.,** The zinc content of epidermal structures in beriberi, *Biochem. J.,* 33, 403, 1939.
452. **Eichhorn, G. L.,** Complexes of polynucleotides and nucleic acids, in *Inorganic Biochemistry,* Eichhorn, G. L., Ed., Elsevier, Amsterdam, 1973, 1210.
453. **Eisemann, J. H., Pond, W. G., and Thonney, M. L.,** Effect of dietary zinc and copper on performance and tissue mineral and cholesterol concentrations in swine, *J. Anim. Sci.,* 48, 1123, 1979.
454. **Elcoate, M., Fischer, I., Mawson, C. A., and Millar, M. J.,** The effect of zinc deficiency on the male genital system, *J. Physiol.,* 129, 53P, 1955.
455. **Ellul-Micallef, R., Galdes, A., and Fenech, F. F.,** Serum zinc levels in corticosteroid-treatment asthmatic patients, *Postgrad. Med. J.,* 52, 148, 1976.
456. **Elmes, M. E. and Jones, J. G.,** Untrastructural studies on Paneth cell apoptosis in zinc deficient rats, *Cell Tissue Res.,* 208, 57, 1980.
457. **Elmes, M. E. and Jones, J. G.,** Untrastructural changes in the intestines of zinc deficient rats, *J. Pathol.,* 130, 37, 1980.
458. **Emdin, S. O., Dodson, G. G., Cutfield, J. M., and Cutfield, S.M.,** Role of zinc in insulin biosynthesis. Some possible zinc insulin interactions in the pancreatic beta cells, *Diabetologia,* 19, 174, 1980.
459. **Emser, W.,** A case of Ehlers-Danlos syndrome and its zinc therapy, *Klin. Paediatr.,* 190, 397, 1978.
460. **Endre, L., Katona, Z., and Gyurkovitis, K.,** Zinc deficiency and cellular immune deficiency in acrodermatitis enteropathica, *Lancet,* i, 1196, 1975.
461. **Engels, L. G. J., Van Den Hamer, C. J. A., and Van Tongeren, J. H. M.,** Iron, zinc and copper balance in short bowel patients on oral nutrition, *Am. J. Clin. Nutr.,* 40, 1038, 1984.
462. **Epand, R. M., Stafford, A. R., Tyers, M., and Nieboer, E.,** Mechanism of action of diabetogenic zinc-chelating agents: model system studies, *Mol. Pharmacol.,* 27, 366, 1985.
463. **Ercan, Z. S., Oner, G., Turker, R. K., and Bor, N.,** Zinc deficiency and lung converting enzyme activity in rats, *Experientia,* 35, 215, 1979.
464. **Erway, L. C.,** Genetic and developmental implications for trace metal metabolism from mutant and inbred strains of animals, in *Metabolism of Trace Metals in Man,* Vol. 1, Rennert, O. M. and Chan, W.-Y., Eds., CRC Press, Boca Raton, Fla., 1984, 17.
465. **Erway, L. C. and Grider, A.,** Zinc metabolism in lethal-milk mice. Otolith, lactation and aging effects, *J. Hered.,* 75, 480, 1984.
466. **Esca, S. A., Brenner, W., Mach, K., and Gschnait, F.,** Kwashiorkor-like zinc deficiency in anorexia nervosa, *Acta Derm. Venereol.,* 59, 361, 1979.
467. **Essatara, M. B., McClain, C. J., Levine, A. S., Elson, M. K., Shafer, R. B., and Morley, J. E.,** Is zinc deficiency anorexia mediated through the endogenous opiates?, *Am. J. Clin. Nutr.,* 35, 832, 1982.
468. **Essatara, M. B., Levine, A. S., Morley, J. E., and McClain, C. J.,** Zinc deficiency and anorexia in rats: normal feeding patterns and stress induced feeding, *Physiol. Behav.,* 32, 469, 1984.
469. **Essatara, M. B., Morley, J. E., Levine, A. S., Elson, M.K., Shafer, R. B., and McClain, C. J.,** The role of the endogenous opiates in zinc deficiency anorexia, *Physiol. Behav.,* 32, 475, 1984.
470. **Essatara, M. B., McClain, C. J., Levine, A. S., and Morley, J. E.,** Zinc deficiency and anorexia in rats: the effect of central administration of norepinephrine, muscimol and bromerogocryptine, *Physiol. Behav.,* 32, 479, 1984.
471. **Ette, S. I., Basu, T. K., and Dickerson, J. W. T.,** Short-term effect of zinc sulphate on plasma and hepatic concentrations of vitamin A and E and normal weanling rats, *Nutr. Metab.,* 23, 11, 1979.
472. **Etzel, K. R., Shapiro, S. G., and Cousins, R. J.,** Regulation of liver metallothionein and plasma zinc by the glucocorticoid dexamethasone, *Biochem. Biophys. Res. Commun.,* 89, 1120, 1979.
473. **Evans, G. W.,** Zinc absorption and transport, in *Trace Elements in Human Health and Disease,* Vol. 1, Prasad, A. S. and Oberleas, D., Eds., Academic Press, New York, 1976, 181.
474. **Evans, G. W., Grace, C. I., and Votava, H. J.,** A proposed mechanim for zinc absorption in the rat, *Am. J. Physiol.,* 228, 501, 1975.
475. **Evans, G. W. and Johnson, E. C.,** Growth stimulatory effect of picolinic acid added to rat diets, *Proc. Soc. Exp. Biol. Med.,* 165, 457, 1980.
476. **Evans, G. W. and Johnson, E. C.,** Zinc concentration of liver and kidneys from rat pups nursing dams fed supplemental zinc dipicolinate or zinc acetate, *J. Nutr.,* 110, 2121, 1980.

477. **Evans, G. W. and Johnson, E. C.**, Effect of iron, vitamin B_6 and picolinic acid on zinc absorption in the rat, *J. Nutr.*, 111, 68, 1981.
478. **Evans, G. W., Johnson, E. C., and Johnson, P. E.**, Zinc absorption in the rat determined by radioisotope dilution, *J. Nutr.*, 109, 1258, 1979.
479. **Evans, G. W. and Johnson, P. E.**, Zinc-binding factor in acrodermatitis enteropathica, *Lancet,* ii, 1310, 1976.
480. **Evans, G. W. and Johnson, P. E.**, Prostaglandin E_2: the zinc-binding ligand in human breast milk, *Clin. Res.*, 25, 536A, 1977.
481. **Evans, G. W. and Johnson, P. E.**, Defective prostaglandin synthesis in acrodermatitis enteropathica, *Lancet,* i, 52, 1977.
482. **Evans, G. W. and Johnson, P. E.**, Copper and zinc binding ligands in the intestinal mucosa, in *Trace Element Metabolism in Man and Animals,* Vol. 3, Kirchgessner, M., Ed., Arbeitskreis fur Tierernahrungs-forschung, Weienstephan, F. R. G., 1978, 98.
483. **Evans, G. W., Majors, P. F., and Cornatzer, W. E.**, Mechanism for cadmium and zinc antagonism of copper metabolism, *Biochem. Biophys. Res. Commun.*, 40, 1142, 1970.
484. **Everett, G. A. and Apgar, J.**, Effect of zinc status on salivary zinc concentrations in the rat, *J. Nutr.*, 109, 406, 1979.
485. **Everett, G. A. and Apgar, J.**, Effect of zinc deficiency on prostaglandin $F_{2\ alpha}$ and E in the rat, in *Trace Element Analytical Chemistry in Medicine and Biology,* Vol. 2, Bratter, P. and Schramel, P., Eds., Walter de Gruyter, New York, 1983, 219.
486. **Everett, G. A. and Apgar, J.**, Effect of zinc deficiency on prostaglandin levels in pregnant rats, *Nutr. Res.*, Suppl. 1, 335, 1985.
487. **Faber, J., Randolph, J. G., Robbins, S., and Smith, J. C., Jr.**, Zinc and copper status in young patients following jejunoileal bypass, *J. Surg. Res.*, 24, 83, 1978.
488. **Fabris, N., Amadio, L., Licastro, F., Mocchegiani, E., Zannoti, M., and Franceshi, C.**, Thymic hormone deficiency in normal aging and Down's syndrome: is there a primary failure of the thymus?, *Lancet,* i, 983, 1984.
489. **Failla, M. L. and Cousins, R. J.**, Zinc accumulation and metabolism in primary cultures of adult rat liver cells, *Biochim. Biophys. Acta,* 543, 293, 1975.
490. **Failla, M. L., van De Veerdonk, M., Morgan, W. T., and Smith, J. C., Jr.**, Characterization of zinc binding proteins in familial hyperzincemia, *J. Lab. Clin. Med.*, 100, 943, 1982.
491. **Fair, W. R. and Heston, W. D. W.**, The relationship of bacterial prostatitis and zinc, in *Zinc Metabolism: Clinical Aspects in Health and Disease,* Prasad, A. S. and Brewer, G. J., Eds., Alan R. Liss, New York, 1977, 129.
492. **Fairweather-Tait, S. J., Wright, A. J. A., Jacqui, C., and Franklin, J.**, Studies of zinc metabolism in pregnant and lactating rats, *Br. J. Nutr.*, 54, 401, 1985.
493. **Fairweather-Tait, S. J., Wright, A. J. A., and Williams, C. M.**, Zinc metabolism in pregnant and lactating rats and the effects of varying iron:zinc in the diet, *Br. J. Nutr.*, 52, 205, 1984.
494. **Falchuk, K. H.**, Effect of acute disease and ACTH on serum zinc proteins, *N. Engl. J. Med.*, 296, 1129, 1977.
495. **Falchuk, K. H., Fawcett, D. W., and Vallee, B. L.**, Role of zinc in cell division of *E. gracilis, J. Cell Sci.*, 17, 57, 1975.
496. **Falchuk, K. H., Hardy, C., Ulpino, L., and Vallee, B. L.**, RNA polymease, manganese and RNA metabolism of zinc sufficient and deficient, *E. gracilis, Biochem. Biophys. Res. Commun.*, 77, 314, 1977.
497. **Falchuk, K. H. and Vallee, B. L.**, Zinc and chromatin: structure composition and function, in *Trace Element Metabolism in Man and Animals,* Vol. 5, Mills, C. F., Ed., Commonwealth Bureaux of Nutrition, Farnham, Slough, U. K., in press.
498. **Faraji, B. and Swendseid, M. E.**, Growth rate, tissue zinc levels and activities of selected enzymes in rats fed a zinc deficient diet by gastric tube, *J. Nutr.*, 113, 447, 1983.
499. **Fargeas, M. J., Fiormonti, J., and Bueno, L.**, Prostaglandin E2: a neuromodulator in the central control of gastrointestinal motility and feeding behaviour by calcitonin, *Science,* 225, 1050, 1984.
500. **Favier, M.**, Metal ions in the amniotic fluid during the last trimester of pregnancy. Significant relationship between zinc level and fetal weight, *Rev. Fr. Gynecol. Obstet.*, 67, 707, 1972.
501. **Feaster, J. P., Hansard, S. L., McCall, J. T., and Davis, G. K.**, Absorption, deposition and placental transfer of zinc-65 in the rat, *Am. J. Physiol.*, 181, 287, 1955.
502. **Feder, J. and Garrett, L. R.**, A rapid method for the removal of zinc from the metalloneutral proteases, *Biochem. Biophys. Res. Commun.*, 43, 943, 1971.
503. **Feeley, R. M., Eitenmiller, R. R., Jones, J. B., and Barnhart, H.**, Copper, iron and zinc contents of human milk at early stages of lactation, *Am. J. Clin. Nutr.*, 37, 443, 1983.
504. **Feinglos, M. N. and Jegasothy, B. V.**, Insulin allergy due to zinc, *Lancet,* 1, 122, 1979.
505. **Fell, G. S., Fleck, A., Cuthbertson, D. P., Queen, K., Morrison, C., Bessent, R. G., and Husain, S. L.**, Urinary zinc levels as an indicator of muscle catabolism, *Lancet,* 1, 280, 1973.

506. **Fell, G. S., Lyon, T. B., Phillips, M., and Fraser, W.,** Assessment of an in vitro serum protein zinc-binding test in human nutrition, *Proc. Nutr. Soc.*, in press.
507. **Fenton, M. R., Burke, J. P., Techner, L. M., and Chinkes, S. L.,** Lipid levels in tumor-bearing mice maintained on a zinc deficient diet, *Nutr. Rep. Int.*, 29, 921, 1984.
508. **Ferguson, H. W. and Leaver, A. G.,** Effects of diets high in zinc and different levels of calcium and vitamin D on the rat humerus and incisor, *Calcif, Tissue Res.*, 8, 265, 1972.
509. **Fernandes, G., Nair, M., Onoe, K., Tanaka, T., Floyd, R., and Good, R. A.,** Impairment of cell mediated immunity function by dietary zinc deficiency in mice, *Proc. Natl. Acad. Sci. U.S.A.*, 76, 457, 1979.
510. **Fernandez, M. A. and O'Dell, B. L.,** Effect of zinc deficiency on plasma glutathione in the rat, *Proc. Soc. Exp. Biol. Med.*, 173, 564, 1983.
511. **Fernandez-Madrid, F., Prasad, A. S., and Oberleas, D.,** Effect of zinc deficiency on collagen metabolism, *J. Lab. Clin. Med.*, 78, 853, 1971.
512. **Fernandez-Madrid, F., Prasad, A. S., and Oberleas, D.,** Effect of zinc deficiency on nucleic acids, collagen and noncollagenous protein of connective tissue, *J. Lab. Clin. Med.*, 82, 951, 1973.
513. **Fernandez-Madrid, F., Prasad, A. S., and Oberleas, D.,** Zinc in collagen metabolism, in *Trace Elements in Human Health and Disease,* Vol. 1, Prasad, A. S. and Oberleas, D., Eds., Academic Press, New York, 1976, 257.
514. **Fernley, R. T.,** Equine angiotensin-converting enzyme: a zinc metalloenzyme, *Clin. Exp. Pharmacol. Physiol.*, 4, 267, 1977.
515. **Festa, M. D., Anderson, H. L., Dowdy, R. P., and Ellerseick, M. R.,** Effect of zinc intake on copper excretion and retention in man, *Am. J. Clin. Nutr.*, 41, 285, 1985.
516. **Fickel, J. J., Freeland-Graves, J. H., and Roby, M. J.,** Zinc tolerance tests in zinc deficient and zinc supplemented diets, *Am. J. Clin. Nutr.*, 43, 47, 1986.
517. **Fiedler, H. and Herrmann, I.,** Changes in thrombocyte aggregation caused by administration of metal salts to rabbits, *Folia Haematol. (Leipzig),* 96, 224, 1971.
518. **Field, H. P. and Kelleher, J.,** A role for zinc in essential fatty acid metabolism, *Proc. Nutr. Soc.*, 43, 54A, 1984.
519. **Figlewicz, D. P., Forman, S. E., Hodgson, A. T., and Grodsky, G. M.,** Zinc-65 and endogenous zinc content and distribution in islets in relationship to insulin content, *Endocrinology,* 115, 877, 1984.
520. **Figlewicz, D. P., Heldt, A., Forhan, S. E., and Grodsky, G. M.,** Effects of exogenous zinc on insulin secretion in vitro, *Endocrinolgy,* 108, 730, 1981.
521. **Fischer, P. W. F. and Collins, M. W.,** Relationship between serum zinc and copper and risk factors associated with cardiovascular disease, *Am. J. Clin. Nutr.*, 34, 595, 1981.
522. **Fischer, P. W. F., Giroux, A., Belonte, B., and Shah, B. G.,** The effect of dietary copper and zinc on cholesterol metabolism, *Am. J. Clin. Nutr.*, 33, 1019, 1980.
523. **Fischer, P. W. F., Giroux, A., and L'Abbé, M. R.,** The effect of dietary zinc on intestinal copper absorption, *Am. J. Clin. Nutr.*, 34, 1670, 1981.
524. **Fischer, P. W. F., Giroux, A., and L'Abbé, M. R.,** Effect of zinc supplementation on copper status in adult men, *Am. J. Clin. Nutr.*, 40, 743, 1984.
525. **Fisher, G. L.,** Effects of disease on serum copper and zinc values in the beagle, *Am. J. Vet. Res.*, 38, 935, 1977.
526. **Fisher, G. L., Byers, V. S., Shifrine, M., and Levin, A. S.,** Copper and zinc levels in serum from human patients with sarcomas, *Cancer,* 37, 356, 1976.
527. **Fitzherbert, J. C.,** Zinc deficiency and acne vulgaris, *Med. J. Aust.*, 2, 273, 1976.
528. **Fjeller, B.,** Drug-induced lupus erythematous aggrevated by oral zinc therapy, *Acta Derm. Venereol.*, 59, 368, 1979.
529. **Flanagan, P. R.,** A model to produce pure zinc deficiency in rats and its use to demonstrate that dietary phytate increases the excretion of endogenous zinc, *J. Nutr.*, 114, 493, 1984.
530. **Flanagan, P. R.,** Absorption of food zinc in human subjects: effect of added iron, *Proc. Can. Fed. Biol. Soc.*, 28, PA26, 1985.
531. **Flanagan, P. R., Cluett, J., Chamberlain, M., and Valberg, L. S.,** Dual isotope method for determination of human zinc absorption: the use of a test meal of turkey meat, *J. Nutr.*, 115, 111, 1985.
532. **Flanagan, P. R., Haist, J., and Valberg, L. S.,** Zinc absorption, intraluminal zinc and intestinal metallothionein in zinc deficient and zinc replete rodents, *J. Nutr.*, 113, 962, 1983.
533. **Fleischman, A. I., Yacowitz, H., Hayton, T., and Bierenbaum, M. L.,** Effect of calcium and vitamin D3 upon fecal excretion of some metals in the mature male rat fed a high fat, cholesterol diet, *J. Nutr.*, 95, 19, 1968.
534. **Fleming, C., Hodges, R. E., Smith, L. M., and Hurley, L. S.,** Essential fatty acids, copper, zinc and tocopherol deficiencies in total parenteral nutrition, *Acta Chir. Scand.*, Suppl. 466, 20, 1976.
535. **Fleming, C. R., Huizenga, K. A., McCall, J. T., Gildea, J., and Dennis, R.,** Zinc nutrition in Crohn's disease, *Dig. Dis. Sci.*, 26, 865, 1981.

536. **Fleming, C. R., Smith, L. M., and Hodges, R. E.,** Essential fatty deficiency in adults receiving total parenteral nutrition, *Am. J. Clin. Nutr.*, 29, 976, 1976.
537. **Floersheim, G. L.,** Influence of zinc, d-penicillamine and oxygen on poisoning with *Amantia phalloides* Zinc accelerates liver regeneration and prevents the depletion of brain noradrenaline caused by the mushroom, *Agents Actions,* 14, 124, 1984.
538. **Floersheim, G. L.,** Protection against ethanol toxicity in mice by zinc aspartate, glycols, levulose and pyritinol, *Agents Actions,* 16, 580, 1985.
539. **Flynn, A. and Franzman, A. W.,** Seasonal variations in hair mineral levels of the Alaskan moose, in *Trace Element Metabolism in Animals,* Vol. 2, Hoekstra, W. G., Suttie, J. W., Ganther, H. E., and Mertz, W., Eds., University Park Press, Baltimore, 1974, 444.
540. **Flynn, A., Martier, S. S., Sokol, R. J., Miller, S. I., Golden, N. I., and Del Villano, B. C.,** Zinc status of pregnant alcoholic women: a determinant of fetal outcome, *Lancet,* i, 572, 1981.
541. **Flynn, A., Pories, W. J., Strain, W. H., and Hill, O. A.,** Zinc deficiency with altered adrenocortical function and its relation to delayed healing, *Lancet,* i, 789, 1973.
542. **Flynn, A., Pories, W. J., and Strain, W. H.,** Rapid serum zinc depletion associated with corticosteroid treatment, *Lancet,* ii, 1169, 1971.
543. **Fogerty, A. C., Ford, G. L., Dreosti, I. E., and Tinsley, I. J.,** Zinc deficiency and fatty acid composition of tissue lipids, *Nutr. Rep. Int.*, 32, 1009, 1985.
544. **Fogerty, A. C., Ford, G. L., Willcox, M. E., and Clancy, S. L.,** Liver fatty acids and the sudden infant death syndrome, *Am. J. Clin. Nutr.*, 39, 201, 1984.
545. **Foley, B., Johnson, S. A., Hackley, B., Smith, J. C., Jr., and Halsted, J. A.,** Zinc content of human platelets, *Proc. Soc. Exp. Biol. Med.*, 128, 265, 1968.
546. **Follis, R. H., Day, H. G., and McCollum, E. V.,** Histological studies of the tissues of rats fed a diet extremely low in zinc, *J. Nutr.*, 22, 223, 1941.
547. **Foote, J. W. and Delves, H. T.,** Measurement of zinc in serum proteins, in *Trace Element Analytical Chemistry in Medicine and Biology,* Vol. 2, Bratter, P. and Schramel, P., Eds., Walter de Gruyter, New York, 1983, 877.
548. **Foote, J. W. and Delves, H. T.,** Distribution of zinc among human serum proteins determined by affinity chromatography and atomic absorption spectrophotometry, *Analyst,* 108, 492, 1983.
549. **Foote, J. W. and Delves, H. T.,** Albumin-bound and alpha (&)2(&)-macroglobulin-bound zinc concentrations in the sera of healthy adults, *J. Clin. Pathol.*, 37, 1050, 1984.
550. **Foote, J. W. and Hinks, L. J.,** Reduced leucocyte zinc and albumin-bound zinc in blood of haemodialysis patients, *Ann. Clin. Biochem.*, 24, 198, 1987.
551. **Forbes, R. M.,** Nutritional interactions of zinc and copper, *Fed. Proc. Fed. Am. Soc. Exp. Biol.*, 19, 643, 1960.
552. **Forbes, R. M., Parker, H. M., and Erdman, J. W.,** Effects of dietary phytate, calcium and magnesium levels on zinc bioavailability to rats, *J. Nutr.*, 114, 1421, 1984.
553. **Fosmire, G. S., Greeley, S., and Sandstead, H. H.,** Maternal and fetal responses to various suboptimal levels of zinc intake during gestation in the rat, *J. Nutr.*, 107, 1543, 1977.
554. **Foster, D. M., Aamodt, R. L., Henkin, R. I., and Berman, M.,** Zinc metabolism in humans: a kinetic model, *Am. J. Physiol.*, 237, R340, 1979.
555. **Foster, D. M., Berman, M., Aamodt, R. L., and Henkin, R. I.,** Steroid-dependent changes in zinc metabolism, *Clin. Res.*, 27, 448A, 1979.
556. **Fraker, P. J.,** Zinc deficiency: a common immunodeficiency state, *Surv. Immunol. Res.*, 2, 155, 1983.
557. **Fraker, P. J., De Pasquele-Jardieu, P., Zwickl, C. M., and Keucke, R. W.,** Regulation of T-cell helper function in zinc deficient adult mice, *Proc. Natl. Acad. Sci. U.S.A.*, 75, 5660, 1978.
558. **Fraker, P. J., Gershwin, M. E., Good, R. A., and Prasad, A. S.,** Interrelationships between zinc and immune function, *Fed. Proc. Fed. Am. Soc. Exp. Biol.*, 45, 1474, 1986.
559. **Fraker, P. J., Zwickl, C. M., and Leucke, R. W.,** Delayed-type hypersensitivity in zinc deficient adult mice: impairment and restoration of responsivity to dinitrofluorbenzene, *J. Nutr.*, 112, 309, 1982.
560. **Fransson, G. B. and Lonnerdal, B.,** Zinc, copper, calcium and magnesium in human milk, *J. Pediatr.*, 101, 504, 1982.
561. **Fransson, G. B. and Lonnerdal, B.,** Distribution of trace elements and minerals in human and cow's milk, *J. Pediatr.*, 17, 912, 1983.
562. **Fransson, G. B. and Lonnerdal, B.,** Iron, copper, zinc calcium and magnesium in human milk fat, *Am. J. Clin. Nutr.*, 39, 185, 1984.
563. **Freeland-Graves, J. H., Ebangit, M. L., and Hendrickson, P. J.,** Alterations in zinc absorption and salivary sediment zinc after a lacto-ovo vegetarian diet, *Am. J. Clin. Nutr.*, 33, 1757, 1980.
564. **Freeland-Graves, J. H., Han, W. H., Friedman, B. J., and Shorey, R. L.,** Effect of dietary zinc-copper ratios on cholesterol and HDL-cholesterol levels in women, *Nutr. Rep. Int.*, 22, 285, 1980.
565. **Freeland-Graves, J. H., Friedman, B. J., Han, W. H., Shorey, R. L., and Young, R.,** Effect of zinc supplementation on plasma high-density lipoprotein cholesterol and zinc, *Am. J. Clin. Nutr.*, 35, 988, 1982.

566. **Freeman, R. M., Richards, C. J., and Rames, L. K.,** Zinc metabolism in aminonucleoside-induced nephrosis, *Am. J. Clin. Nutr.*, 28, 699, 1975.
567. **Friberg, J. and Nilsson, O.,** The amount of zinc detected in washed human spermatozoa, *Upsala J. Med. Sci.*, 79, 63, 1973.
568. **Friedlander, B.,** Selective inhibition of HSV type 1 DNA polymerase by zinc ions, *Virology*, 84, 551, 1978.
569. **Friel, J. K., Gibson, R. S., Balassa, R., and Watts, J. L.,** A comparison of the zinc, copper and manganese status of very low birth weight pre-term and full term infants during the first twelve months, *Acta Paediatr. Scand.*, 73, 596, 1984.
570. **Friel, J. K., Gibson, R. S., Kawash, G. F., and Watts, J.,** Dietary zinc intake and growth during infancy, *J. Pediatr. Gastroenterol. Nutr.*, 4, 746, 1985.
571. **Freil, J. K., Gibson, R. S., Peliowski, A., and Watts, J.,** Serum zinc, copper and selenium concentrations in preterm infants receiving enteral nutrition or parenteral nutrition supplemented with zinc and copper, *J. Pediatr.*, 104, 763, 1984.
572. **Frithz, G. and Ronquist, G.,** Increased red cell content of zinc in essential hypertension, *Acta Med. Scand.*, 205, 647, 1979.
573. **Frommer, D. J.,** The healing of gastric ulcers by zinc sulphate, *Med. J. Aust.*, 2, 793, 1975.
574. **Fujii, T.,** Presence of zinc in nucleoli and its possible role in mitosis, *Nature (London)*, 174, 1108, 1954.
575. **Fujii, T., Utida, S., and Mizuno, T.,** Reaction of starfish spermatozoa to histidine and certain other substances considered in relation to zinc, *Nature (London)*, 176, 1068, 1955.
576. **Gabriel, G. N., Schrager, T. F., and Newberne, P. M.,** Zinc deficiency, alcohol and retinoid: association with esophageal cancer in rats, *JNCI*, 68, 785, 1982.
577. **Gallant, K. R. and Cherian, M. G.,** Influence of maternal mineral deficiency on hepatic metallothionein and zinc in newborn rats, *Biochem. Cell Biol.*, 64, 8, 1986.
578. **Gardiner, P. E., Gessner, H., Bratter, P., Stoeppler, M., and Nurnberg, H. W.,** The distribution of zinc in human erythrocytes, *J. Clin. Chem. Clin. Biochem.*, 22, 159, 1984.
579. **Garafolo, J. A., Ashikari, H., Lesser, M. L., Menendez-Botet, C., Cunningham-Rundles, S., Schwartz, M. K., and Good, R. A.,** Serum zinc, copper and the copper/zinc ratio in patients with benign and malignant breast lesions, *Cancer*, 46, 2682, 1980.
580. **Garofolo, J. A., Strong, E., and Good, R. A.,** Zinc deficiency in intestinal bypass procedures, *Ann. Intern. Med.*, 90, 990, 1979.
581. **Garretts, M. and Molokhia, M.,** Acrodermatitis enteropathica without hypozincemia, *J. Pediatr.*, 91, 492, 1977.
582. **Gates, R. R., Craig-Schmidt, M. C., and Faircloth, S. A.,** Effect of zinc and essential fatty acid deficiencies on prostaglandin production by rat lung and liver, *Fed. Proc. Fed. Am. Soc. Exp. Biol.*, 43, 478, 1984.
583. **Gebhard, R. L., Karouani, R., Prigge, W. F., and McClain, C. J.,** The effect of severe zinc deficiency on activity of intestinal disaccharidases and 3-hydroxy-3-methylglutaryl Coenzyme A reductase in the rat, *J. Nutr.*, 113, 855, 1983.
584. **Geissler, A. H., Turnlund, J. R., and Cohen, R. D.,** Effect of chlorthalidone on zinc levels, testosterone and sexual function in man, *Drug Nutr. Interact.*, 4, 275, 1986.
585. **Geist, F. C., Bateman, J. A., and Hayden, F. G.,** *In vitro* activity of zinc salts against human rhinoviruses, *Antimicrob. Agents Chemother.*, 31, 622, 1987.
586. **Geller, B. L. and Winge, D. R.,** Rat liver copper, zinc superoxide dismutase, *J. Biol. Chem.*, 257, 8945, 1982.
587. **Gentile, P. S., Trentalange, M. J., and Coleman, M.,** The relationship of hair zinc concentration to height, weight, age and sex in the normal population, *Pediatr. Res.*, 15, 123, 1981.
588. **Ghavami-Maibodi, S., Collipp, P. J., Castro-Magana, M., Stewart, C., and Chen, S. Y.,** Effect of oral zinc supplements on growth, hormonal levels and zinc in healthy short children, *Ann. Nutr. Metab.*, 27, 214, 1983.
589. **Ghishan, F. K.,** Fetal alcohol syndrome: failure of zinc supplementation to reverse the effect of ethanol on placental transport of zinc, *Pediatr. Res.*, 17, 529, 1983.
590. **Ghishan, F. K. and Greene, H. L.,** Intestinal transport of zinc in the diabetic rat, *Life Sci.*, 32, 1735, 1984.
591. **Ghishan, F. K., Patwardhan, R., and Greene, H. L.,** Fetal alcohol syndrome: inhibition of placental zinc transport as a potential mechanism for fetal growth retardation in the rat, *J. Lab. Clin. Med.*, 100, 45, 1982.
592. **Ghishan, F. K., Said, H. M., Wilson, P. C., Murrell, J. E., and Greene, H. L.,** Intestinal transport of zinc and folic acid: a mutual inhibitory effect, *Am. J. Clin. Nutr.*, 43, 258, 1986.
593. **Ghosh, A., Fong, L. Y. Y., Wan, C. W., Liang, S. T., Woo, J. S. K., and Wong, V.,** Zinc deficiency is not a cause for abortion, congenital abnormality and small-for-gestational-age infants in Chinese women, *Br. J. Obstet. Gynecol.*, 92, 886, 1985.

594. **Gibson, R. S., Anderson, B. M., and Scythes, C. A.,** Regional differences in hair zinc concentrations: a possible effect of water hardness, *Am. J. Clin. Nutr.*, 37, 37, 1983.

595. **Gibson, R. S. and deWolfe, M. S.,** Copper, zinc, manganese, vanadium and iodine concentration in the hair of Canadian low birth-weight neonates, *Am. J. Clin. Nutr.*, 32, 1728, 1979.

596. **Gibson, R. S. and deWolfe, M. S.,** Changes in serum zinc concentrations of some Canadian full term and low birth weight infants from birth to six months, *Acta Paediatr. Scand.*, 70, 497, 1981.

597. **Gierdoc, D. P. and Coleman, J. E.,** Structural and function differences between the two intrinsic zinc ions of *E. coli* RNA polymerase, *Biochemistry,* 25, 4969, 1986.

598. **Giovetti, A. C., Russell, R. M., and Iber, F. L.,** Effect of ethanol ingestion on serum and urine zinc and serum copper, *Clin. Res.*, 27, 232A, 1979.

599. **Gipp, W. F., Pond, W. G., and Kallfelz, F. A.,** Effect of dietary copper, iron and ascorbic acid levels on hematology, blood and tissue copper, iron and zinc concentrations, *J. Nutr.*, 104, 532, 1974.

600. **Giroux, E. L.,** Determination of zinc distribution between albumin and alpha 2-macroglobulin in human serum, *Biochem. Med.*, 12, 258, 1975.

601. **Giroux, E. L., Durieux, M., and Schechter, P. J.,** A study of zinc distribution in serum, *Bioinorg. Chem.*, 5, 211, 1976.

602. **Giroux, E. L. and Henkin, R. I.,** Competition for zinc among serum albumin and amino acids, *Biochim. Biophys. Acta,* 273, 64, 1972.

603. **Giroux, E. L., Schechter, P. J., Schoun, J., and Sjoerdama, A.,** Reduced binding of added zinc in the serum of patients with decompensated hepatic cirrhosis, *Eur. J. Clin. Invest.*, 7, 71, 1977.

604. **Glover, S. C. and White, M.,** Zinc again, *Br. Med. J.*, ii, 640, 1977.

605. **Goette, D. K.,** Zinc deficiency, pellegra or both, *Arch. Dermatol.*, 115, 507, 1979.

606. **Gold, G. and Grodsky, G. M.,** Kinetic aspects of compartmental storage and secretion of insulin and zinc, *Experientia,* 40, 1105, 1984.

607. **Goldberg, H. J. and Sheehy, E. M.,** Fifth day fits: an acute zinc deficiency syndrome? *Arch. Dis. Child.*, 57, 633, 1982.

608. **Golden, B. E. and Golden, M. H. N.,** Plasma zinc and the clinical features of malnutrition, *Am. J. Clin. Nutr.*, 32, 2490, 1979.

609. **Golden, B. E. and Golden, M. H. N.,** Plasma zinc, rate of weight gain, and the energy cost of tissue deposition in children recovering from severe malnutrition on a cow's milk or soy protein-based diet, *Am. J. Clin. Nutr.*, 34, 892, 1981.

610. **Golden, B. E. and Golden, M. H. N.,** Effect of zinc supplementation on the composition of newly synthesized tissue in children recovering from malnutrition, *Proc. Soc. Nutr.*, in press.

611. **Golden, M. H. N. and Golden, B. E.,** Effect of zinc supplementation on the dietary intake, rate of weight gain and energy cost of tissue deposition in children recovering from severe malnutrition, *Am. J. Clin. Nutr.*, 34, 900, 1981.

612. **Golden, M. H. N., Golden, B. E., Harland, P. S. E. G., and Jackson, A. A.,** Zinc and immunocompetence in protein-energy malnutrition, *Lancet,* i, 1226, 1978.

613. **Golden, M. H. N., Golden, B. E., and Jackson, A. A.,** Skin breakdown in kwashiorkor responds to zinc, *Lancet,* i, 1256, 1980.

614. **Golden, M. H. N., Jackson, A. A., and Golden, B. E.,** Effect of zinc on thymus of recently malnourished children, *Lancet,* ii, 1057, 1977.

615. **Goldey, D. H., Mansmann, H. C., and Rasmussen, A. I.,** Zinc status of asthmatic, prednisone-treated asthmatic, and non-asthmatic children, *J. Am. Diet. Assoc.*, 84, 157, 1984.

616. **Goldstein, L. and Pfeiffer, C. C.,** Effects of single oral doses of trace elements on the normal quantitated EEG of normal subjects and chronic schizophrenics, *Psychopharmacol. Bull.*, 14, 55, 1978.

617. **Golub, M. S., Gershwin, M. E., Hurley, L. S., Baly, D. L., and Hendrickx, A. G.,** Studies of marginal zinc deprivation in Rhesus monkeys. I. Influence on pregnant dams, *Am. J. Clin. Nutr.*, 39, 265, 1984.

618. **Golub, M. S., Gershwin, M. E., Hurley, L. S., Baly, D. L., and Hendrickx, A. G.,** Studies of marginal zinc deprivation in Rhesus monkeys. II. Pregnancy outcome, *Am. J. Clin. Nutr.*, 39, 879, 1984.

619. **Golub, M. S., Gershwin, M. E., Hurley, L. S., Hendrickx, A. G., and Saito, W. Y.,** Studies of marginal zinc deprivation in Rhesus monkeys: infant behaviour, *Am. J. Clin. Nutr.*, 42, 1229, 1985.

620. **Golub, M. S., Gershwin, M. E., Hurley, L. S., Saito, W. Y., and Hendrickx, A. G.,** Studies of marginal zinc deprivation in Rhesus monkeys. IV. Growth of infants in the first year, *Am. J. Clin. Nutr.*, 40, 192, 1984.

621. **Good, R. A., Fernandes, G., Garofolo, J. A., Cunningham-Rundles, C., Iwata, T., and West, A.,** Zinc and immunity, in *Clinical, Biochemical and Nutritional Aspects of Trace Elements,* Prasad, A. S., Ed., Alan R. Liss, New York, 1982, 189.

622. **Goodman, L. S. and Gilman, A.,** *The Pharmacological Basis of Therapeutics,* 4th ed., Macmillan, London, 1970.

623. **Goodwin, J. S., Hunt, W. C., Hooper, P., and Garry, P. J.,** Relationship between zinc intake, physical activity and blood levels of high density lipoprotein cholesterol in a healthy elderly population, *Metabolism,* 34, 519, 1985.
624. **Gordon, J., Morlet, J. E., and Hershman, J. M.,** Thyroid function and zinc deficiency, *Clin. Res.,* 27, 20A, 1979.
625. **Gordon, P. R. and O'Dell, B. L.,** Rat platelet aggregation impaired by short term zinc deficiency, *J. Nutr.,* 110, 2125, 1980.
626. **Gordon, P. R. and O'Dell, B. L.,** Short term zinc deficiency and hemostasis in the rat, *Proc. Soc. Exp. Biol. Med.,* 163, 240, 1980.
627. **Gordon, P. R. and O'Dell, B. L.,** Zinc deficiency and impaired platelet aggregation in guinea pigs, *J. Nutr.,* 113, 239, 1983.
628. **Gorodetsky, R., Fuks, Z., Sulkes, A., Ginsberg, H., and Weshler, Z.,** Correlation of erythrocyte and plasma levels of zinc, copper and iron with evidence of metastatic spread in cancer patients, *Cancer,* 55, 779, 1985.
629. **Graham, C. W. M. S.,** On the internal use of zinc in glett and leucorrhea, *Edinb. Med. Surg. J.,* 26, 107, 1826.
630. **Graham, J. R.,** Zinc deficiency in Crohn's disease, *Med. J. Aust.,* 2, 484, 1979.
631. **Graig, F. A.,** Role of zinc and other trace elements in diabetes mellitus, *N.Y. State J. Med.,* 1, 75, 1962.
632. **Grant, P. T., Coombs, T. L., and Frank, B. H.,** Differences in the nature of the interaction of insulin and proinsulin with zinc, *Biochem. J.,* 126, 433, 1972.
633. **Grant-Frost, D. R. and Underwood, E. J.,** Zinc toxicity in the rat and interrelation with copper, *Aust. J. Exp. Biol. Med. Sci.,* 36, 339, 1958.
634. **Gray, L. F. and Ellis, G. H.,** Some interrelationships of copper, molybdenum, zinc and lead in the nutrition of the rat, *J. Nutr.,* 40, 441, 1950.
635. **Greaves, M. W.,** Zinc in cutaneous ulceration due to vascular insufficiency, *Am. Heart J.,* 83, 716, 1972.
636. **Greaves, M. W. and Boyde, T. R. C.,** Plasma zinc concentrations in patients with psoriasis, other dermatoses and venous leg ulceration, *Lancet,* ii, 1019, 1967.
637. **Greaves, M. W. and Skillen, A. W.,** Effect of continued ingestion of zinc sulphate in patients with venous leg ulceration, *Lancet,* ii, 889, 1970.
638. **Greeley, S., Fosmire, G. J., and Sandstead, H. H.,** Nitrogen retention during late gestation in the rat in response to marginal zinc intake, *Am. J. Physiol.,* 239, E113, 1980.
639. **Greene, H. L.,** Trace metals in parenteral nutrition, in *Zinc Metabolism: Current Aspects in Health and Disease,* Prasad, A. S. and Brewer, G. J., Eds., Alan R. Liss, New York, 1977, 87.
640. **Greger, J. L. and Sickles, V. S.,** Saliva zinc levels: potential indicators of zinc status, *Am. J. Clin. Nutr.,* 32, 1859, 1979.
641. **Greiner, A. C., Chan, S. C., and Nicolson, G. A.,** Human brain contents of calcium, copper, magnesium, and zinc in some neurological pathologies, *Clin. Chim. Acta,* 54, 211, 1975.
642. **Grider, A. and Erway, L. C.,** Intestinal metallothionein in lethal milk mice with systemic zinc deficiency, *Biochem. Genet.,* 24, 635, 1986.
643. **Gross, G., Mayr, U., Stuber, D., Westphal, W., Zacher, M., Frank, R., and Blocker, H.,** Stabilization of human interferon-beta synthesis in *E. coli* by zinc ions, *Biochim. Biophys. Acta,* 825, 207, 1985.
644. **Gross, R. L., Osdin, N., Fong, L., and Newberne, P. M.,** Depressed immunological function in zinc-deprived rats as measured by mitogen response of spleen, thymus and peripheral blood, *Am. J. Clin. Nutr.,* 32, 1260, 1979.
645. **Guigliano, R. and Millward, D. J.,** Growth and zinc homeostasis in the severely zinc deficient rat, *Br. J. Nutr.,* 52, 545, 1984.
646. **Guigliano, R. and Millward, D. J.,** The effects of severe zinc deficiency on protein turnover in muscle and thymus, *Br. J. Nutr.,* 57, 139, 1987.
647. **Guiraldes, E., Sorensen, R., Gutierrez, C., Cofre, P., and Gonzalez, B.,** Zinc sulphate for acrodermatitis enteropathica, *Lancet,* ii, 710, 1975.
648. **Guja, A.,** Gastric disorders and uropepsin level in persons subjected to zinc oxides, *Wiad. Lek.,* 26, 141, 1973.
649. **Gunn, S. A., Gould, T. C., and Anderson, W. A. D.,** The effect of growth hormone and prolactin preparations on the control by ICSH of uptake of zinc-65 by the rat dorsolateral prostate, *J. Endocrinol.,* 32, 205, 1965.
650. **Gupta, B. D.,** Hair zinc in cases of Indian childhood cirrhosis, *Indian Pediatr.,* 15, 827, 1978.
651. **Gupta, R. P., Verma, P. C., and Gupta, R. K. P.,** Experimental zinc deficiency in guinea pigs. Clinical signs and some haematological studies, *Br. J. Nutr.,* 54, 421, 1985.
652. **Gupta, R. P., Verma, P. C., and Gupta, R. K. P.,** Experimental zinc deficiency in guinea pigs: biochemical changes, *Br. J. Nutr.,* 55, 613, 1986.
653. **Gvozdanovic, S., Gvozdanovic, D., Crofton, R. W., Aggett, P. J., Mowat, N. A., and Brunt, P. W.,** Study of zinc kinetics in liver and skeleton in patients with cirrhosis, *Nucl. Med. Commun.,* 3, 127, 1982.

654. **Haarakangas, H., Hyvarinen, H., and Ojanen, M.,** Seasonal variations and the effects of nesting and moulting on liver mineral content in the house sparrow, *Passer domesticus L., Comp. Biochem. Physiol.,* 47A, 153, 1974.
655. **Haas, S., Fraker, P. J., and Luecke, R. W.,** The effect of zinc deficiency on the immune response of A/J mice, *Fed. Proc. Fed. Am. Soc. Exp. Biol.,* 35, 659, 1976.
656. **Haavikko, K., Antilla, A., Helle, A., and Pesonen, E.,** Atherosclerosis precursors in Finnish children and adolescents. XIV. Zinc and copper concentrations in deciduous teeth, *Acta Paediatr. Scand.,* S318, 213, 1985.
657. **Habib, F. K., Hammond, G. L., Lee, I. R., Dawson, J. B., Mason, M. K., Smith, P. H., and Stitch, S. R.,** Metal androgeninterrelations in carcinoma and hyperplasia of the human prostate, *J. Endocrinol.,* 71, 133, 1976.
658. **Habib, F. K., Smith, P. H., and Stitch, S. R.,** Cancer of the prostate-early diagnosis by zinc and hormone analysis, *Br. J. Cancer,* 59, 700, 1979.
659. **Hackman, M. and Hurley, L. S.,** Interactions of salicylate, dietary zinc and genetic strain on teratogenesis in rats, *Teratology,* 30, 225, 1984.
660. **Haeger, K. and Lanne, E.,** Oral zinc sulphate and ischemic leg ulcers, *J. Vasc. Dis.,* 3, 77, 1974.
661. **Haeger, K., Lanner, E., and Magnusson, P.-O.,** Oral zinc sulphate in the treatment of venous leg ulcers, in *Clinical Applications of Zinc Metabolism,* Pories, W. J., Strain, W. H., Hsu, J. M., and Woolsey, R. L., Eds., Academic Press, New York, 1974, 158.
662. **Hager, M. H.,** Zinc deficiency compromises the adrenal response to sodium deprivation in rats, *Nutr. Rep. Int.,* 34, 141, 1986.
663. **Hahn, C. and Evans, G. W.,** Identification of a low molecular weight zinc-65 complex in rat intestine, *Proc. Soc. Exp. Biol. Med.,* 144, 793, 1973.
664. **Halas, E. S.,** Behavioural changes accompanying zinc deficiency in animals, in *Neurobiology of the Trace Elements,* Vol. 1, Dreosti, I. E. and Smith, R. M., Eds., Humana Press, Clifton, N.J., 1983, 213.
665. **Halas, E. S., Hunt, C. D., and Eberhardt, M. J.,** Learning and memory disabilities in young adult rats from mildly deficient dams, *Physiol. Behav.,* 37, 451, 1986.
666. **Halevy, O. and Sklan, D.,** A low molecular weight zinc-copper lipolytic protein from chick liver, *Life Sci.,* 34, 1945, 1984.
667. **Halevy, O. and Sklan, D.,** Effect of copper and zinc depletion on vitamin A and triglyceride metabolism in chick liver, *Nutr. Rep. Int.,* 33, 723, 1986.
668. **Haley, J. V.,** Zinc sulphate and wound healing, *J. Surg. Res.,* 27, 168, 1979.
669. **Hallbook, T.,** Changes in serum zinc and copper induced by operative trauma and effects of pre- and post-operative zinc infusion, *Acta Chir. Scand.,* 144, 423, 1978.
670. **Hallbook, T. and Lanner, E.,** Serum zinc and healing of venous leg ulcers, *Lancet,* ii, 780, 1972.
671. **Hallmans, G. and Liden, S.,** Penetration of zinc-65 through the skin of rats, *Acta Derm. Venerol.,* 59, 105, 1979.
672. **Halsted, J. A., Ronghy, H. A., Abadi, P., Hagnshenass, M., Barakat, R., and Reinhold, J. G.,** Zinc deficiency in man: the Shiraz experiment, *Am. J. Med.,* 53, 277, 1972.
673. **Halsted, J. A. and Smith, J. C., Jr.,** Plasma zinc in health and disease, *Lancet,* i, 322, 1970.
674. **Halsted, J. A., Smith, J. C., Jr., and Irwin, M. I.,** A conspectus of research of zinc requirements of man, *J. Nutr.,* 104, 345, 1974.
675. **Hambidge, K. M.,** Hair analysis: worthless for vitamins, limited for minerals, *Am. J. Clin. Nutr.,* 36, 943, 1982.
676. **Hambidge, K. M.,** Trace element nutritional requirements during infancy, in *Trace Element Analytical Chemistry in Medicine and Biology,* Vol. 2, Bratter, P. and Schramel, P., Eds., Walter de Gruyter, New York, 1983, 3.
677. **Hambidge, K. M.,** Zinc deficiency in the weanling — how important?, *Acta Paediatr. Scand.,* 75(Suppl. 323), 52, 1986.
678. **Hambidge, K. M. and Droegemueller, W.,** Changes in plasma and hair concentration of zinc, copper, chromium and manganese during pregnancy, *Obstet. Gynecol.,* 44, 666, 1974.
679. **Hambidge, K. M., Hambidge, C., Jacobs, M., and Baum, J. D.,** Low levels of zinc in hair, anorexia, poor growth and hypogeusia in children, *Pediatr. Res.,* 6, 868, 1972.
680. **Hambidge, K. M., Krebs, N. F., Jacobs, M. A., Favier, A., Guyette, L., and Ikle, D. N.,** Zinc nutritional status during pregnancy: a longitudinal study, *Am. J. Clin. Nutr.,* 37, 429, 1983.
681. **Hambidge, K. M., Neldner, K. H., and Walravens, P. A.,** Zinc acrodermatitis enteropathica and congenital malformations, *Lancet,* i, 577, 1975.
682. **Hambidge, K. M., Neldner, K. H., Weston, W. L., Silverman, A., Sabol, J. L., and Brown, R. M.,** Zinc and acrodermatitis enteropathica, in *Zinc and Copper in Clinical Medicine,* Hambidge, K. M. and Nicholls, B. L., Eds., S. P. Medical and Scientific Books, Jamaica, N.Y., 1977, 81.
683. **Hambidge, K. M. and Silverman, A.,** Pica with rapid improvement after dietary zinc supplementation, *Arch. Dis. Child.,* 48, 567, 1973.

684. **Hambidge, K. M. and Walravens, P. A.,** Zinc deficiency in infants and pre-adolescent children, in *Trace Elements in Human Health and Disease,* Vol. 1, Prasad, A. S. and Oberleas, D., Eds., Academic Press, New York, 1976, 21.
685. **Hambidge, K. M., Walravens, P. A., Casey, C. E., Brown, R. M., and Bender, C.,** Plasma zinc concentrations of breast-fed infants, *J. Pediatr.*, 94, 607, 1979.
686. **Hamesmaki, E., Ylikorkala, O., and Alfthan, G.,** Concentrations of zinc and copper in pregnant problem drinkers and their newborn infants, *Br. Med. J.*, 291, 1470, 1985.
687. **Hamilton, R. M., Gillespie, C. T., and Cook, H. W.,** Relationships between levels of essential fatty acids in plasma of cystic fibrosis patients, *Lipids,* 16, 374, 1981.
688. **Handy, R. W.,** Zinc concentration in vacutainer tubes, *Clin. Chem.*, 25, 197, 1979.
689. **Hansard, S. L. and Itoh, H.,** Influence of limited dietary calcium upon zinc absorption, placental transfer and utilization by swine, *J. Nutr.*, 95, 23, 1968.
690. **Hansen, R. C., Lemen, R., and Revsin, B.,** Cystic fibrosis manifesting with acrodermatitis enteropathica-like eruption: association with essential fatty acid and zinc deficiencies, *Arch. Dermatol.*, 119, 51, 1983.
691. **Hanson, L. J., Sorenson, D. K., and Kernkamp, H. C. H.,** Essential fatty acid deficiency — its role in parakeratosis, *Am. J. Vet. Res.*, 18, 921, 1958.
692. **Harper, M. E., Danutra, V., Chanduer, J. A., and Griffiths, K.,** The effect of 2-bromo-alpha-ergocryptine (CB154) administration on the hormone levels, organ weights, prostatic morphology and zinc concentrations in the male rat, *Acta Endocrinol.*, 83, 211, 1976.
693. **Harpey, J. P., Jaudon, M.-C., Clavel, J.-P., Galli, A., and Darbois, Y.,** *Cutis laxa* and low serum zinc after antinatal exposure to penicillamine, *Lancet,* ii, 858, 1983.
694. **Harrap, G. J., Best, J. S., and Saxton, C. A.,** Human oral retention of zinc from mouthwashes containing zinc salts and its relevance to dental plaque control, *Arch. Oral Biol.*, 29, 87, 1984.
695. **Harrap, G. J., Saxton, C. A., and Best, J. S.,** Inhibition of plaque growth by zinc salts, *J. Peridontal Res.*, 18, 634, 1983.
696. **Harrison, M. F.,** Composition of the liver cell, *Biochem. J.*, 55, 203, 1953.
697. **Hartoma, I. R., Nahoul, K., and Netter, A.,** Zinc, plasma androgens and sterility, *Lancet,* ii, 1125, 1977.
698. **Hartoma, T. R., Sotaniemi, E. A., and Maatanen, J.,** Effect of zinc on some biochemical indices of metabolism, *Nutr. Metab.*, 23, 294, 1979.
699. **Hartoma, T. R., Soteniemi, E. A., Pelkonen, O., and Ahlquist, J.,** Serum zinc and serum copper and indices of drug metabolism in alcoholics, *Eur. J. Clin. Pharmacol.*, 12, 147, 1977.
700. **Haschke, F., Singer, P., Baumgartner, D., Steffan, I., Schilling, R., and Lothaller, H.,** Growth and zinc and copper nutritional status of male premature infants with different zinc intake, *Ann. Nutr. Metab.*, 29, 95, 1985.
701. **Haskins, K. M., Zombola, R. R., Boling, J. M., Lee, Y. C., and Himes, R. H.,** Tubulin assembly induced by cobalt and zinc, *Biochem. Biophys. Res. Commun.*, 95, 1703, 1980.
702. **Haxthausen, H.,** Some remarks on the bactericidal properties of zinc oxide, *Br. J. Dermatol. Syph.*, 40, 497, 1928.
703. **Heath, J. C. and Liquier-Milward, J.,** The distribution and function of zinc in normal and malignant tissues. I. Uptake and distribution of radioactive zinc, *Biochim. Biophys. Acta,* 5, 404, 1950.
704. **Heinitz, M.,** Clinical and biochemical aspects of the prophylaxis and therapy of senile cataract with zinc sulphate aspartate, *Klin. Monatsbl. Augenheilkd.*, 172, 778, 1978.
705. **Helvig, B. S. and Brady, F. O.,** Effects of glucagon, arginine vasopressin and angiotensin II on rat hepatic zinc thionein levels, *Life Sci.*, 35, 2513, 1984.
706. **Henderson, G. I., Hoyumpa, A. M., McClain, C. J., and Schenker, S.,** The effects of chronic and acute alcohol administration on fetal development in the rat, *Alcoholism: Clin. Exp. Res.*, 3, 99, 1979.
707. **Hendricks, D. G. and Mahoney, A. W.,** Glucose tolerance in zinc deficient rats, *J. Nutr.*, 102, 1079, 1972.
708. **Henkin, R. I.,** Growth hormone-dependent changes in zinc and copper metabolism in man, in *Trace Element Metabolism in Animals,* Vol. 2, Hoekstra, W. G., Suttie, J. W., Ganther, H. E., and Mertz, W., Eds., University Park Press, Baltimore, 1974, 653.
709. **Henkin, R. I.,** On the role of adrenocorticosteroids in the control of zinc and copper metabolism, in *Trace Element Metabolism in Animals,* Vol. 2, Hoekstra, W. G., Suttie, J. W., Ganther, H. E., and Mertz, W., Eds., University Park Press, Baltimore, 1974, 647.
710. **Henkin, R. I.,** New aspects in the control of food intake and appetite, *Ann. N.Y. Acad. Sci.*, 300, 321, 1977.
711. **Henkin, R. I.,** Zinc, saliva and taste: interrelationships of gustin, nerve growth factor, saliva and zinc, in *Zinc and Copper in Clinical Medicine,* Hambidge, K. M. and Nichols, B. L., Eds., S. P. Medical and Scientific Books, Jamaica, N.Y., 1977, 35.

712. **Henkin, R. I.,** Zinc dependent control of food intake, taste and smell function, in *Trace Element Metabolism in Man and Animals,* Vol. 3, Kirchgessner, M., Ed., Arbeitkreis fur Tierernahrungsforschung, Weinstephan, F. R. G., 1978, 190.
713. **Henkin, R. I.,** Zinc in taste function. A critical review, *Biol. Trace Elem. Res.,* 6, 263, 1984.
714. **Henkin, R. I. and Aamodt, R. L.,** Zinc absorption in acrouermatitis enteropathica and in hypogeusia and hyposomia, *Lancet,* i, 1379, 1975.
715. **Henkin, R. I. and Bradley, D. F.,** Hypogeusia corrected by nickel and zinc, *Life Sci.,* 9, 701, 1970.
716. **Henkin, R. I., Foster, D. M., Aamodt, R. L., and Berman, M.,** Zinc metabolism in adrenal cortical insufficiency: effects of carbohydrate active steroids, *Metabolism,* 33, 491, 1984.
717. **Henkin, R. I., Meret, S., and Jacobs, J.,** Steroid-dependent changes in copper and zinc metabolism, *J. Clin. Invest.,* 48, 38c, 1969.
718. **Henkin, R. I., Mueller, C., and Wolf, R.,** Estimation of zinc concentration of parotid saliva by flameless atomic absorption spectrophotometry in normal subjects and in patients with idiopathic hypogeusia, *J. Lab. Clin. Med.,* 86, 175, 1975.
719. **Henkin, R. I., Patten, B. M., Re, P. K., and Bronzert, D. A.,** A syndrome of acute zinc loss. Cerebellar dysfunction, mental changes, anorexia and taste and smell dysfunction, *Arch. Neurol.,* 32, 745, 1975.
720. **Henkin, R. I., Schechter, P. J., and Hoye, R.,** Idiopathic hypogeusia with dysgeusia, hyposmia and dysosmia. A new syndrome, *JAMA,* 217, 434, 1971.
721. **Henkin, R. I., Talal, I., Larson, A. L., and Mattern, C. F. T.,** Abnormalities of taste and smell in Sjogren's syndrome, *Ann. Intern. Med.,* 76, 375, 1972.
722. **Henry, R. W. and Elmes, M. E.,** Plasma zinc and acute starvation, *Br. Med. J.,* i, 625, 1975.
723. **Henzel, J. H., De Weese, M. S., and Lichti, E. L.,** Zinc concentrations within healing wounds: significance of post-operative zincuria on availability and requirements during tissue repair, *Arch. Surg.,* 349, 357, 1970.
724. **Henzel, J. H., Keitzer, F. W., Lichti, E. L., and De Weese, M.,** Efficacy of zinc medication as a therapeutic modality in atherosclerosis: follow-up observations on patients medicated over prolonged periods, *Trace Subst. Environ. Health,* 13, 336, 1971.
725. **Henzel, J. H., Lichti, E. L., Shepard, D. W., and Paone, J.,** Longterm oral zinc sulphate in the treatment of atherosclerotic peripheral vascular disease: efficacy of possible mechanisms of action, in *Clinical Aspects of Zinc Metabolism,* Pories, W. J., Strain, W. H., Hsu, J. M., and Woolsey, R. L., Eds., Academic Press, New York, 1974, 243.
726. **Herbert, V.,** The five possible causes of all nutrient deficiency: illustrated by deficiencies of vitamin B12 and folic acid, *Am. J. Clin. Nutr.,* 26, 77, 1973.
727. **Herington, A. C.,** Effect of zinc on insulin binding to rat adipocytes and hepatic membranes and to human placental membranes and IM-9 lymphocytes, *Horm. Metab. Res.,* 17, 328, 1985.
728. **Herman, Z., Greeley, S., and King, J. C.,** Placenta and maternal effects of marginal zinc deficiency during gestation in rats, *Nutr. Res.,* 5, 211, 1985.
729. **Herman, Z., Wada, L. L., and King, J. C.,** The effects of zinc intake in men on serum alkaline phosphatase and its isoenzymes, *Nutr. Rep. Int.,* 29, 1253, 1984.
730. **Herry, R. and Keil-Dlouha, V.,** Inhibition of Achomobactes collagenase by bromoacetone and by zinc ions, *FEBS Lett.,* 85, 65, 1978.
731. **Herson, V. C., Phillips, A. F., and Zimmerman, A.,** Acute zinc deficiency in a premature infant after bowel resection and intravenous alimentation, *Am. J. Dis. Child.,* 135, 968, 1981.
732. **Hesketh, J. E.,** Impaired microtubule assembly in brain from zinc deficient pigs, *Int. J. Biochem.,* 13, 921, 1981.
733. **Hesketh, J. E.,** Zinc-stimulated microtubule assembly and evidence for zinc binding to tubulin, *Int. J. Biochem.,* 14, 983, 1982.
734. **Hesketh, J. E.,** Effects of dietary zinc deficiency on Leydig cell ultrastructure in the boar, *J. Comp. Pathol.,* 92, 239, 1982.
735. **Hesketh, J. E.,** Zinc binding to tubulin, *Int. J. Biochem.,* 15, 743, 1983.
736. **Hesketh, J. E.,** Microtubule assembly in rat brain extracts. Further characterization of the effects of zinc on assembly and cold stability, *Int. J. Biochem.,* 16, 1331, 1985.
737. **Hess, F., King, J., and Margen, S.,** The effect of a low zinc intake on zinc excretion in healthy young women, *Fed. Proc. Fed. Am. Soc. Exp. Biol.,* 35, 658, 1976.
738. **Hesse, G. W.,** Chronic zinc deficiency alters neuronal functional of hippocampal mossy fibres, *Science,* 205, 1005, 1979.
739. **Hesse, G. W., Frank Hesse, K. A., and Catalanotto, F. A.,** Behavioural characteristics of rats experiencing chronic zinc deficiency, *Physiol. Behav.,* 22, 211, 1979.
740. **Hetland, O. and Brubakk, E.,** Diurnal variations in serum zinc concentrations, *Scand. J. Clin. Lab. Invest.,* 32, 225, 1973.
741. **Hew, C. L. and Penner, P. E.,** Cell-free synthesis of zinc thionein, *Can. J. Biochem.,* 57, 1030, 1979.

742. **Heyns, A. du P., Eldor, A., Yarom, D., and Marx, G.,** Zinc-induced platelet aggregation is mediated by the fibrinogen receptor and is not accompanied by release or by thromboxane synthesis, *Blood,* 66, 213, 1985.
743. **Hill, C. H. and Matrone, G.,** Chemical parameters in the study of in vivo and in vitro interaction of transition metals, *Fed. Proc. Fed. Am. Soc. Exp. Biol.,* 29, 1474, 1970.
744. **Hill, G. M., Brewer, G. J., Hogikyan, N. D., and Stellini, M. A.,** The effect of depot panteral zinc on copper metabolism in the rat, *J. Nutr.,* 114, 2283, 1984.
745. **Hill, G. M., Brewer, G. J., Juni, J. E., Prasad, A. S., and Dick, R. S.,** Treatment of Wilson's disease with zinc. II. Validation of oral copper with copper balance, *Am. J. Med. Sci.,* 292, 344, 1986.
746. **Hill, G. M., Ku, P. K., Miller, E. R., Ullrey, D. E., Losty, F. A., and O'Dell, B. L.,** A copper deficiency in neonatal pigs induced by a high zinc maternal diet, *J. Nutr.,* 113, 867, 1983.
747. **Hillstrom, L., Pettersson, L., Hellbe, L., Kjellin, A., Leczinsky, C. G., and Nordwall, C.,** Comparison of oral treatments with zinc sulphate and placebo in acne vulgaris, *Br. J. Dermatol.,* 97, 679, 1977.
748. **Hine, R. J., Karan, O. C., and Pringle, D. J.,** Zinc and copper nutriture of institutionalized mentally retarded adults before and after transfer to a group home, *Nutr. Res.,* 4, 185, 1984.
749. **Hinks, L. J., Clayton, B. E., and Lloyd, R. S.,** Zinc and copper concentrations in leucocytes and erythrocytes in healthy adults and the effect of oral contraceptives, *J. Clin. Pathol.,* 36, 1016, 1983.
750. **Hinks, L. J., Colmsee, M., and Delves, H. T.,** Determination of zinc and copper in isolated leucocytes, *Analyst,* 107, 815, 1982.
751. **Hirschberg, R., von Herrath, D., Voss, K., Bosaller, K., Mauelshagen, U., Pauls, A., and Schaefer, K.,** Parathyroid hormone and 1,25-dihydroxyvitamin D3 affect the tissue concentrations of zinc in uremic rats, *Nephron,* 39, 277, 1985.
752. **Ho, P. P. K., Walters, P., and Sullivan, H. R.,** Biosynthesis of thromboxane B_2: assay, isolation and properties of the enzyme system in human platelets, *Prostaglandins,* 12, 951, 1976.
753. **Ho, S.-Y., Catalanotto, F. A., and Dore-Duffy, P.,** Erythrocyte bound zinc in multiple sclerosis, *Neurology,* 33, 194, 1983.
754. **Ho, S.-Y., Catalanotto, F. A., Lisak, R. P., and Dore-Duffy, P.,** Zinc in multiple sclerosis. II. Correlation with disease activity and elevated plasma and membrane-bound zinc in erythrocytes from patients with multiple sclerosis, *Ann. Neurol.,* 20, 712, 1986.
755. **Hoekstra, W. G.,** Recent observations on mineral interrelationships, *Fed. Proc. Fed. Am. Soc. Exp. Biol.,* 23, 1068, 1964.
756. **Hogberg, B. and Uvnas, B.,** Further observation on the disruption of rat mesentery mast cells caused by compound 48/80, antigen-antibody reaction, lecithinase A and decylamine, *Acta Physiol. Scand.,* 48, 133, 1960.
757. **Holman, R. T.,** Essential fatty acid deficiency, *Prog. Chem. Fats Other Lipids,* 9, 275, 1966.
758. **Holman, R. T.,** Polyunsaturated fatty acid profiles in human disease, *Curr. Top. Nutr. Dis.,* 5, 25, 1981.
759. **Holmberg, C. G.,** Uricase purification and properties, *Biochem. J.,* 33, 1901, 1939.
760. **Holterman, H., Heier, A., and Bergh, H.,** Zinc in ACTH, *Lancet,* ii, 1308, 1952.
761. **Homa, S. T., Belin, J., Smith, A. D., Monro, J. A., and Zilkha, K. J.,** Levels of linoleate and arachidonate in red blood cells of healthy individuals and in patients with multiple sclerosis, *J. Neurol. Neurosurg. Psychiatr.,* 43, 106, 1980.
762. **Homan, J. D., Overbeek, G. A., Neutelings, J. P. T., Booij, C. J., and Van der Vies, J.,** Corticotrpohin zinc phosphate and hydroxide, *Lancet,* i, 541, 1954.
763. **Hooda, A., Mehta, U., and Bhat, C. M.,** Effect of different levels of dietary zinc and protein on nitrogen retention in rat, *Nutr. Rep. Int.,* 30, 1183, 1984.
764. **Hoogenraad, T. U.,** Effective treatment of Wilson's diasease with oral zinc, *Arch. Neurol.,* 39, 672, 1982.
765. **Hoogenraad, T. U.,** Luna fixata Lindemanni or the introduction of oral zinc therapy in official medicine, *Trace Elem. Med.,* 1, 47, 1984.
766. **Hoogenraad, T. U., Koevoet, R., and De Ruyter Korver, E. G. W. M.,** Oral zinc sulphate as long term treatment in Wilson's disease, *Eur. Neurol.,* 18, 205, 1979.
767. **Hoogenraad, T. U., Dekker, A. W., and Van den Hamer, C. J. A.,** Copper-responsive anemia, induced by oral zinc therapy in a patient with acrodermatitis enteropathica, *Sci. Tot. Environ.,* 42, 37, 1985.
768. **Hoogenraad, T. U. and Sindram, J. W.,** Oral zinc in primary biliary cirrhosis, *N. Engl. J. Med.,* 307, 122, 1982.
768. **Hoogenraad, T. U. and Sindram, J. W.,** Oral zinc in primary biliary cirrhosis, *N. Engl. J. Med.,* 307, 122, 1982.
769. **Hoogenraad, T. U. and Van den Hamer, C. J. A.,** Three years of continous oral therapy in four patients with Wilson's disease, *Acta Neurol. Scand.,* 67, 356, 1983.
770. **Hoogenraad, T. U., Van den Hamer, C. J. A., Koevert, R., and de Ruyter Korver, E. G. W. M.,** Oral zinc in Wilson's disease, *Lancet,* ii, 1262, 1978.
771. **Hoogenraad, T. U., Van den Hamer, C. J. A., and Van Hattum, J.,** Effective treatment of Wilson's disease with oral zinc sulphate: two case reports, *Br. Med. J.,* 289, 273, 1984.

772. **Hoogenraad, T. U., Van Hattum, J., and Van den Hamer, C. J. A.**, Management of Wilson's disease with zinc sulphate. Experience in a series of 27 patients, *J. Neurol. Sci.*, 77, 137, 1987.

773. **Hooper, P. L., Visconti, L., Garry, P. J., and Johnson, G. E.**, Zinc lowers high density lipoprotein cholesterol levels, *JAMA*, 244, 1960, 1980.

774. **Horrobin, D. F.**, *Prostaglandins: Physiology, Pharmacology and Clinical Significance*, Eden Press, Montreal, 1978.

775. **Horrobin, D. F. and Cunnane, S. C.**, Zinc, essential fatty acids and prostaglandins, *Arch. Dermatol.*, 115, 640, 1979.

776. **Horrobin, D. F. and Cunnane, S. C.**, Interactions between zinc, essential fatty acids and prostaglandins: relevance to the mechanism of acrodermatitis enteropathica, total parenteral nutrition, glucagonoma syndrome, diabetes, anorexia nervosa and sickle cell anemia, *Med. Hypoth.*, 6, 277, 1980.

777. **Horrobin, D. F. and Morgan, R. D.**, Myotonic dystrophy: a disease caused by functional zinc deficiency due to an abnormal zinc-binding ligand, *Med. Hypoth.*, 6, 375, 1980.

778. **Horrobin, D. F., Huang, Y. S., Cunnane, S. C., and Manku, M. S.**, Essential fatty acids in plasma, red blood cells and liver phospholipids in common laboratory animals as compared to humans, *Lipids*, 19, 806, 1984.

779. **Horrobin, D. F., Karmazyn, M., Manku, M. S., Karmali, R. A., Morgan, R. D., and Ally, A. I.**, Zinc acrodermatitis, acne and prostaglandins, *Br. Med. J.*, ii, 190, 1977.

780. **Horrobin, D. F., Manku, M. S., Cunnane, S. C., Karmazyn, M., Ally, A. I., Morgan, R. D., and Karmali, R. A.**, Zinc, penicillamine and prostaglandin E_1, *Arthritis Rheum.*, 21, 492, 1978.

781. **Hosokawa, S., Nishitani, H., Umemura, K., Tomoyoshi. T., Sawanishi, K., and Yoshida, O.**, Serum and corpuscular nickel and zinc in chronic hemodialysis patients, *Nephron*, 45, 151, 1987.

782. **Houle, R. E. and Grant, W. M.**, Zinc chloride, keratography and cataracts, *Am. J. Ophthalmol.*, 75, 992, 1973.

783. **Hove, E., Elvehjem, C. A., and Hart, E. B.**, The physiology of zinc in the nutrition of the rat, *Am. J. Physiol.*, 119, 768, 1937.

784. **Hove, E., Elvehjem, C. A., and Hart, E. B.**, Further studies on zinc deficiency in rats, *Am. J. Physiol.*, 124, 750, 1938.

785. **Howell, G. A., Welch, M. G., and Fredrickson, C. J.**, Stimulation induced uptake and release of zinc in hippocampal slices, *Nature (London)*, 308, 736, 1984.

786. **Howell, S. L., Tyhurst, M., Duvefelt, H., Andesson, A., and Hellerstrom, C.**, Role of zinc and calcium in the formation and storage of insulin in the pancreatic betacell, *Cell Tissue Res.*, 188, 107, 1978.

787. **Hoyer, H. and Weismann, K.**, Effect of oral zinc loading on the absorption of zinc-65 in the rat, *Arch. Dermatol. Res.*, 254, 327, 1979.

788. **Hsu, J. M.**, Zinc content in pyridoxine deficient rats, *Proc. Soc. Exp. Biol. Med.*, 119, 177, 1965.

789. **Hsu, J. M.**, Zinc as related to cysteine metabolism, in *Trace Elements in Human Health and Disease*, Prasad, A. S. and Oberleas, D., Eds., Academic Press, New York, 1976, 295.

790. **Hsu, J. M.**, The role of zinc in amino acid metabolism, in *Zinc and Copper in Clinical Medicine*, Hambidge, K. M. and Nicholls, B. L., Eds., Academic Press, New York, 1976, 295.

791. **Hsu, J. M.**, Current knowledge on zinc, copper and chromium in aging, *World Rev. Nutr. Diet.*, 33, 42, 1979.

792. **Hsu, J. M., Aniline, J. K., and Scalon, D. E.**, Pancreatic carboxypeptidase: activities in zinc deficient rats, *Science*, 153, 882, 1966.

793. **Hsu, J. M. and Anthony, W. L.**, Impairment of cysteine sulphur-35 incorporation into skin protein by zinc deficient rats, *J. Nutr.*, 101, 445, 1971.

794. **Hsu, J. M. and Anthony, W. L.**, Zinc deficiency and collagen metabolism, *Trace Subst. Environ. Health*, 6, 137, 1973.

795. **Hsu, J. M. and Anthony, W. L.**, Incorporation of glycine into skin collagen in zinc deficient rats, in *Trace Element Metabolism in Animals*, Vol. 2, Hoekstra, W. G., Suttie, J. W., Ganther, H. E., and Mertz, W., Eds., University Park Press, Baltimore, 1974, 733.

796. **Hsu, J. M. and Anthony, W. L.**, Effect of zinc deficiency on urinary excretion of nitrogenous compounds and liver amino acid catabolizing enzymes in rats, *J. Nutr.*, 105, 26, 1975.

797. **Hsu, J. M., Anthony, W. L., and Buchanan, P. J.**, Zinc deficiency and incorporation of labelled methionine into tissue protein in rats, *J. Nutr.*, 99, 425, 1969.

798. **Hsu, J. M., Kim, K. M., and Anthony, W. L.**, Biochemical and electron microscopic studies of rat skin during zinc deficiency, *Adv. Exp. Biol. Med.*, 48, 347, 1974.

799. **Huang, Y.-S., Cunnane, S. C., Horrobin, D. F., and Davignon, J.**, Most biological effects of zinc deficiency corrected by gamma-linolenic acid but not by linoleic acid, *Atherosclerosis*, 41, 193, 1982.

800. **Huang, Y.-S., Manku, M. S., Kent, E. T., Nassar, B. A., and Horrobin, D. F.**, A possible new mechanism of action of aspirin and other non-steroidal anti-inflammatory drugs (NSAID): inhibition of essential fatty acid metabolism, *Prog. Lipid Res.*, 25, 633, 1986.

801. **Huber, A. M. and Gershoff, S. N.,** Effect of zinc deficiency in rats on insulin release from the pancreas, *J. Nutr.*, 103, 1739, 1973.
802. **Huber, A. M. and Gershoff, S. N.,** Effects of zinc deficiency on the oxidation of retinol and ethanol in rats, *J. Nutr.*, 105, 1486, 1975.
803. **Hughes, M. A., Smith, G. L., and Williams, D. R.,** The binding of metal ions by captopril. I. Complexation of zinc (II), cadmium (II), and lead (II), *Inorg. Chim. Acta,* 107, 247, 1985.
804. **Hulseboch, H. J. and Ponec-Waelsch, M.,** The interaction of anthralin, salicylic acid and zinc oxide in pastes, *Dermatologica,* 144, 287, 1972.
805. **Hunt, I. F., Murphy, N. J., Cleaver, A. E., Faraji, B., Swendseid, M. E., Coulson, A. H., Clark, V. A., Laine, N., Davis, C. A., and Smith, J. C., Jr.,** Zinc supplementation during pregnancy: zinc concentration of serum and hair from low-income women of Mexican descent, *Am. J. Clin. Nutr.*, 37, 572, 1983.
806. **Hunt, I. F., Murphy, N. J., Cleaver, A. E., Faraji, B., Swendseid, M. E., Coulson, A. H., Clark, V. A., Browdy, B. L., Cabalum, M. T., and Smith, J. C., Jr.,** Zinc supplementation during pregnancy: effects on selected blood constituents and in progress and outcome of pregnancy in low-income women of Mexican descent, *Am. J. Clin. Nutr.*, 40, 508, 1984.
807. **Hunter, F. E. and Ford, L.,** Inactivation of oxidative and phosphorylative systems in mitochondria by pre-incubation with phosphate and other ions, *J. Biol. Chem.*, 216, 357, 1955.
808. **Hurd, R. W., Wilder, B. J., and Van Rinsvelt, H. A.,** Valproate, birth defects and zinc, *Lancet,* i, 181, 1985.
809. **Hurley, L. S.,** Perinatal effects of trace element deficiencies, in *Trace Elements in Human Health and Disease,* Vol. 2, Prasad, A. S. and Oberleas, D., Eds., Academic Press, New York, 1976, 301.
810. **Hurley, L. S.,** Teratogenic aspects of manganese, zinc, and copper nutrition, *Physiol. Rev.*, 61, 249, 1981.
811. **Hurley, L. S., Dreosti, I. E., and Swenerton, H.,** Studies on increased enzymes, and nucleic acid synthesis in relation to congenital malformations in zinc deficient rats, Proc. Western Hemisphere Nutr. Congr., San Juan, Puerto Rico, 1968.
812. **Hurley, L. S., Duncan, J. R., Sloan, M. V., and Eckhert, C. D.,** Zinc binding ligands in milk and intestine. A role in neonatal nutrition?, *Proc. Natl. Acad. Sci. U.S.A.*, 74, 3457, 1977.
813. **Hurley, L. S., Golub, M. S., Gershwin, M. E., and Hendrickx, A. G.,** Marginal zinc deprivation in pregnant monkeys and effects on offspring, in *Trace Element Metabolism in Man and Animals,* Vol. 5, Mills, C. F., Ed., Commonwealth Bureaux of Nutrition, Farnham, Slough, U.K., 1986, in press.
814. **Hurley, L. S. and Lonnerdal, B.,** Zinc binding in human milk: citrate versus picolinate, *Nutr. Rev.*, 40, 65, 1982.
815. **Hurley, L. S. and Shrader, R. E.,** Congenital malformations of nervous system in zinc deficient rats, in *Neurobiology of the Trace Elements Zinc and Copper,* Pfeiffer, C. C., Ed., Academic Press, New York, 1972, 7.
816. **Hurley, L. S. and Shrader, R. E.,** Abnormal development of preimplantiation rat eggs after three days of maternal dietary zinc deficiency, *Nature (London),* 254, 427, 1975.
817. **Hurley, L. S. and Swenerton, H.,** Congenital malformations resulting from zinc deficiency in rats, *Proc. Soc. Exp. Biol. Med.*, 123, 692, 1966.
818. **Hurley, L. S. and Swenerton, H.,** Lack of mobilization of bone and liver zinc under teratogenic conditions of zinc deficiency in rats, *J. Nutr.*, 101, 597, 1971.
819. **Hurley, L. S. and Tao, S.-H.,** Alleviation of teratogenic effects of zinc deficiency by simultaneous lack of calcium, *Am. J. Physiol.*, 222, 322, 1972.
820. **Husain, S. L. and Bessant, R. G.,** Oral zinc sulphate in the treatment of leg ulcers, in *Clinical Aspects of Zinc Metabolism,* Pories, W. J., Strain, W. H., Hsu, J. M., and Woolsey, R. L., Eds., Academic Press, New York, 1974, 168.
821. **Hwang, D. H., Chanmugam, P., and Wheeler, C.,** Zinc deficiency affects neither platelet arachidonic acid metabolism nor platelet aggregation in rats, *J. Nutr.*, 114, 398, 1984.
822. **Hytten, F. E.,** Do pregnant women need zinc supplements?, *Br. J. Obstet. Gynecol.*, 92, 873, 1985.
823. **Hyvarinen, H., Helle, T., Niemeinen, M., Vayrynen, P., and Vayrynen, R.,** The influence of nutrition and seasonal conditions on mineral status in the reindeer, *Can. J. Zool.*, 55, 648, 1977.
824. **Hyvarinen, H. and Valtonen, T.,** Seasonal changes in the liver mineral content of *Coregonus nasus* (Pallas), in the bay of Bothnia, *Comp. Biochem. Physiol.*, 45B, 875, 1973.
825. **Ikeda, M., Hosotani, T., Ueda, T., Kotake, Y., and Sakaibara, B.,** Observations of the concentration of zinc and iron in tissues of vitamin B_6 deficient germ-free rats, *J. Nutr. Sci. Vitaminol.*, 25, 151, 1979.
826. **Ikeda, T., Kimura, K., Morioka, S., and Tamaki, N.,** Inhibitory effects of zinc on muscle glycolysis and their reversal by histidine, *J. Nutr. Sci. Vitaminol.*, 26, 351, 1980.
827. **Ilchyshyn, A. and Mendelsohn, S.,** Zinc deficiency due to alcoholic cirrhosis mimicking acrodermatitis enteropathica, *Br. Med. J.*, 284, 1676, 1982.
828. **Innes, C.,** Affective illness and zinc deficiency, *Lancet,* i, 645, 1985.
829. **Iolascon, A. and Perrone, L.,** Erythrocyte zinc during childhood, *Acta Haematol.*, 73, 114, 1985.

830. **Iqbal, M.,** Activity of alkaline phosphatase and carbonic anhydrase in male and female zinc deficient rats, *Enzyme,* 12, 33, 1971.

831. **Ishizaka, A., Tsuchida, F., and Ishii, T.,** Clinical zinc deficiency during zinc supplemented parenteral nutrition, *J. Pediatr.*, 99, 339, 1981.

832. **Issacson, A. and Sandow, A.,** Effects of zinc on responses of skeletal muscle, *J. Gen. Physiol.*, 46, 655, 1963.

833. **Issacson, A. and Sandow, A.,** Zinc content of muscle and tendon in normal and dystrophic mouse and chicken, *Life Sci.*, 7, 369, 1968.

834. **Issell, B. F., MacFayden, B. V., Gum, E. T., Valdivieso, M., Dudrick, S. J., and Bodey, G. P.,** Serum zinc levels in lung cancer patients, *Cancer,* 47, 1845, 1981.

835. **Itoh, M. and Ebadi, M.,** The selective inhibition of hippocampal glutamic acid decarboxylase in zinc-induced epileptic seizures, *Neurochem. Res.*, 7, 1287, 1982.

836. **Iwata, I., Incefy, G. S., Tanaka, T., Fernandes, G., Menendez-Botet, C. J., Pih, K., and Good, R. A.,** Circulating thymic hormone levels in zinc deficiency, *Cell. Immunol.*, 47, 100, 1979.

837. **Jackson, A. J. and Schumacher, H. J.,** The teratogenic activity of a thalidomide analogue (EM 12) in rats on a low zinc diet, *Teratology,* 19, 341, 1979.

838. **Jackson, M. J.,** Zinc and di-iodohydroxyquinoline therapy in acrodermatitis enteropathica, *J. Clin. Pathol.*, 30, 284, 1977.

839. **Jackson, M. J. and Edwards, R. H. T.,** Zinc excretion in patients with muscular disorders, *Muscle Nerve,* 5, 661, 1982.

840. **Jackson, M. J. and Garrod, P. J.,** Plasma zinc, copper and amino acid levels in the blood of autistic children, *J. Autism Child. Schizophr.*, 8, 203, 1978.

841. **Jackson, M. J., Jones, D. A., and Edwards, R. H. T.,** Tissue zinc level as an index of body zinc status, *Clin. Physiol.*, 2, 333, 1982.

842. **Jackson, M. J., Jones, D. A., and Liliburn, M. F.,** Demonstration of zinc homeostasis in man, *J. Physiol.*, 305, 53P, 1980.

843. **Jacob, M., Chan, J. C. M., and Smith, J. C., Jr.,** Effect of prednisone on growth and zinc metabolism in rats, *Nutr. Res.*, 4, 877, 1984.

844. **Jacob, R. A., Sandstead, H. H., Solomons, N. W., Rieger, C., and Rothberg, R.,** Zinc status and vitamin A transport in cystic fibrosis, *Am. J. Clin. Nutr.*, 31, 638, 1978.

845. **Jacobs, L. S. and Lorenson, M. Y.,** Cysteamine, zinc and thiols modify detectibility of rat pituitary prolactin: a comparison with effects on bovine prolactin suggests differences in hormone storage, *Metab. Clin. Exp.*, 35, 209, 1986.

846. **Jacobs, R. A., Winter, T. W., and Sandstead, H. H.,** Mesenteric lymph proteins in zinc deficient rats, *Am. J. Physiol.*, 236, E180, 1979.

847. **Jacobson, S. G., Keeling, P. W. N., Meadows, N. J., and Thompson, R. P. H.,** The electroretinogram in cats with zinc depletion, *J. Physiol.*, 338, 37P, 1983.

848. **Jagell, S., Hallmans, G., and Gustavson, K.-H.,** Zinc and copper in serum of patients with congenital ichthyoses, spastic di- or tetraplagia and mental retardation (Sjogren-Larssen syndrome), *Upsala J. Med. Sci.*, 86, 291, 1981.

849. **Jain, V. K. and Chandra, R. K.,** Does nutritional deficiency predispose to acquired immunodeficiency syndrome?, *Nutr. Res.*, 4, 537, 1984.

850. **Jakinovich, W. and Osborn, D. W.,** Zinc nutrition and salt preference in rats, *Am. J. Physiol.*, 241, R233, 1981.

851. **Jamall, I. S., Mignand, J. E., Lynch, V. D., Bidanset, J. H., Lau-Cam, C., and Greening, M.,** Protective effects of zinc sulphate and l-lysine on acute ethanol toxicity in mice, *Environ. Res.*, 19, 112, 1979.

852. **Jameson, S.,** Effects of zinc deficiency in human reproduction, *Acta Med. Scand. Suppl.* 593, 1, 1976.

853. **Janghorbani, M. and Young, V. R.,** Stable isotopes in studies of dietary mineral bioavailability in humans with special reference to zinc, in *Clinical, Biochemical and Nutritional Aspects of Trace Elements,* Prasad, A. S., Ed., Alan R. Liss, New York, 1982, 447.

854. **Jayakumari, N., Nampoothiri, V. R., Nambisan, B., and Kurup, P. A.,** Lowering of aortic cholesterol in hypercholesterolemic rats: effect of vitamin A, ascorbic acid, protein fraction from blackgrain, bovine aortic and intestinal mucosa MPS and zinc salts, *Indian J. Exp. Biol.*, 16, 1289, 1978.

855. **Jeffery, E. H.,** The effect of zinc on NADPH oxidation and monooxygenase activity in rat hepatic microsomes, *Mol. Pharmacol.*, 23, 467, 1983.

856. **Jeffery, J., Chesters, J., Mills, C. F., Sadler, P. J., and Jornvall, H.,** Sorbitol dehydrogenase is a zinc enzyme, *EMBO J.*, 3, 357, 1984.

857. **Jensen, R., Clark, R., and Ferris, A.,** Composition of the lipids in human milk: a review, *Lipids,* 15, 345, 1980.

858. **Johnson, M. A. and Flagg, E. W.,** Effect of sucrose and corn starch on the development of copper deficiency in rats fed high levels of zinc, *Nutr. Res.*, 6, 1307, 1986.

859. **Johnson, P. E. and Evans, G. W.,** Relative zinc availability in human breast milk, infant formulae and cow's milk, *Am. J. Clin. Nutr.*, 31, 416, 1978.
860. **Johnson, R. C. and Shah, S. N.,** Effect of feeding zinc deficient diet and restricted food intake during early post-weaning period on rat brain development. Myelin and synaptosome content and lipid composition, *Biochem. Arch.*, 3, 77, 1987.
861. **Johnson, S. B. and Holman, R. T.,** Influence of reduced food intake on polyunsaturated fatty acid metabolism in zinc deficient rats, *J. Am. Oil Chem. Soc.*, 61, 679, 1984.
862. **Johnson, W. T. and Canfield, W. W.,** Intestinal absorption and excretion of zinc in streptozotocin-diabetic rats as affected by dietary zinc and protein, *J. Nutr.*, 115, 1217, 1985.
863. **Johnson, W. T. and Evans, G. W.,** Tissue uptake of zinc in rats following the administration of zinc dipicolinate or zinc histidinate, *J. Nutr.*, 112, 914, 1982.
864. **Jones, J. G., Elmes, M. E., Aggett, P. J., and Harries, J. T.,** The effect of zinc therapy on lysosomal inclusion bodies in intestinal epithelial cells in acrodermatitis enteropathica, *Pediatr. Res.*, 17, 354, 1983.
865. **Jones, K. L. and Smith, D. W.,** Recognition of the fetal alcohol syndrome in early pregnancy, *Lancet*, ii, 999, 1973.
866. **Jones, R. B., Hilton, P. J., Michael, J., Patrick, J., and Johnson, V. E.,** Zinc transport in normal human leucocytes — dependence on media composition, *Clin. Sci.*, 59, 351, 1980.
867. **Jones, R. B., Keeling, P. W. N., Hilton, P. J., and Thompson, R. P. H.,** The relationship between leucocyte and muscle zinc in health and disease, *Clin. Sci.*, 60, 237, 1981.
868. **Judd, A. M., MacLeod, R. M., and Logain, I. S.,** Zinc acutely, selectively and reversibly inhibits pituitary prolactin secretion, *Brain Res.*, 294, 190, 1984.
869. **Julius, R., Schulkind, M., Sprinkle, T., and Rennert, O.,** Acrodermatitis enteropathica with immune deficiency, *J. Pediatr.*, 83, 1007, 1973.
870. **Kabat, A. I., Niedworok, J., and Blaszczyk, J.,** Effects of zinc ions on selected osmotic characteristics of human erythrocytes *in vitro, Zentralbl. Bakteriol.*, 166, 375, 1978.
871. **Kabat, A. I., Niedworok, J., Kediora, J., Blaszczyk, J., and Bartosz, G.,** Effect of zinc ions on the oxygen affinity of hemoglobin and the level of 2,3-diphosphyglycerate in normal red cells in vitro, *Zentralbl. Bakteriol.*, 169, 436, 1979.
872. **Kahn, A. M. and Ozerman, R. S.,** Liver and serum zinc abnormalities in rats with cirrhosis, *Gastroenterology*, 53, 193, 1967.
873. **Kalinowski, J. and Chavez, E. R.,** Effect of low dietary zinc during late gestation and early lactation on the sow and neonatal piglet, *Can. J. Anim. Sci.*, 64, 749, 1984.
874. **Kampschmidt, R. F. and Pulliam, L. A.,** Effect of delayed hypersensitivity on plasma iron and zinc concentration and blood leucocytes, *Proc. Soc. Exp. Biol. Med.*, 147, 242, 1974.
875. **Kang, Y.-J., Olson, M. O. J., and Busch, H.,** Phosphorylation of acid-soluble proteins in isolated nucleoli of Novikoff hepatoma ascites cells, *J. Biol. Chem.*, 249, 5580, 1974.
876. **Kasarskis, E. J.,** Zinc metabolism in normal and zinc deficient rat brain, *Exp. Neurol.*, 85, 114, 1984.
877. **Kasarskis, E. J., Sparks, D. L., and Slevin, J. T.,** Changes in hypothalamic noradrenergic systems during the anorexia of zinc deficiency, *Biol. Trace Elem. Res.*, 9, 25, 1986.
878. **Katya-Katya, M., Ensminger, A., Mejean, L., and Debry, G.,** The effect of zinc supplementation on plasma cholesterol levels, *Nutr. Res.*, 4, 633, 1984.
879. **Kawa, K.,** Zinc-dependent action potentials in giant neurons of the snail *Enhadra quaestia, J. Membr. Biol.*, 49, 325, 1979.
880. **Kay, R. G. and Tasman-Jones, C.,** Zinc deficiency and intravenous feeding, *Lancet*, ii, 605, 1975.
881. **Kayden, H. J. and Cox, R. P.,** Evidence for normal metabolism and interconversions of unsaturated fatty acids in acrodermatitis enteropathica, *J. Pediatr.*, 83, 993, 1973.
882. **Kazimierczak, W.,** The action of the complexes of lidocain with zinc on histamine release from isolated rat mast cells, *Biochem. Pharmacol.*, 27, 243, 1978.
883. **Kazimierczak, W., Adamas, B., and Maslinski, C.,** Inhibition of anaphylctic histamine release by complexes of lidocaine with zinc, *Biochem. Pharmacol.*, 28, 2843, 1979.
884. **Kazimierczak, W., Bankowska, K., Adamas, B., and Maslinski, C.,** The inhibitory effects of complexes of lidocaine with zinc, copper and cobalt on histamine release from rat mast cells, *Agents Actions*, 9, 65, 1979.
885. **Kazimierczak, W. and Maslinski, C.,** The effect of zinc ions on selective and non-selective histamine release in vitro, *Agents Actions*, 4, 1, 1974.
886. **Keeling, P. W. N., Jones, R. B., Hilton, P. J., and Thompson, R. P. H.,** Reduced leucocyte zinc in liver disease, *Gut.*, 21, 561, 1980.
887. **Keeling, P. W. N., Ruse, W., Bull, J., Hannigan, B., and Thompson, R. P. H.,** Direct measurement of hepatointestinal extraction of zinc in cirrhosis and hepatitis, *Clin. Sci.*, 61, 441, 1981.
888. **Keen, C. L.,** Molecular localization of copper and zinc in rat fetal liver in dietary and drug-induced copper deficiency, *Biochem. Biophys. Res. Commun.*, 118, 697, 1984.
889. **Keilin, D. and Mann, T.,** Carbonic anhydrase, *Nature (London)*, 144, 442, 1939.

890. **Kelly, R. W. and Abel, M. H.,** Copper and zinc inhibit the metabolism of prostaglandins by the human uterus, *Biol. Reprod.*, 28, 883, 1983.

891. **Kelly, R., Davidson, G. P., Kownley, R. R. W., and Campbell, P. E.,** Reversible intestinal mucosal abnormalities, *Arch. Dis. Child.*, 51, 219, 1976.

892. **Kelsey, J. L. and Prather, E. S.,** Mineral balances of human subjects consuming a low fiber diet and a diet containing fruits and vegetables, *Am. J. Clin. Nutr.*, 38, 12, 1983.

893. **Kenney, M. A., Ritchey, S. J., Culley, P., Sandovak, W., Moak, S., and Schilling, P.,** Erythrocyte and dietary zinc in adolescent females, *Am. J. Clin. Nutr.*, 39, 446, 1980.

894. **Kennedy, A. C., Bessant, R. G., Davis, P., and Reynolds, P. M. G.,** The estimation of whole body zinc and zinc turnover in rheumatoid and osteoarthritis using tracer zinc, *Br. J. Nutr.*, 40, 115, 1978.

895. **Kennedy, A. C., Fell, G. S., Rooney, P. J., Stevens, W. H., Dick, W. C., and Buchanan, W. W.,** Zinc: its relationship to osteoporosis in rheumatoid arthritis, *Scand. J. Rheumatol.*, 4, 243, 1975.

896. **Kennedy, M. L. and Failla, M. L.,** Chronic obesity alters essential trace metal metabolism in C57BL/6J (ob/ob) mice, *J. Am. Coll. Nutr.*, 4, 358, 1985.

897. **Keppen, L. D., Pysher, T., and Rennert, O. M.,** Zinc deficiency acts as a co-teratogen with alcohol in fetal alcohol syndrome, *Pediatr. Res.*, 19, 944, 1985.

898. **Kfoury, G. A., Reinhold, J. G., and Simonian, S. J.,** Enzyme activities in tissues of zinc deficient rats, *J. Nutr.*, 95, 102, 1968.

899. **Khalil, M., Kabiel, A., El-Khateab, S., Aref, M., El Kozy, S., Jahnin, S., and Nasr, F.,** Plasma and red cell water and elements in protein-calorie malnutrition, *Am. J. Clin. Nutr.*, 27, 260, 1974.

900. **Khera, K. S. and Shah, B. G.,** Failure of zinc acetate to reduce ethylene thiouria-induced fetal anomalies in rats, *Toxicol. Appl. Pharmacol.*, 48, 229, 1979.

901. **Kiely, M.,** Zinc status and pregnancy outcome, *Lancet,* i, 893, 1981.

902. **Kiilerich, S. and Christiansen, C.,** Distribution of serum zinc between albumin and alpha$_2$-macroglobulin in patients with different zinc metabolic disorders, *Clin. Chim. Acta,* 154, 1, 1986.

903. **Kiilholma, P., Gronroos, M., Nanto, V., and Paul, R.,** Pregnancy and delivery in Ehlers-Danlos syndrome. Role of copper and zinc, *Acta Obstet. Gynecol. Scand.*, 63, 437, 1984.

904. **King, A., Sica, D., Chan, W., Centor, R., Chan, J., Davis, J., and Miller, G.,** Zinc absorption in uremia is vitamin-D dependent, *Am. J. Clin. Nutr.*, 41, 872, 1985.

905. **King, G. C., Martin, C. T., Pham, T. T., and Coleman, J. E.,** Transcription by T7 RNA polymerase is not zinc dependent and is abolished on amidomethylation of cysteine-347, *Biochemistry,* 25, 36, 1986.

906. **King, J. C., Raynolds, W. L., and Margen, S.,** Absorption of stable isotopes of iron, copper and zinc during oral contraceptive use, *Am. J. Clin. Nutr.*, 31, 1198, 1978.

907. **King, J. C., Stein, T., and Doyle, M.,** Effect of vegetarianism on the zinc status of pregnant women, *Am. J. Clin. Nutr.*, 34, 1049, 1981.

908. **Kinlaw, W. B., Levine, A. S., Morley, J. E., Silvis, S. E., and McClain, C. J.,** Abnormal zinc metabolism in type II diabetes mellitus, *Am. J. Med.*, 75, 273, 1983.

909. **Kirchgessner, M., Roth, H.-P., Spoerl, R., Schnegg, A., Kellner, R. J., and Weigand, E.,** A comparative view on trace elements and growth, *Nutr. Metab.*, 21, 199, 1977.

910. **Kirchgessner, M., Roth, H.-P., and Weigand, E.,** Biochemical changes in zinc deficiency, in *Trace Element Metabolism in Animals,* Vol. 2, Hoekstra, W. G., Suttie, J. W., Ganther, H. E., and Mertz, W., Eds., University Park Press, Baltimore, 1976, 189.

911. **Kirchgessner, M., Schwarz, F. J., and Schnegg, A.,** Interactions of essential metals in human physiology, in *Clinical, Biochemical and Nutritional Aspects of Trace Elements,* Prasad, A. S., Ed., Alan R. Liss, New York, 1982, 477.

912. **Klasing, K. C.,** Effect of inflammatory agents and interleukin I on iron and zinc metabolism, *Am. J. Physiol.*, 247, R901, 1984.

913. **Kleimola, V., Salmi, T. T., Andersson, A., Nanto, V., Jarnstrom, S., and Lindholm, A.,** The zinc, copper and iron status in children with chronic diseases, in *Trace Element Analytical Chemistry in Medicine and Biology,* Bratter, P. and Schramel, P., Eds., Walter de Gruyter, New York, 1983, 627.

914. **Klevay, L. M.,** Hair as a biopsy material. I. Assessment of zinc nutriture, *Am. J. Clin. Nutr.*, 23, 284, 1970.

915. **Klevay, L. M.,** Interactions amoung dietary copper, zinc and the metabolism of cholesterol and phospholipids, in *Trace Element Metabolism in Animals,* Vol. 2, Hoekstra, W. G., Suttie, J. W., Ganther, H. E., and Mertz, W., Eds., University Park Press, Baltimore, 1974, 553.

916. **Klevay, L. M.,** The ratio of zinc to copper in milk and mortality due to coronary heart disease: an association, *Trace Subst. Environ. Health,* 8, 9, 1974.

917. **Klevay, L. M.,** Coronary heart disease: the zinc/copper hypothesis, *Am. J. Clin. Nutr.*, 28, 764, 1975.

918. **Klevay, L. M. and Hyg, S. D.,** Hypercholesterolemis in rats produced by an increase in the ratio of zinc/copper ingested, *Am. J. Clin. Nutr.*, 26, 1060, 1973.

919. **Klingberg, W. G., Prasad, A. S., and Oberleas, D.,** Zinc deficiency following penicillamine therapy, in *Trace Elements in Human Health and Disease,* Vol. 1, Prasad, A. S. and Oberleas, D., Eds., Academic Press, new York, 1976, 51.
920. **Kocsis, J. J., Walaszek, E. J., Graham, C. E., and Geiling, E. M. K.,** Zinc content of various pituitary fractions, *Fed. Proc. Fed. Am. Soc. Exp. Biol.,* 12, 336, 1953.
921. **Kolaric, K., Roguljic, A., Ivankovic, G., and Vukas, D.,** Serum zinc levels in patients with malignant lymphoma, *Acta Med. Jugosl.,* 29, 331, 1975.
922. **Koletzko, B., Bretschneider, A., and Bremer, H. J.,** Fatty acid composition of plasma lipids in acrodermatitis enteropathica before and after zinc supplementation, *Eur. J. Pediatr.,* 143, 310, 1984.
923. **Koletzko, B., Abiodun, P. D., Laryea, M., and Bremer, H. J.,** Deficiency of linoleic acid metabolites in Nigerian children with protein-energy malnutrition, presented at the 13th Int. Congr. Nutrition, Brighton, 1985.
924. **Komulainen, H.,** Enhancement of 5-hydroxytryptamine uptake in rabbit hypothalamic synaptosomes but not in blood platelets by zinc and lead ex vivo, *Acta Pharmacol., Toxicol.,* 53, 166, 1983.
925. **Konczewska, Z.,** Zinc deficiency in Klinefelter's syndrome, *Pol. Tyg. Lek.,* 26, 431, 1971.
926. **Koo, S. I., Algilani, K., Norvell, J. E., and Henderson, D. A.,** Delayed plasma clearance and hepatic uptake of lymph chylomicron C-14 cholesterol in marginally zinc deficient rats, *Am. J. Clin. Nutr.,* 43, 429, 1986.
927. **Koo, S. I., Fullmer, S., and Wasserman, R. H.,** Effect of cholecalciferol and 1,25-dihydroxy cholecalciferol on the intestinal absorption of zinc in the chick, *J. Nutr.,* 110, 1813, 1980.
928. **Koo, S. I., Henderson, D. A., Algiani, K., and Norvell, J. E.,** Effect of marginal zinc deficiency on the morphological characteristics of intestinal nascent chylomicrons and distribution of soluble apoprotein of lymph chylomicrons, *Am. J. Clin. Nutr.,* 42, 671, 1985.
929. **Koo, S. I., Norvell, J. E., Algiani, K., and Chow, J.,** Effect of marginal zinc deficiency on the lymphatic absorption of C-14 cholesterol, *J. Nutr.,* 116, 2363, 1986.
930. **Koo, S. I. and Ramlet, J. S.,** Dietary cholesterol decreases the serum level of zinc: further evidence for the positive relationship between zinc and high-density lipoproteins, *Am. J. Clin. Nutr.,* 37, 918, 1983.
931. **Koo, S. I. and Ramlet, J. S.,** Effects of dietary linoleic acid on the tissue levels of zinc and copper and serum high density lipoprotein cholesterol, *Atherosclerosis,* 50, 123, 1984.
932. **Koo, S. I. and Turk, D. E.,** Effect of zinc deficiency on the ultrastructure of the pancreatic acinar cell and intestinal epithelium in the rat, *J. Nutr.,* 107, 896, 1977.
933. **Koo, S. I. and Turk, D. E.,** Effect of zinc deficiency on intestinal transport of triglyceride in the rat, *J. Nutr.,* 107, 909, 1977.
934. **Koo, S. I. and Williams, D. A.,** Relationship between the nutritional status of zinc and cholesterol concentration of serum lipoproteins in adult male rats, *Am. J. Clin. Nutr.,* 34, 2376, 1981.
935. **Kosman, D. J. and Henkin, R. I.,** Plasma and serum zinc concentration, *Lancet,* i, 1410, 1979.
936. **Kotlarek, F. and Berg, W.,** Copper and zinc in cerebrospinal fluid of children with neurological diseases, *Monatsschr., Kinderheilkd.,* 126, 718, 1978.
937. **Kowarsky, S., Blair-Stanek, C. S., and Schachter, D.,** Active transport of zinc and identification of zinc binding protein in rat jejunal mucosa, *Am. J. Physiol.,* 226, 401, 1974.
938. **Kozma, M. and Szerdahelyi, P.,** Zinc deficiency-induced trace element concentration and localization changes in the central nervous system of albino rats during post-natal development. I. Optical microscope histochemical observations, *Acta Histochem.,* 70, 54, 1982.
939. **Kramer, L. B., Osis, D., Coffey, J., and Spencer, H.,** Mineral and trace element content of vegetarian diets, *J. Am. Coll. Nutr.,* 3, 3, 1984.
940. **Kramer, T. R., Briske-Anderson, M., Johnson, S. B., and Holman, R. T.,** Influence of reduced food intake on polyunsaturated fatty acid metabolism in zinc deficient rats, *J. Nutr.,* 114, 122, 1984.
941. **Kravich, M. E., Meyer, J., and Waterhouse, J. P.,** Increased numbers of mast cells in the hyperplastic buccal mucosa of the zinc deficient rat, *J. Oral Pathol.,* 10, 22, 1981.
942. **Krebs, N. F. and Hambidge, K. M.,** Zinc requirements and zinc intakes of breast-fed infants, *Am. J. Clin. Nutr.,* 43, 288, 1986.
943. **Krebs, N. F., Hambidge, K. M., Jacobs, M. A., and Rasbach, J. O.,** The effects of a dietary zinc supplement during lactation on logitudinal changes in maternal zinc status and milk zinc concentrations, *Am. J. Clin. Nutr.,* 41, 560, 1985.
944. **Krieger, I., Alpern, B. E., and Cunnane, S. C.,** Transient neonatal zinc deficiency, *Am. J. Clin. Nutr.,* 43, 955, 1986.
945. **Krieger, I. and Evans, G. W.,** Acrodermatitis enteropathica without hypozincemia: therapeutic effect of a pancreatic preparation due to a zinc-binding ligand, *J. Pediatr.,* 96, 32, 1980.
946. **Krieger, I., Evans, G. W., and Zelkowitz, P. S.,** Zinc dependency as a cause of chronic diarrhea in variant acrodermatitis enteropathica, *Pediatrics,* 69, 773, 1982.
947. **Krischer, K. N.,** Copper and zinc in childhood behavior, *Psychopharmacol. Bull.,* 14, 58, 1978.

948. **Kroneman, J., Mey, G. J. W. V. D., and Helder, A.,** Hereditary zinc deficiency in Dutch Freisian cattle, *Zentralbl. Veterinaermed.*, 22A, 201, 1975.
949. **Krotkiewski, M., Gudmandsson, M., Backstrom, P., and Mandrouka, K.,** Zinc and muscle strength and endurance, *Acta Physiol. Scand.*, 116, 309, 1983.
950. **Kruckeberg, W. C., Bargal, R., and Brewer, G. J.,** The membrane activity of zinc: ATPase inhibition, *Prog. Clin. Biol. Res.*, 20, 135, 1978.
951. **Kruckeberg, W. C. and Brewer, G. J.,** The mechanism and control of human erythrocyte zinc uptake, *Med. Biol.*, 56, 5, 1978.
952. **Kruckeberg, W. C., Knutsen, C., and Brewer, G. J.,** Mechanisms of red cell zinc uptake with a note on zinc and red cell metabolism, in *Zinc Metabolism: Current Aspects in Health and Disease,* Prasad, A. S. and Brewer, G. J., Eds., Alan R. Liss, New York, 1977, 259.
953. **Kruis, W., Rindfleisch, G. E., and Weinzierl, M.,** Zinc deficiency as a problem in patients with Crohn's disease and fistula formation, *Hepatolgastroenterol.*, 32, 133, 1985.
954. **Kubena, K. S., Landmann, W. A., Young, C. R., and Carpenter, Z. L.,** Influence of magnesium deficiency and soy protein on magnesium and zinc status in rats, *Nutr. Res.*, 5, 317, 1985.
955. **Kumar, S. P. and Anday, E. K.,** Edema, hypoproteinemia and zinc deficiency in low birth weight infants, *Pediatrics,* 73, 327, 1984.
956. **Kumar, S., Mangal, B. D., Srivastava, D. K., Agarwal, K., and Seth, O. N.,** Plasma zinc in relation to creatinine, electrolytes and albumin in renal failure, *Indian J. Med. Res.*, 75, 417, 1982.
957. **Kumar, S. and Rao, K. S.,** Plasma and erythrocyte zinc levels in protein-calorie malnutrition, *Nutr. Res.*, 15, 364, 1973.
958. **Kumar, V. and Kapoor, A. C.,** Availability of zinc as affected by phytate, *Nutr. Rep. Int.*, 28, 103, 1983.
959. **Kuramoto, Y., Igarashi, Y., Kato, S., and Tagami, H.,** Acquired zinc deficiency in two breast-fed mature infants, *Acta Dermatol. Venereol.*, 66, 359, 1986.
960. **Kuribayashi, R.,** Effects of manganese and zinc ions on the contraction of smooth muscle of guinea pig taenia coli, Tohuku *J. Exp. Med.*, 98, 241, 1969.
961. **Kurioka, S. and Matsuda, M.,** Phospholipase C assay using *p*-nitrophenylphosphoryl-choline together with sorbitol and its application to studying the metal and detergent requirement of the enzyme, *Anal. Biochem.*, 75, 281, 1976.
962. **Kvist, U. and Bjorndahl, L.,** Zinc preserves an inherent capacity for human sperm chromatin decondensation, *Acta Physiol. Scand.*, 124, 195, 1985.
963. **Kynest, G. and Saling, E.,** Effect of oral zinc application during pregnancy, *Gynecol. Obstet. Invest.*, 21, 117, 1986.
964. **Kynest, G., Saling, E., and Wagner, N.,** The relevance of zinc determination in amniotic fluid. II. Zinc in cases of high fetal risk, *J. Pediatr. Med.*, 7, 69, 1979.
965. **Labadie, H., Verneau, A., Trinchet, J. C., and Beaugrand, M.,** Is oral zinc supplementation beneficial on the cellular immune response of patients with alcoholic cirrhosis?, *Gastroenterol. Clin. Biol.*, 10, 799, 1986.
966. **Ladefoged, K., Nicolaidou, P., and Jarnum, S.,** Calcium, phosphorus, magnesium, zinc and nitrogen balance in patients with severe short bowel syndrome, *Am. J. Clin. Nutr.*, 33, 2137, 1980.
967. **Laditan, A. O. and Ette, S. I.,** Plasma zinc and copper during the acute phase of protein-energy malnutrition (PEM) and after recovery, *Trop. Geogr. Med.*, 34, 77, 1982.
968. **Laitinen, R., Jalanko, H., Kolho, K.-L., Von Koskull, H., and Vuori, E.,** Zinc and alpha-feto-protein in amniotic fluid from early pregnancies with fetal malformations, *Am. J. Obstet. Gynecol.*, 152, 561, 1985.
969. **Laitinen, R., Siimes, A. S. I., Vuori, E., and Salmela, S. S.,** Amniotic fluid zinc in risk pregnancies, *Biol. Trace Elem. Res.*, 6, 415, 1984.
970. **Lambert, J. M., Boocock, M. R., and Coggins, J. R.,** The 3-dehydro quintate synthase activity of the pentafunctional *arom* enzyme complex of *N. crassa* is zinc dependent, *Biochem. J.*, 226, 817, 1985.
971. **Lanfranchi, G. A., Brignola, C., Campiere, M., Bazzoochi, G., and Rossi, M. S.,** Serum zinc concentration in Crohn's disease, *Dig. Dis. Sci.*, 27, 1141, 1982.
972. **Larson, D. L., Maxwell, R., and Abston, S.,** Zinc deficiency in burned children, *Plast. Reconstr. Surg.*, 46, 13, 1970.
973. **Latimer, J. S., McClain, C. J., and Sharp, H. L.,** Clinical zinc deficiency during zinc-supplemented parenteral nutrition, *J. Pediatr.*, 97, 434, 1980.
974. **Latta, D. and Liebman, M.,** Iron and zinc status of vegetarian and non-vegetarian males, *Nutr. Rep. Int.*, 30, 141, 1984.
975. **Laussac, J.-P., Haran, R., Dardenne, M., Lefrancier, P., and Binet, J.-F.,** Nuclear magnetic resonance study of the interaction of zinc with thymulin *C. R. Acad. Sci. Ser. C.*, 301, 471, 1985.
976. **Lazaris, J. A. and Bavelskyi, Z. E.,** Primary insulin insufficiency after blocking of zinc in pancreatic beta-cells, *Endocrinol. Exp.*, 15, 99, 1981.

977. **Leake, A., Chisholm, G. D., Busuttil, A., and Habib, F. K.,** Subcellular distribution of zinc in the benign and malignant human prostate. Evidence for a direct zinc-androgen interaction, *Acta Endocrinol.*, 105, 281, 1984.
978. **Leake, A., Chisholm, G. D., and Habib, F. K.,** Interaction between prolactin and zinc in the human prostate, *J. Endocrinol.*, 102, 73, 1984.
979. **Lease, J. G.,** Effect of a soluble fraction of oilseed meals on the uptake of zinc-65 from calcium-magnesium-zinc-65-phytate complexes by the chick, *J. Nutr.*, 96, 126, 1968.
980. **Lease, J. G., Barnett, B. D., Lease, E. J., and Turk, D. E.,** The biological unavailability to the chick of zinc in a sesame meal ration, *J. Nutr.*, 72, 66, 1960.
981. **Leathem, J. H.,** Gonadotrophic activity of equine gonadotrophin in combination with zinc, *Am. J. Physiol.*, 145, 28, 1945.
982. **Lee, D. and Matrone, G.,** Iron and copper effects on serum caruloplasmin activity of rats with zinc-induced copper deficiency, *Proc. Soc. Exp. Biol. med.*, 130, 1190, 1969.
983. **Lee-Chuan, C. and Cerklewski, F. L.,** Interaction between ethanol and low dietary zinc during gestation and lactation in the rat, *J. Nutr.*, 114, 2027, 1984.
984. **Leek, J. C., Volger, J. B., Gershwin, M. E., Golub, M. S., Hurley, L. S., and Hendrickx, A. G.,** Studies of marginal zinc deprivation in Rhesus monkeys. V. Fetal and infant skeletal effects, *Am. J. Clin. Nutr.*, 40, 1203, 1984.
985. **Lefevre, M., Keen, C. L., Lonnerdal, B., Hurley, L. S., and Schneeman, B. O.,** Different effects of copper and zinc deficiency on composition of plasma high-density lipoproteins in rats, *J. Nutr.*, 115, 359, 1985.
986. **Lei, K. Y., Abbasi, A., and Prasad, A. S.,** Function of the pituitary-gonadal axis in zinc deficient rats, *Am. J. Physiol.*, 230, 1730, 1976.
987. **Leitch, G. J. and Rosemond, R.,** Failure of zinc supplement to reverse teratogenic effects of in vitro alcohol, *Alcoholism: Clin. Exp. Res.*, 5, 159, 1981.
988. **Lema, O. and Sandstead, H. H.,** Zinc deficiency: effect on epiphysis growth, *Clin. Res.*, 18, 458, 1970.
989. **Lenard, H. G. and Lombeck, I.,** Treatment of Ehlers-Danlos syndrome with zinc, *Klin. Paediatr.*, 191, 578, 1979.
990. **Lennard, E., Bjornson, A. B., Petering, H., and Alexander, J.,** An immunologic and nutritional evaluation of burn neutrophil function, *J. Surg. Res.*, 16, 286, 1974.
991. **Lentz, D. and Gershwin, M. E.,** Is transient hypogammaglobulinemia of infancy a manifestation of zinc deficiency? A review, *Dev. Comp. Immunol.*, 8, 1, 1984.
992. **Leonard, A., Gerber, G. B., and Leonard, F.,** Mutagenicity, carcinogenicity and teratogenicity of zinc, *Mutat. Res.*, 168, 343, 1987.
993. **Lerman-Sagie, T., Statter, M., Szabo, G., and Lerman, P.,** Effect of valproic acid therapy on zinc metabolism in children with primary epilepsy, *Clin. Neuropharmacol.*, 10, 80, 1987.
994. **Leure-duPree, A. E.,** Vascularization of the rat cornea after prolonged zinc deficiency, *Anat. Rec.*, 216, 27, 1986.
995. **Leure-duPree, A. E. and McClain, C. J.,** Effect of severe zinc deficiency on the morphology of the rat pigment epithelium, *Invest. Ophthalmol.*, 23, 425, 1982.
996. **Leure-duPree, A. E., Rothman, R. J., and Fosmire, G. J.,** Effect of zinc deficiency on the ultrastructure of the rat adrenal cortex, *Am. J. Anat.*, 165, 295, 1982.
997. **Levine, A. S., McClain, C. J., Handwerger, B. S., Brown, D. M., and Morley, J. E.,** Tissue zinc status of genetically diabetic and streptozotocin-induced diabetic mice, *Am. J. Clin. Nutr.*, 36, 382, 1983.
998. **Levine, J. B., Aamodt, R. L., Tschudy, P., and Henkin, R. I.,** Histidine-mediated decreases in total body zinc and in urinary porphyrins and porphyria, *J. Clin. Invest.*, 52, 52A, 1973.
999. **Lewis, P. K., Hoekstra, W. G., Grummer, R. H., and Phillips, P. H.,** Effect of certain nutritional factors including calcium, phosphorus, and zinc on parakeratosis in swine, *J. Anim. Sci.*, 15, 741, 1956.
1000. **Lewis-Jones, M. S., Evans, S., and Culshaw, M. A.,** Cutaneous manifestations of zinc deficiency during treatment with anticonvulsants, *Br. Med. J.*, i, 603, 1985.
1001. **Li, E. T. S. and O'Dell, B. L.,** Prostaglandin $F_{2\alpha}$ binding to ovarian membranes of zinc deficient pregnant rats, *Fed. Proc. Fed. Am. Soc. Exp. Biol.*, 44, 768, 1985.
1002. **Lifschitz, M. D. and Henkin, R. I.,** Circadian variation in copper and zinc in man, *J. Appl. Physiol.*, 31, 88, 1971.
1003. **Lindeman, R. D., Clark, M. L., and Colmore, J. P.,** Influence of age and sex on plasma and red cell zinc concentrations, *J. Gerontol.*, 26, 358, 1971.
1004. **Lindeman, R. D., Yunice, A. A., and Baxter, D. J.,** Zinc metabolism in acute myocardial infarction, in *Trace Elements in Human Health and Disease,* Vol. 1, Prasad, A. S. and Oberleas, D., Eds., Academic Press, New York, 1976, 143.
1005. **Lindeman, R. D., Yunice, A. A., Baxter, D. J., Miller, L. R., and Nordquist, J.,** Myocardial zinc metabolism in experimental myocardial infarction, *J. Lab. Clin. Med.*, 81, 194, 1973.
1006. **Liptrap, D. O.,** Sex influence on the zinc requirement of developing swine, *J. Anim. Sci.*, 30, 736, 1970.

1007. **Little, C. and Otnass, A.,** The metal ion dependence of phospholipase C from *Bacillis cereus, Biochim. Biophys. Acta,* 391, 326, 1975.

1008. **Lockett, C. J., Reyes, A. J., Leary, W. P., Alcocer, L., and Olhaberry, J. V.,** Zinc angiotensin-I-converting enzyme and hypertension, *S. Afr. Med. J.,* 64, 1022, 1983.

1009. **Lockitch, G., Pendray, M. R., Godolphin, W. J., and Quigley, G.,** Serial changes in selected serum constituents in low birth weight infants on peripheral parenteral nutrition with different zinc and copper supplements, *Am. J. Clin. Nutr.,* 42, 24, 1985.

1010. **Logan, I. S., Thorner, M. O., and Maclead, R. M.,** Zinc may have a physiological role in regulating pituitary prolactin secretion, *Neuroendocrinology,* 37, 317, 1983.

1011. **Lombeck, I., Schnippering, H. G., Kasperek, K., Ritzl, F., Kastner, H., Feinendegen, L. E., and Bremer, H. J.,** Akrodermatitis enteropathica. Zinkstoffwechselstorung mit Zink malabsorption, *Z. Kinderheilk.,* 120, 181, 1975.

1012. **Lombeck, I., Schnippering, H. G., Ritzl, F., Feinendegen, L. E., and Bremer, H. J.,** Absorption of zinc in acrodermatitis enteropathica, *Lancet,* i, 855, 1975.

1013. **Lomeo, F., Khokher, M. A., and Dandona, P.,** Dihomo-gamma-linolenic acid and linolenic acid potentiate the stimulatory effect of insulin on adipocyte lipogenesis, *Prog. Lipid Res.,* 25, 511, 1986.

1014. **Londesborough, J.,** The high Km cyclic AMP phosphodiesterase of baker's yeast is a zinc metalloenzyme, *Biochem. Soc. Trans.* 6, 1218, 1978.

1015. **Lonnerdal, B., Cederblad, A., Davidsson, L., and Sandstrom, B. M.,** The effect of individual components of soy formulae and cow's milk formulae on zinc bioavailability, *Am. J. Clin. Nutr.,* 40, 1964, 1984.

1016. **Lonnerdal, B., Hoffman, B., and Hurley, L. S.,** Zinc and copper binding proteins of human milk, *Am. J. Clin. Nutr.,* 36, 1170, 1982.

1017. **Lonnerdal, B., Keen, C. L., Sloan, M. V., and Hurley, L. S.,** Molecular localization of zinc in rat milk and neonatal intestine, *J. Nutr.,* 110, 2414, 1980.

1018. **Love, A. H. G., Elmes, M., Golden, M. K., and McMaster, D.,** Zinc deficiency and coeliac disease, in *Trace Element Metabolism in Man and Animals,* Vol. 3, Kirchgessner, M., Ed., Arbeitskreis fur tierernahrungsforschung, Weinstephan, F. R. G., 1977, 357.

1019. **Low, W. I. and Ikram, H.,** Plasma zinc in acute myocardial infarction, *Br. Heart J.,* 38, 1339, 1976.

1020. **Lowry, S. F., Goodgame, J. T., Smith, J. C., Jr., Mahar, M. M., Makuch, R. W., Henkin, R. I., and Brennan, M. F.,** Abnormalities of zinc and copper during total parenteral nutrition, *Ann. Surg.,* 189, 120, 1979.

1021. **Lucis, O. J., Lucis, R., and Shaikh, Z. A.,** Cadmium and zinc in pregnancy and lactation, *Arch. Environ. Health,* 25, 14, 1972.

1022. **Ludwig, J. C. and Chvapil, M.,** Effects of metal ions on lysosomes, in *Trace Elements in the Pathogenesis and Treatment of Inflammation,* Rainsford, K. D., Brune, K., and Whitehouse, M. W., Eds., Birkhausen Verlag, Basel, 1981, 65.

1023. **Ludwig, J. C., Misiorowski, R. L., Chvapil, M., and Seymour, M. D.,** Interaction of zinc ions with electron carrying coenzymes NADPH and NADH, *Chem. Biol. Interact.,* 30, 25, 1980.

1024. **Ludvigsen, C., McDaniel, M., and Lacy, P. E.,** The mechanism of zinc uptake in isolated islets of Langerhans, *Diabetes,* 28, 570, 1979.

1025. **Luecke, R. W.,** Domestic animals in the elucidation of zinc's role in nutrition, *Fed. Proc. Fed. Am. Soc. Exp. Biol.,* 43, 2823, 1984.

1026. **Luecke, R. W., Baltzer, B. V., and Whitenack, D. L.,** The effect of supplementary lysosome on zinc deficiency in the rat, in *Trace Element Metabolism in Animals,* Vol. 2, Hoekstra, W. G., Suttie, J. W., Ganther, H. E., and Mertz, W., Eds., University Park Press, Baltimore, 1974, 739.

1027. **Luecke, R. W., Hoefer, J. A., Brammell, W. S., and Schmidt, D. A.,** Calcium and zinc in parakeratosis of swine, *J. Anim. Sci.,* 16, 3, 1957.

1028. **Lui, E. M. K., Gauther, T., and Cherian, M. G.,** Effects of dexamethasone injection on body retention and hepatic distribution of zinc, cadmium and metallothionein in newborn rats, *Toxicology,* 41, 267, 1986.

1029. **Lukaski, H. C., Bolonchuk, W. W., Klevay, L. M., Milne, D. B., and Sandstead, H. H.,** Changes in plasma zinc content after exercise in men fed a low zinc diet, *Am. J. Physiol.,* 247, E88, 1984.

1030. **Lutz, R. E.,** The normal occurrence of zinc in biological materials: a review of the literature and a study of the normal distribution of zinc in the rat, cat and man, *J. Ind. Hyg.,* 8, 177, 1926.

1031. **Macalpinlac, M. P., Pearson, W. N., Barney, G. H., and Darby, W. J.,** Protein and nucleic acid metabolism in the testes of zinc deficient rats, *J. Nutr.,* 95, 569, 1968.

1032. **Macalpinlac, M. P., Pearson, W. N., and Darby, W. J.,** Some characteristics of zinc deficiency in the albino rat, in *Zinc Metabolism,* Prasad, A. S., Ed., Charles C. Thomas, Springfield, Ill., 1966, 142.

1033. **MacDonald, L. D., Gibson, R. S., and Miles, J. E.,** Changes in hair zinc and copper concentrations of breast-fed and bottle-fed infants during the first six months, *Acta Paediatr. Scand.,* 71, 785, 1982.

1034. **MacLean, W. C.,** Plasma zinc concentration of formula-fed infants, *Am. J. Clin. Nutr.,* 40, 1304, 1984.

1035. **Madding, C. I., Jacob, M., Ramsay, V. P., and Sokol, R. Z.,** Serum and semen zinc levels in normospermic and oligospermic men, *Ann. Nutr. Metab.*, 30, 213, 1986.

1036. **MAFF,** Ministry of Agriculture, Foods and Fisheries, Food Surveillance Paper no. 5, Survey of Copper and Zinc in Food, Her Majesty's Stationery Office, 1981, 10.

1037. **Magee, A. C. and Matrone, G.,** Studies on growth, copper metabolism and iron metabolism of rats fed high levels of zinc, *J. Nutr.*, 72, 233, 1960.

1038. **Magee, W. L., Gallai-Hatchard, J., Sanders, H., and Thompson, R. H. S.,** The purification and properties of phospholipase A from human pancreas, *Biochem. J.*, 83, 17, 1962.

1039. **Mahajan, S. K., Hamburger, R. J., Flamenbaum, W., Prasad, A. S., and McDonald, F. D.,** Effect of zinc supplementation on hyperprolactinemia in uremic men, *Lancet*, ii, 750, 1985.

1040. **Mahajan, S. K., Prasad, A. S., and McDonald, F. D.,** Sexual dysfunction in uremic males: improvement following oral zinc supplementation, *Contrib. Nephrol.*, 38, 103, 1984.

1041. **Mahajan, S. K., Prasad, A. S., Rabbini, P., Briggs, W. A., and McDonald, F. D.,** Zinc deficiency in uremia, *Clin. Res.*, 27, 226A, 1979.

1042. **Mahajan, S. K., Prasad, A. S., Rabbini, P., Briggs, W. A., and McDonald, F. D.,** Zinc deficiency: a reversible complication of uremia, *Am. J. Clin. Nutr.*, 36, 1177, 1982.

1043. **Main, A. N. H., Hall, M. J., Russell, M. I., Fell, G. S., Mills, P. R., and Shenkin, A.,** Clinical experience of zinc supplementation during intravenous nutrition in Crohn's disease: value of serum and urine zinc measurements, *Gut*, 23, 984, 1982.

1044. **Majumdar, S. K., Shaw, G. K., and Thomson, A. D.,** Serum zinc, magnesium and calcium status in the Wernicke-Korsakoff syndrome, *Drug Alcohol Dependence*, 12, 403, 1983.

1045. **Makino, T.,** A potential problem on comparison of plasma with serum zinc concentration, *Clin. Chem.*, 29, 1313, 1983.

1046. **Malette, L. E. and Henkin, R. I.,** Altered copper and zinc metabolism in primary hyperparathyroidism, *Am. J. Med. Sci.*, 272, 167, 1976.

1047. **Mankad, V. N., Ronnlund, R. D., and Suskind, R. M.,** Increased immune function in sickle cell disease patients after zinc therapy, *Pediatr. Res.*, 17, 237A, 1982.

1048. **Manku, M. S., Horrobin, D. F., Karmazyn, M., and Cunnane, S. C.,** Prolactin and zinc effects on rat vascular reactivity: possible relationship to dihomo-gamma-linolenic acid and to prostaglandin synthesis, *Endocrinology*, 104, 774, 1979.

1049. **Manku, M. S., Horrobin, D. F., Morse, N., Wright, S., and Burton, J. L.,** Essential fatty acids in the plasma phospholipids of patients with atopic eczema, *Br. J. Dermatol.*, 110, 643, 1984.

1050. **Manku, M. S., Horrobin, D. F., Seidah, N., and Chretien, M.,** Beta-endorphin at physiological concentrations blocks prolactin and zinc-induced synthesis of a prostaglandin E_1 like substance, presented at the Int. Conf. Central Nervous System Effects of Hypothalamic Hormones and Other Peptides, Montreal, 1978.

1051. **Mann, S. O., Fell, B. F., and Dalgarno, A. L.,** Observations on the bacterial flora and pathology of the tongue of sheep deficient in zinc, *Res. Vet. Sci.*, 17, 91, 1974.

1052. **Mansouri, K., Halsted, J. A., and Gombos, E. A.,** Zinc, copper magnesium and calcium in dialysed and non-dialysed uremic patients, *Arch. Intern. Med.*, 125, 88, 1970.

1053. **Mapes, C. A., Bailey, P. T., Matson, C. F., Hauer, E. C., and Sobocinski, P. Z.,** In vitro and in vivo actions of zinc ion affecting cellular substances which influence host metabolic responses to inflammation, *J. Cell Physiol.*, 95, 115, 1978.

1054. **Margraf, H. W. and Covey, T. H.,** A trial of a silver-zinc allantoinate in the treatment of leg ulcers, *Arch. Surg.*, 112, 699, 1977.

1055. **Markowitz, M. E., Rosen, J. F., and Mizruchi, M.,** Circadian variations in serum zinc concentrations: correlation with blood ionized calcium, serum total calcium and phosphate in humans, *Am. J. Clin. Nutr.*, 41, 689, 1985.

1056. **Marks, R., Pearse, A. D., and Walker, A. P.,** The effects of a shampoo containing zinc pyrithione on the control of dandruff, *Br. J. Dermatol.*, 112, 415, 1985.

1057. **Marmar, J. L., Katz, S., Praiss, D. E., and Debendictis, T. J.,** Semen zinc levels in infertile and post-vasectomy patients with prostatitis, *Fertil. Steril.*, 26, 1057, 1975.

1058. **Marone, G., Columbo, M., De Paulis, A., Cirillo, R., Giugliano, R., and Condorelli, M.,** Physiological concentrations of zinc inhibit the release of histamine from human basophils and lung mast cells, *Agents Actions*, 18, 103, 1986.

1059. **Marone, G., Findlay, S. R., and Lichtenstein, L. M.,** Modulation of histamine release from human basophils in vitro by physiological concentrations of zinc, *J. Pharmacol. Exp. Ther.*, 217, 292, 1981.

1060. **Martin, C., Wallum, B., Krom, B., Hall, L., and Gerich, J.,** Effect of a zinc phosphate suspension of a long-acting somatostatin analogue on postprandial plasma glucose, triglyceride and glucagon concentrations in alloxan-diabetic dogs, *Life Sci.*, 35, 2627, 1984.

1061. **Martinez-Escalera, G., Clapp, C., Morales, M. T., Lorensen, M. Y., and Mena, F.,** Reversal by thiols of dopamine-, stalk median eminence- and zinc-induced inhibition of prolactin transformation in adenohypophysis of lactating rats, *Endocrinology,* 118, 1803, 1986.
1062. **Mashimo, H. and Washio, H.,** The effect of zinc on the electrical properties of membranes and the twitch tension in frog muscle fibres, *Jpn. J. Physiol.,* 14, 538, 1964.
1063. **Masters, D. G., Keen, C. L., Lonnerdal, B., and Hurley, L. S.,** Release of zinc from maternal tissues during zinc deficiency or simultaneous zinc and calcium deficiency in the pregnant rat, *J. Nutr.,* 116, 2148, 1986.
1064. **Mateo, M. C. M., Bustamente, J. B., and Cantalapiedra, M. A. G. I.,** Serum zinc, copper and insulin in diabetes mellitus, *Biomedicine,* 29, 56, 1978.
1065. **Mateo, M. C. M., Bustaments, J. B., De Quiros, J. F. B., and Manchado, O. O.,** A study of metabolism of zinc and its metalloenzymes in diabetes mellitus, *Biomedicine,* 23, 134, 1975.
1066. **Mathur, N. K. and Bumb, R. A.,** Oral zinc in the trophic ulsers of leprosy, *Int. J. Leprosy,* 51, 410, 1983.
1067. **Mathur, N. K., Bumb, R. A., Mangal, H. N., and Sharma, M. L.,** Oral zinc as an adjunct to Dapsone in lepromatous leprosy, *Int. J. Leprosy,* 52, 331, 1984.
1068. **Matin, M. A., Sylvester, P. E., Edwards, D., and Dickerson, J. W. T.,** Vitamins and zinc status in Down's syndrome, *J. Ment. Defic. Res.,* 25, 121, 1981.
1069. **Matesesche, J. W., Phillips, S. F., Malagelada, J.-R., and McCall, J. T.,** Recovery of dietary iron and zinc from the proximal intestine of healthy man. Studies of different meals and supplements, *Am. J. Clin. Nutr.,* 33, 1946, 1980.
1070. **Matustik, M. C., Chausmer, A. B., and Meyer, W. J.,** The effect of sodium intake on zinc excretion in patients with sickle cell anemia, *J. Am. Coll. Nutr.,* 1, 331, 1982.
1071. **Mauras, Y. and Allan, P.,** Inhibition of delta-aminolevulinic acid dehydratase in human red blood cells by lead and activation by zinc or cysteine, *Enzyme,* 24, 181, 1979.
1072. **Mawson, C. A. and Fisher, M. I.,** Zinc and carbonic anhydrase in human semen, *Biochem. J.,* 55, 696, 1953.
1073. **May, J. M. and Contoreggi, C. S.,** The mechanism of the insulin-like effect of ionic zinc, *J. Biol. Chem.,* 257, 4362, 1982.
1074. **Mayer, J.,** Zinc deficiency: a cause of growth retardation?, *Postgrad. med.,* 35, 206, 1964.
1075. **Maze, P.,** Influences respectives des elements de la solution mineral et sur le development di mais, *Ann. Inst. Pasteur Paris,* 28, 21, 1914.
1076. **McBean, L. D., Dove, J. T., Halsted, J. A., and Smith, J. C., Jr.,** Zinc concentrations in human tissues, *Am. J. Clin. Nutr.,* 25, 672, 1972.
1077. **McBean, L. D., Mahloudji, M., Reinhold, J. G., and Halsted, J. A.,** Correlation of zinc concentrations in human plasma and hair, *Am. J. Clin. Nutr.,* 24, 506, 1971.
1078. **McBean, L. D., Smith, J. C., Jr., Berne, B. H., and Halstad, J. A.,** Serum zinc and alpha$_2$-macroglobulin concentration in myocardial infarction, multiple myeloma, decubitis ulcer, prostatic carcinoma, Down's syndrome and nephrotic syndrome, *Clin. Chim. Acta,* 50, 43, 1974.
1079. **McCall, J. T., McLennan, K. G., Goldstein, M., and Randall, R. V.,** Copper and zinc homeostasis during chelation therapy, *Trace Subst. Environ. Health,* 2, 127, 1969.
1080. **McCance, R. A. and Widdowson, E. M.,** The absorption and excretion of zinc, *Biochem. J.,* 36, 692, 1942.
1081. **McClain, C. J.,** Zinc metaboism in malabsorption syndromes, *J. Am. Coll. Nutr.,* 4, 49, 1985.
1082. **McClain, C. J., Gavaler, J. S., and Van Thiel, D. H.,** Hypogonadism in the zinc deficient rat: localization of the functional abnormalities, *J. Lab. Clin. Med.,* 104, 1007, 1984.
1083. **McClain, C. J., Soutor, C., Steele, N., Levine, A. S., and Silvis, S. E.,** Severe zinc deficiency presenting with acroderatitia enteropathica during hyperalimentation: diagnosis, pathogenesis and treatment, *J. Clin. Gastroenterol.,* 2, 125, 1980.
1084. **McClain, C. J., Soutor, C., and Zieve, L.,** Zinc deficiency: a complication of Crohn's disease, *Gastroenterology,* 78, 272, 1980.
1085. **McClain, C. J. and Su, L.-C.,** Zinc deficiency in the alcoholic: a review, *Alcoholism: Clin. Exp. Res.,* 7, 5, 1983.
1086. **McClain, C. J., Van Thiel, D. H., Parker, S., Badzin, L. K., and Gilbert, H.,** Alterations in zinc, vitamin A and retinol-binding protein in chronic alcoholics: a possible mechanism for night blindness and hypogonadism, *Alcoholism: Clin. Exp. Res.,* 3, 135, 1979.
1087. **McClain, P. E., Wiley, E. R., Beecher, G. R., Anthony, W. L., and Hsu, J. M.,** Influence of zinc deficiency on synthesis and cross-linking of rat skin collagens, *Biochim. Biophys. Acta,* 304, 457, 1973.
1088. **McConnell, R. J., Blair-Stanek, C. S., and Rivlin, R. S.,** Decreased intestinal transport of zinc in hypothyroidism, *Clin. Res.,* 25, 658A, 1977.
1089. **McConnell, S. D. and Henkin, R. I.,** Altered preference of sodium chloride, anorexia and changes in plasma and urinary zinc in rats fed a zinc deficient diet, *J. Nutr.,* 104, 1108, 1974.

1090. **McCormick, D. B., Gregory, M. E., and Snell, E. E.,** Pyridoxal phosphokinases. I. Assay, distribution, purification and properties, *J. Biol. Chem.*, 236, 2076, 1961.

1091. **McCormick, D. B. and Snell, E. E.,** Pyridoxal kinase of human brain and its inhibition by hydrazine derivatives, *Proc. Natl. Acad. Sci. U.S.A.*, 45, 1371, 1959.

1092. **McKenzie, J. M.,** Content of zinc in serum, urine, hair and toe nails of New Zealand adults, *Am. J. Clin. Nutr.*, 32, 570, 1979.

1093. **McKenzie, J. M., Fosmire, G. J., and Sandstead, H. H.,** Zinc deficiency during the latter third of pregnancy: effects on fetal rat brain, liver, and placenta, *J. Nutr.*, 105, 1466, 1975.

1094. **McKenzie, J. M. and Kay, D. L.,** Urinary excretion of cadmium, zinc and copper in normotensive and hypertensive women, *N. Z. J. Med.*, 78, 68, 1973.

1095. **McMahon, R. A., Parker, M. L. M., and McKinnon, M. C.,** Zinc treatment in malabsorption, *Med. J. Aust.*, 2, 210, 1968.

1096. **McMichael, A. J., Dreosti, I. E., Gibson, G. T., Hartshorne, J. M., Buckley, R. A., and Colley, D. P.,** A prospective study of serial maternal serum zinc levels and pregnancy outcome, *Early Hum. Dev.*, 7, 59, 1982.

1097. **McMillan, E. M. and Rowe, D.,** Plasma zinc in psoriasis. Relation to surface area involvement, *Br. J. Dermatol.*, 108, 301, 1983.

1098. **McQuitty, J. T., De Wys, W. D., Monaco, L., Strain, W. H., Rob, C. G., Apgar, J., and Pories, W. J.,** Inhibition of tumor growth by dietary zinc deficiency, *Cancer Res.*, 30, 1387, 1970.

1099. **Meadows, N. J., Grainger, S. L., Ruse, W., Keeling, P. W. N., and Thompson, R. P. H.,** Oral iron and the bioavailability of zinc, *Br. Med. J.*, 287, 1013, 1983.

1100. **Meadows, N. J., Ruse, W., Keeling, P. W. N., Scopes, J. W., and Thompson, R. P. H.,** Peripheral blood leucocyte zinc depletion in babies with intrauterine growth retardation, *Arch. Dis. Child.*, 58, 807, 1984.

1101. **Meadows, N. J., Smith, M. J., Keeling, P. W. N., Ruse, W., Day, J., Scopes, J. W., Thompson, R. P. H., and Bloxam, D. L.,** Zinc and small babies, *Lancet*, ii, 1135, 1981.

1102. **McWilliams, P. L., Agarwal R. P., and Henkin, R. I.,** Zinc concentration in erythrocyte membranes in normal volunteers and in patients with taste and smell dysfunction, *Biol. Trace Elem. Res.*, 5, 1, 1983.

1103. **Medeiros, D. M. and Brown, B. J.,** Blood pressure in young adults as influenced by copper and zinc intake, *Biol. Trace Elem. Res.*, 5, 165, 1983.

1104. **Medeiros, D. M., Brown, B. J., and Pellum, L. K.,** Blood pressure in young adult normotensives as associated with anthropometrics and copper and zinc status, *Fed. Proc. Fed. Am. Soc. Exp. Biol.*, 42, 817, 1983.

1105. **Medeiros, D. M. and Pellum, L. K.,** Elevation of cadmium, lead and zinc in the hair of adult black female hypertensives, *Bull. Environ. Contam. Toxicol.*, 32, 525, 1984.

1106. **Meftah, S. P., Prasad, A. S., Dumouchelle, E., Cossack, Z. T., and Rabbini, P.,** Testicular androgen binding protein in zinc deficient rats, *Nutr. Res.*, 4, 437, 1984.

1107. **Mellow, M. H., Layne, E. A., Lipton, T. O., Kaushik, M., Hoestetler, C., and Smith, J. C., Jr.,** Plasma zinc and vitamin A in human squamous carcinoma of the esophagus, *Cancer*, 51, 1615, 1983.

1108. **Menard, M. P. and Cousins, R. J.,** Zinc transport by brush border membrane vesicles from rat intestine, *J. Nutr.*, 113, 1434, 1983.

1109. **Mendelson, R. A., Anderson, G. H., and Bryan, M. H.,** Zinc, copper and iron content of milk from mothers of preterm and fullterm infants, *Early Hum. Dev.*, 6, 145, 1982.

1110. **Mendelson, R. A., Bryan, M. H., and Anderson, G. H.,** Trace mineral balances in preterm infants fed their own mother's milk, *J. Pediatr. Gastroenterol. Nutr.*, 2, 256, 1983.

1111. **Mendelson, R. A. and Huber, A. M.,** The effect of ethanol consumption on trace elements in the fetal rat, in *Currents in Alcoholism*, Vol. 7, Galanter, M., Ed., Grune & Stratton, New York, 1980, 39.

1112. **Mercalli, M. E., Seri, S., and Aquilio, E.,** Zinc deficiency and thymus ultrastructure in rats, *Nutr. Res.*, 4, 665, 1984.

1113. **Merchant, H. W., Gangarosa, L. P., Glassman, A. B., and Sobel, R. E.,** Zinc sulphate supplementation for treatment of recurring oral ulcers, *S. Afr. Med. J.*, 70, 559, 1977.

1114. **Mertz, W.,** The effects of zinc in man: nutritional considerations, in *Clinical Applications of Zinc Metabolism*, Pories, W. J., Strain, W. H., Hsu, J. M., and Woolesy, R. L., Eds., Charles C. Thomas, Springfield, Ill., 1974.

1115. **Messing, B., Poitras, P., and Bernier, J. J.,** Zinc deficiency in total parenteral nutrition, *Lancet*, ii, 97, 1977.

1116. **Meves, H.,** The effect of zinc on the late displacement current in squid giant axons, *J. Physiol.*, 254, 787, 1976.

1117. **Meydani, S. N. and Dupont, J.,** Effect of zinc deficiency on prostaglandin synthesis in different organs of the rat, *J. Nutr.*, 112, 1098, 1982.

1118. **Meydani, S. N., Meydani, M., and Dupont, J.,** Effects of prostaglandin modifiers and zinc deficiency on possibly related functions in rats, *J. Nutr.*, 113, 494, 1983.

1119. **Michael, J., Hilton, P. J., and Jones, N. F.**, Zinc and the sodium pump in uremia, *Am. J. Clin. Nutr.*, 31, 1945, 1978.
1120. **Michaelsson, G.**, Zinc — a new and successful therapy for acrodermatitis enteropathica, *Lakartidingen*, 71, 1959, 1974.
1121. **Michaelsson, G., Juhlin, L., and Valquist, A.**, Effects of oral zinc and vitamin A in acne, *Arch Dermatol.*, 113, 31, 1977.
1122. **Michaelsson, G., Valquist, A., and Lennart, J.**, Serum zinc and retinol-binding protein in acne, *Br. J. Dermatol.*, 96, 283, 1977.
1123. **Mikac-Devic, D.**, Methodology of zinc determinations and the role of zinc in biochemical processes, in *Advances in Clinical Chemistry*, Vol. 13, Bodansky, O. and Stewart, S. P., Eds., Academic Press, New York, 1970, 271.
1124. **Millar, M. J., Elcoate, P. V., and Mawson, C. A.**, Sex hormone control of the zinc content of the prostate, *Can. J. Biochem. Physiol.*, 35, 865, 1957.
1125. **Miller, E. R., Luecke, R. W., Ullrey, D. E., Baltzer, B. V., Bradley, B. L., and Hoefer, J. A.**, Biochemical, skeletal and allometric changes due to zinc deficiency in the baby pig, *J. Nutr.*, 95, 278, 1968.
1126. **Miller, J., McLaughlin, A. D., and Klug, A.**, Repetitive zinc-binding domains in the protein transcription factor IIIA from *Xenopus* oocytes, *EMBO J.*, 4, 1609, 1985.
1127. **Miller, S. I., Villano, B. C. D., Flynn, A., and Krumhansl, M.**, Interaction of alcohol and zinc in fetal dysmorphogenesis, *Pharmacol. Biochem. Behav.*, 18(Suppl 1), 311, 1983.
1128. **Miller, W. J.**, Absorption, tissue distribution, endogenous excretion and homeostatic control of zinc in ruminants, *Am. J. Clin. Nutr.*, 22, 1323, 1969.
1129. **Mills, B. J., Broghamer, W. L., Higgins, P. J., and Lindeman, R. D.**, Inhibition of tumor growth by zinc depletion of rats, *J. Nutr.*, 114, 746, 1984.
1130. **Mills, B. J., Broghamer, W. L., Higgins, P. J., and Lindeman, R. D.**, A specific dietary zinc requirement for the growth of Walker 256/MI tumors in the rat, *Am. J. Clin. Nutr.*, 34, 1661, 1981.
1131. **Mills, P. R., Fell, G. S., Bessent, R. G., Nelson, L. M., and Russell, R. I.**, A study of zinc metabolism in alcoholic cirrhosis, *Clin. Sci.*, 64, 527, 1983.
1132. **Milman, N., Hvid-Jacobsen, K., Hegnhoj, J., and Solsten Sorensen, S.**, Zinc absorption in patients with compensated alcoholic cirrhosis, *Scand. J. Gastroenterol.*, 18, 871, 1984.
1133. **Milne, D. B., Canfield, W. K., Mahalko, J. R., and Sandstead, H. H.**, Effect of dietary zinc on whole body surface loss of zinc: impact on estimation of zinc retention by balance method, *Am. J. Clin. Nutr.*, 38, 181, 1983.
1134. **Milne, D. B., Canfield, W. K., Mahalko, J. R., and Sandstead, H. H.**, Effect of oral folic acid supplements on zinc copper and iron absorption and excretion, *Am. J. Clin. Nutr.*, 39, 535, 1984.
1135. **Milne, D. B. and Gallagher, S. B.**, Microbiological and radioimmunological assays for folic acid in whole blood compared: effect of zinc nutriture, *Clin. Chem.*, 29, 2117, 1983.
1136. **Milne, D. B., Ralston, N. V. C., and Wallwork, J. C.**, Zinc content of blood cellular components and lymph node and spleen lymphocytes in severely zinc deficient rats, *J. Nutr.*, 115, 1073, 1985.
1137. **Minkel, D. T., Dolhun, P. J., Calhoun, B. L., Saryan, L. A., and Petering, D. H.**, Zinc deficiency and growth of Erhlich's ascites tumor, *Cancer Res.*, 39, 2451, 1979.
1138. **Mjor-Grimsrud, M., Soli, N. E., and Silversen, T.**, The distribution of soluble copper and zinc binding proteins in goat liver, *Acta Pharmacol. Toxicol.*, 44, 319, 1979.
1139. **Mobarhan, S., Russell, R. M., Newberne, P. M., and Ahmed, S. B.**, The effect of zinc deficiency and alcohol feeding on esophageal epithelium of rats, *Nutr. Rep. Int.*, 29, 639, 1984.
1140. **Moffitt, A. E., Dixon, J. R., Phipps, F. C., and Stokinger, H. E.**, The effect of benzpyrene, phenobarbital and carbon tetrachloride on subcellular metal distribution and microsomal enzyme activity, *Cancer Res.*, 32, 1148, 1972.
1141. **Moger, W. H. and Geschwind, I. I.**, The action of prolactin on the sex accessory glands of the male rat, *Proc. Soc. Exp. Biol. Med.*, 141, 1017, 1972.
1142. **Molokhia, M. M. and Portnoy, B.**, Zinc and copper in dermatology, in *Zinc and Copper in Medicine*, Karcioglu, Z. A. and Sarper, R. M., Eds., Charles C. Thomas, Springfield, Ill., 1980, 634.
1143. **Montgomery, M. L., Sheline, G. E., and Chaikoff, I. L.**, The elimination of administered zinc in pancreatic juice, duodenal juice and bile of the dog as measured by its radioactive isotope (zinc-65), *J. Exp. Med.*, 78, 151, 1943.
1144. **Moore, M. E. C., Moran, J. R., and Greene, H. L.**, Zinc supplementation in lactating women — evidence for mammary control of zinc secretion, *J. Pediatr.*, 105, 600, 1984.
1145. **Moore, R.**, Bleeding gastric erosion (oral zinc sulphate), *Br. Med. J.*, i, 754, 1978.
1146. **Moran, J. R. and Lewis, J. C.**, The effects of severe zinc deficiency on intestinal permeability — an ultrastructural study, *Pediatr. Res.*, 19, 968, 1985.
1147. **Morley, J. E., Gordon, J., and Hershman, J. M.**, Zinc deficiency, chronic starvation and hypothalmic-pituitary-thyroid function, *Am. J. Clin. Nutr.*, 33, 1767, 1980.

1148. **Morley, J. E., Russell, R. M., Reed, A., Carney, E. A., and Hershman, J. M.,** The interrelationship of thyroid hormones with vitamin A and zinc nutritional status in patients with chronic hepatitis and gastrointestinal disorders, *Am. J. Clin. Nutr.*, 34, 1489, 1981.
1149. **Morris, E. R. and Ellis, R.,** Bioavailability to rats of zinc and iron in wheat bran. Response to low phytate bran and effect of the phytate/zinc molar ratio, *J. Nutr.*, 110, 2000, 1980.
1150. **Morrison, S. A., Russell, R. M., Carney, E. A., and Oaks, E. V.,** Zinc deficiency: a cause of abnormal dark adaptation in cirrhotics, *Am. J. Clin. Nutr.*, 31, 276, 1978.
1151. **Mortimer, P. S., Gough, P., Newbold, P. C. H., Dawber, R. P. R., and Ryan, T. J.,** Acrodermatitis enteropathica, *J. R. Soc. Med.*, 77, 67, 1984.
1152. **Morton, J. J. P. and Malone, M. H.,** Evaluation of vulnerary activity by an open wound procedure in rats, *Arch. Int. Pharmacodyn. Ther.*, 196, 117, 1972.
1153. **Moser, P. R., Borel, J., Majerus, T., and Anderson, R. A.,** Serum zinc and urinary zinc excretion of trauma patients, *Nutr. Res.*, 5, 253, 1985.
1154. **Moser, P. B. and Reynolds, R. D.,** Dietary zinc intake and zinc concentration of plasma, erythrocytes and breast milk in antepartum and post-partum lactating and nonlactating women: a longitudinal study, *Am. J. Clin. Nutr.*, 38, 101, 1983.
1155. **Moynahan, E. J.,** Acrodermatitis enteropathica: a lethal inherited zinc deficiency disorder, *Lancet,* ii, 399, 1974.
1156. **Moynahan, E. J.,** Zinc deficiency and disturbances of mood and visual behaviour, *Lancet,* i, 91, 1976.
1157. **Moynahan, E. J. and Barnes, P. M.,** Zinc deficiency and a synthetic diet for lactose intolerance, *Lancet,* i, 676, 1973.
1158. **Mozha, I. B.,** Levels of various trace elements in the blood of patients with various types of retinal pathology, *Vestn. Oftalmol.*, 5, 59, 1974.
1159. **Mozzillo, N., Ayala, F., and Federici, G.,** Zinc deficiency in patients on long term total parenteral nutrition, *Lancet,* i, 744, 1982.
1160. **Mtabaji, J. P., Kihara, M., and Yamori, Y.,** Zinc and vascular reactivity in rat mesenteric vessels: possible altered dihomo-gamma-linolenic acid metabolism in spontaneously hypertensive rats, *Prostagl. Leukotr. Med.*, 18, 235, 1985.
1161. **Mukerjee, M. D., Sandstead, H. H., Ratnaparki, M. V., Johnson, L. K., Milne, D. B., and Stelling, H. P.,** Maternal zinc, iron folic acid and protein nutriture and outcome of human pregnancy, *Am. J. Clin. Nutr.*, 40, 496, 1984.
1162. **Muneoka, Y., Twarog, B. M., and Kanno, Y.,** The effects of zinc ion on the mechanical responses of *Mytilus* smooth muscle, *Comp. Biochem. Physiol.*, 62C, 35, 1979.
1163. **Murer, H. and Kinne, R.,** The use of isolated membrane vesicles to study epithelial transport processes, *J. Membr. Biol.*, 55, 81, 1980.
1164. **Murphy, J. F., Gray, O. P., Rendall, J. R., and Hann, S.,** Zinc deficiency: a problem with preterm breast milk, *Early Hum. Dev.*, 10, 303, 1985.
1165. **Murphy, J. Y.,** Intoxication following ingestion of elemental zinc, *JAMA,* 212, 2119, 1976.
1166. **Murray, M. J., Erickson, M. L., and Fisher, G. L.,** Effects of dietary zinc on melanoma growth and experimental metastasis, *Cancer Lett.*, 21, 183, 1983.
1167. **Murthy, L., Klevay, L. M., and Petering, H. G.,** Interrelationships of zinc and copper, *J. Nutr.*, 104, 1458, 1974.
1168. **Murthy, L. and Petering, H. G.,** Effect of dietary zinc and copper interrelationships on blood parameters of the rat, *J. Agric. Food Chem.*, 24, 808, 1976.
1169. **Muskiet, F. D. and Muskiet, F. A. J.,** Lipids, fatty acids, and trace elements in plasma and erythrocytes of pediatric patients with homozygous sickle cell disease, *Clin. Chim. Acta,* 142, 1, 1984.
1170. **Mutch, P. B. and Hurley, L. S.,** Effect of zinc deficiency during lactation on postnatal growth and development of rats, *J. Nutr.*, 104, 828, 1974.
1171. **Muto, Y., Smith, J. E., Milch, P. O., and Goodman, D. S.,** Regulation of retinol-binding protein metabolism by vitamin A status in the rat, *J. Biochem.*, 247, 2542, 1977.
1172. **Naess, K.,** Sink til behandling av ulcus ventriculi, *Tidsskr. Nor. Laegeforen.*, 96, 1334, 1976.
1173. **Nanji, A. A.,** Relationship between zinc and alkaline phosphatase, *Hum. Nutr. Clin. Nutr.*, 37, 461, 1984.
1174. **Nanji, A. A. and Anderson, F. H.,** Alkaline phosphatase is not a relaible indicator of serum zinc levels, *Hum. Nutr. Clin. Nutr.*, 37C, 461, 1983.
1175. **Nanto-Salonen, K., Halme, T., Penttinen, R., Langevelde, F. V., Vis, R. D., and Alftan, C.,** Disturbed metabolism of copper and zinc in aspartylglycosaminuria. Possible involvement with connective tissue changes, *J. Inherit. Metab. Dis.*, 8, 212, 1985.
1176. **Nassar, B. A., Manku, M. S., Tynan, N., and Horrobin, D. F.,** Seasonal and sexual variations in the response of rabbit hearts to prolactin, *Endocrinology,* 97, 1008, 1975.
1177. **Nassi, L., Poggini, G., Nassi, P. A., Vecchi, C., and Galvan, P.,** Notes on zinc metabolism. Note V. Biochemical fractionation of zinc and its distribution in human, cow and cow's milk colostrum and milk proteins, *Minerva Pediatr.*, 28, 591, 1976.

1178. **National Research Council, U. S. A.,** Recommended Dietary Allowances, 9th ed., National Academy of Sciences, Washington, D.C., 1980.

1179. **Naveh, Y., Lightman, A., and Zinder, O.,** Effect of diarrhea on serum zinc concentrations in infants and children, *J. Pediatr.*, 101, 730, 1982.

1180. **Naveh, Y., Lightman, A., and Zinder, O.,** A prospective study of serum zinc concentration in children with celiac diseases, *J. Pediatr.*, 102, 734, 1983.

1181. **Navert, B., Sandstrom, B. M., and Cederblad, A.,** Reduction of the phytate content of bran by leavening in bread and its effect on zinc absorption in man, *Br. J. Nutr.*, 53, 47, 1985.

1182. **Naylor, W. G. and Anderson, J. E.,** Effects of zinc on cardiac muscle contraction, *Am. J. Physiol.*, 209, 17, 1965.

1183. **Neary, J. T. and Divan, W. F.,** Purification, properties and a possible mechanism for pyridoxal kinase from bovine brain, *J. Biol. Chem.*, 245, 5585, 1970.

1184. **Neldner, K. H., Hagler, L., Wise, W. R., Stifel, F. B., Lufkin, E. G., and Herman, R. H.,** Acrodermatitis enteropathica: a clinical and biochemical survey, *Arch. Dermatol.*, 110, 711, 1974.

1185. **Neldner, K. H. and Hambidge, K. M.,** Zinc therapy for acrodermatitis enteropathica, *N. Engl. J. Med.*, 292, 879, 1975.

1186. **Neve, J., Sinet, P. M., Molle, L., and Nicole, A.,** Selenium, zinc and copper in Down's syndrome (Trisomy 21): blood levels and relation with glutathione peroxidase and superoxide dismutase, *Clin. Chim. Acta*, 133, 209, 1983.

1187. **Neve, J., Van Geffel, R., Hanocq, M., and Molle, L.,** Plasma and erythrocyte zinc, copper and selenium and cystic fibrosis, *Acta Pediatr. Scand.*, 72, 437, 1983.

1188. **Ng, W. L., Fong, L. Y. Y., and Newberne, P. M.,** Forestomach squamous papillomas in the rat: effect of dietary zinc deficiency on induction, *Cancer Lett.*, 22, 329, 1984.

1189. **Nigi, V., Chierci, R., Osti, L., Fagioli, F., and Rescazzi, R.,** Serum zinc concentration in exclusively breast-fed infants and in infants fed an adapted formula, *Eur. J. Pediatr.*, 142, 245, 1984.

1190. **Nickerson, V. J. and Veldstra, H.,** The influence of various cations on the binding of colchicine by rat brain homogenates: stabilization of intact microtubules by zinc and cadmium ions, *FEBS Lett.*, 23, 309, 1972.

1191. **Niedermeier, W. and Griggs, J. H.,** Trace metal composition of synovial fluid and blood serum of patients with rheumatoid arthritis, *J. Chronic Dis.*, 23, 527, 1979.

1192. **Niell, H. B., Leach, B. E., and Kraus, A. P.,** Zinc metabolism in sickle cell anemia, *JAMA*, 242, 2686, 1979.

1193. **Nielson, J. P. and Jemec, B.,** Zinc metabolism in patients with severe burns, *Scand. J. Plast. Reconstr. Surg.*, 2, 47, 1968.

1194. **Nielsen, F. H., Sunde, M. L., and Hoekstra, W. G.,** Effect of some dietary synthetic and natural chelating agents on the zinc deficiency syndrome in the chick, *J. Nutr.*, 89, 35, 1966.

1195. **Nielsen, F. H., Sunde, M. L., and Hoekstra, W. G.,** Effect of histamine, histidine and some related compounds on the zinc deficient chick, *Proc. Soc. Exp. Biol. Med.*, 124, 1106, 1967.

1196. **Nielsen, F. H., Sunde, M. L., and Hoekstra, W. G.,** Alleviation of the leg abnormality in zinc deficient chicks by histamine and various anti-arthritic agents, *J. Nutr.*, 99, 527, 1968.

1197. **Nishi, Y., Hatano, S., Aihara, K., and Usui, T.,** Role of zinc in testicular function of chronic renal failure, *Pediatrics*, 73, 740, 1984.

1198. **Nishi, Y., Hatino, S., Horino, N., Sakano, T., and Usui, T.,** Zinc concentration in leucocytes, mononuclear cells, granulocytes, T-lymphocytes, non-T lymphocytes and monocytes, *Hiroshima J. Med. Sci.*, 30, 65, 1981.

1199. **Nishi, Y., Lifshitz, F., Bayne, M. A., Daum, F., Silverberg, M., and Aiges, H.,** Zinc status and its relation to growth retardation in children with chronic inflammatory bowel disease, *Am. J. Clin. Nutr.*, 33, 2613, 1980.

1200. **Noordin, R. W., Krook, L., Pond, W. G., and Walker, E. F.,** Experimental zinc deficiency in weanling pigs on high and low calcium diets, *Cornell Vet.*, 63, 264, 1973.

1201. **Norris, D.,** Zinc and cutaneous inflammation, *Arch. Dermatol.*, 121, 985, 1985.

1202. **Nystrom, A., Hallmans, G., and Lithner, F.,** Zinc metabolism in long-term alloxan diabetic rats after thermal injury, *Acta Med. Scand. Suppl.*, 687, 101, 1984.

1203. **Oba, T., Takagi, V., and Hotta, K.,** Effect of temperature and zinc on isometric contractile properties and electrical phenomena of frog (*Rana* and *Xenopus*) skeletal muscle fibres, *Can. J. Phyisol. Pharmacol.*, 62, 1511, 1984.

1204. **Oberleas, D. and Prasad, A. S.,** Growth as affected by zinc and protein nutrition, *Am. J. Clin. Nutr.*, 22, 1304, 1969.

1205. **O'Dell, B. L.,** Effect of dietary components upon zinc availability, *Am. J. Clin. Nutr.*, 22, 1315, 1969.

1206. **O'Dell, B. L.,** Biochemical basis of the clinical effects of copper deficiency, in *Clinical, Biochemical and Nutritional Aspects of Trace Elements*, Prasad, A. S., Ed., Alan R. Liss, New York, 1982, 301.

1207. **O'Dell, B. L., Browning, J. D., and Reeves, P. G.,** Plasma levels of prostaglandin metabolites in zinc deficient female rats near term, *J. Nutr.*, 113, 760, 1983.

1208. **O'Dell, B. L., Burpo, C. E., and Savage, J. E.,** Evaluation of zinc availability in foodstuffs of plant and animal origin, *J. Nutr.*, 102, 653, 1972.

1209. **O'Dell, B. L. and Reeves, P. G.,** Metabolic function of zinc — a new look, in *Trace Element Metabolism in Man and Animals,* Vol. 4, Howell, J. McC., Gawthorne, J. M., and White, C. L., Eds., Australian Academy of Sciences, Canberra, 1981, 319.

1210. **O'Dell, B. L., Reeves, P. G., and Morgan, R. F.,** Interrelationship of tissue copper and zinc concentrations in rat nutritionally deficient in one or other of these elements, *Trace Subst. Environ. Health,* 10, 411, 1976.

1211. **O'Dell, B. L., Reynolds, G., and Reeves, P. G.,** Analogous effects of zinc deficiency and aspirin toxicity in the pregnant rat, *J. Nutr.*, 107, 1222, 1977.

1212. **O'Dell, B. L. and Savage, J. E.,** Potassium, zinc and distillers dried solubles as supplements to a purified diet, *Poult. Sci.*, 36, 459, 1957.

1213. **O'Dell, B. L. and Savage, J. E.,** Effects of phytic acid on zinc availability, *Proc. Soc. Exp. Biol. Med.*, 103, 304, 1960.

1214. **Odutunga, A. A.,** Effects of low zinc status and essential fatty acid deficiency on bone development and mineralization, *Comp. Biochem. Physiol.*, 71A, 383, 1982.

1215. **Oelshlegel, F. J. and Brewer, G. J.,** Factors affecting absorption of pharmacologically administered zinc, *Clin. Res.*, 23, 222A, 1975.

1216. **Oelshlegel, F. J. and Brewer, G. J.,** Absorption of pharmacological doses of zinc, in *Zinc Metabolism: Current Aspects in Health and Disease,* Prasad, A. S. and Brewer, G. J., Eds., Alan R. Liss, New York, 1977, 299.

1217. **Oelshlegel, F. J., Brewer, G. J., Knutsen, C., Prasad, A. S., and Schoomaker, E. B.,** Studies on the interaction of zinc with hemoglobin, *Arch. Biochem. Biophys.*, 163, 742, 1974.

1218. **Oelshlegel, F. J., Brewer, G. J., Prasad, A. S., Knutsen, C., and Schoomaker, E. B.,** Effect of zinc on increasing oxygen affinity of sickle and normal red blood cells, *Biochem. Biophys. Res. Commun.*, 53, 560, 1973.

1219. **Oestreicher, P. and Cousins, R. J.,** Copper and zinc absorption in the rat: mechanism of mutual antagonism, *J. Nutr.*, 115, 159, 1985.

1220. **Ohno, H., Doi, R., Yamamura, K., Yamashita, K., Izuka, S., and Taniguchi, N.,** A study of zinc distribution in erythrocytes of normal humans, *Blut,* 50, 113, 1985.

1221. **Ohtaka, Y., Uchida, K., and Sakai, T.,** Purification and properties of ribonuclease from yeast, *J. Biochem. (Tokyo),* 54, 322, 1963.

1222. **Okahata, H., Muraki, K., Hatano, S., Aihara, K., Miyachi, Y., and Usui, T.,** The effect of zinc ion on adenylate cyclase in rat testicular tissue, *Horm. Metab. Res.*, 16, 327, 1984.

1223. **Okayasu, T., Nagao, M., Ishibashi, T., and Imai, Y.,** Purification and partial characterization of linoleoyl-CoA desaturase from rat liver microsomes, *Arch. Biochem. Biophys.*, 206, 21, 1981.

1224. **Okumura, M. and Funakoshi, Y.,** Anomaly of zinc and copper metabolism in hepatic diseases, *Jpn. J. Clin. Pathol.*, 19, 63, 1971.

1225. **Okuyama, S., Mishina, H., Hasegawa, K., Nakano, N., and Ise, K.,** Probable atherogenic role of zinc and copper as studied in chronic hemodialysis, *Tohoku J. Exp. Med.*, 138, 227, 1982.

1226. **Olafson, R. W.,** Thymic metallothione in: regulation of zinc-thionein in the aging mouse, *Can. J. Biochem.*, 63, 91, 1985.

1227. **Olsson, R.,** Oral zinc treatment in primary biliary cirrhosis, *Acta Med. Scand.*, 212, 191, 1982.

1228. **Oner, G., Bhaumick, B., and Bala, R. M.,** Effect of zinc deficiency on serum somatomedin levels and skeletal growth in young rats, *Endocrinology,* 114, 1860, 1984.

1229. **Ota, D. M., MacFayden, B. V., Gum, E. T., and Didrick, S. J.,** Zinc and copper deficiencies in man during intravenous hyperalimentation, in *Zinc and Copper in Clinical Medicine,* Hambidge, K. M. and Nicholls, B. L., Eds., S. P. Medical and Scientific Books, Jamaica, N.Y., 1977, 99.

1230. **Ottolenghi, A. C.,** Phospholipase C from *Bacillus cereus*, a zinc requiring metalloenzyme, *Biochim. Biophys. Acta,* 106, 510, 1965.

1231. **Owens, C. W. I., Al-Khader, A. A., Jackson, M. J., and Prichard, B. N.,** A severe 'stasis eczema' associated with a low plasma zinc, successfully treated with oral zinc, *Br. J. Dermatol.*, 105, 461, 1981.

1232. **Pak, C. Y. C., Ruskin, B., and Diller, E.,** Enhancement of renal excretion of zinc by hydrochlorthiazide, *Clin. Chim. Acta,* 39, 511, 1973.

1233. **Palin, H. D., Underwood, B. A., and Denning, C. R.,** The effect of oral zinc sulfate supplementation on plasma levels of vitamin A and retinol-binding protein in cystic fibrosis, *Pediatr. Res.*, 10, 358, 1976.

1234. **Palin, D., Underwood, B. A., and Denning, C. R.,** The effect of oral zinc supplementation on plasma levels of vitamin A and retinol-binding protein in cystic fibrosis, *Am. J. Clin. Nutr.*, 32, 1253, 1979.

1235. **Palm, R. and Hallmans, G.,** Zinc and copper in multiple sclerosis, *J. Neurol. Neurosurg. Psychiatr.*, 45, 691, 1982.

1236. **Palma, P. A., Conley, S. B., Crandell, S. S., and Denson, S. E.**, Zinc deficiency following surgery in zinc-supplemented infants, *Pediatr. Res.*, 69, 801, 1982.

1237. **Pangaro, J. A., Weinstein, M., Devetak, M. C., and Soto, R. J.**, Red cell zinc and red cell zinc metalloenzymes in hypethyroidism, *Acta Endocrinol.*, 76, 645, 1974.

1238. **Parisi, A. F. and Vallee, B. L.**, isolation of zinc-alpha$_2$-macroglobulin from human serum, *Biochemistry*, 9, 2421, 1970.

1239. **Park, J. H. Y., Grandjean, C. T., Hart, M. H., Erdman, S. H., Pour, P., and Vanderhof, J. A.**, Effect of pure zinc deficiency on glucose tolerance and insulin and glucagon levels, *Am. J. Physiol.*, 251, E273, 1986.

1240. **Parker, P. H., Helenik, G. L., Meneely, R. L., Stroop, S., Ghishan, F. K., and Greene, H. L.**, Zinc deficiency in a premature infant fed exclusively on breast milk, *Am. J. Dis. Child.*, 136, 77, 1982.

1241. **Parkinson, C. E., Tan, J. C. Y., Lewis, P. J., and Bennett, M. J.**, Amniotic fluid zinc and copper and neural tube defects, *J. Obstet. Gynecol.*, 1, 207, 1981.

1242. **Parrish, R. F. and Fair, W. R.**, Selective binding of zinc to heparin rather than to other glycosaminoglycans, *Biochem. J.*, 193, 407, 1981.

1243. **Pasanen, S. and Koskela, P.**, Seasonal changes in calcium, magnesium, copper and zinc content in the liver of the common frog *Rana temporaria* L., *Comp. Biochem. Physiol.*, 48A, 27, 1974.

1244. **Pasentes-Morales, H. and Cruz, C.**, Protective effect of taurine and zinc on peroxidation-induced damage in photoreceptor outer segments, *J. Neurosci. Res.*, 11, 303, 1984.

1245. **Patel, P. B., Chang, R. A., and Lu, J. Y.**, Effect of zinc deficiency on serum and liver cholesterol in the femal rat, *Nutr. Rep. Int.*, 12, 205, 1975.

1246. **Patrick, J. and Dervish, C.**, Leukocyte zinc in the assessment of zinc status, *CRC Crit. Rev. Clin. Lab. Sci.*, 20, 95, 1984.

1247. **Patrick, J., Golden, B. E., and Golden, M. H. N.**, Leucocyte sodium transport and dietary zinc in protein-energy malnutrition, *Am. J. Clin. Nutr.*, 33, 617, 1980.

1248. **Patterson, P. G. and Bettger, W. J.**, Effect of dietary zinc intake on the hematological profile of the rat, *Comp. Biochem. Physiol.*, 83, 721, 1986.

1249. **Patterson, W. P., Winkelman, M., and Perry, M. C.**, Zinc-induced copper deficiency — megamineral sideroblastic anemia, *Ann. Intern. Med.*, 103, 385, 1985.

1250. **Pattison, S. E. and Cousins, R. J.**, Kinetics of zinc uptake and exchange by primary cultures of rat hepatocytes, *Am. J. Physiol.*, 250, E677, 1986.

1251. **Pattison, S. E. and Dunn, M. F.**, On the relationship of zinc ion to the structure and function of the 7S nerve growth factor protein, *Biochemistry*, 14, 2733, 1975.

1252. **Patton, S. and Keenan, T. W.**, The milk fat globule membrane, *Biochim. Biophys. Acta*, 415, 273, 1975.

1253. **Paul, A. A. and Southgate, D. A. T.**, *McCance and Widdowson's The Composition of Foods*, Her Majesty's Stationery Office, London, 1978.

1254. **Pecoud, A., Donzel, P., and Schelling, J. L.**, Effects of foodstuffs on the absorption of zinc sulphate, *Clin. Pharmacol. Ther.*, 17, 469, 1975.

1255. **Pei, Y., Zhao, D., Huang, J., and Cao, L.**, Zinc-induced seizures: a new experimental model of epilepsy, *Epilepsia*, 24, 169, 1983.

1256. **Peirce, P., Jackson, M., Tomkins, A., and Millward, D. J.**, Zinc is conserved in the severely zinc deficient rat, *Proc. Nutr. Soc.*, in press.

1257. **Pekarek, R. S., Burghen, G. A., Bartelloni, P. J., Calia, F. M., Bostian, K. A., and Beisel, W. R.**, The effect of live attenuated Venezuelian equine encephalomyelitis virus vaccine on serum iron, zinc and copper concentrations in man, *J. Lab. Clin. Med.*, 76, 293, 1970.

1258. **Pekarek, R. S. and Evans, G. W.**, Effect of acute infection and endotoxemia on zinc absorption in the rat, *Proc. Soc. Exp. Biol. Med.*, 150, 755, 1975.

1259. **Pekarek, R. S. and Evans, G. W.**, Effect of leucocytic endogenous mediator on zinc absorption in the rat, *Proc. Soc. Exp. Biol. Med.*, 152, 573, 1976.

1260. **Pekarek, R. S., Jacob, R. A., Barcome, D. F., and Sandstead, H. H.**, Effect of acquired zinc deficiency on the cellular immune response, *Am. J. Clin. Nutr.*, 30, 612, 1977.

1261. **Pekarek, R. S., Kluge, R. M., Dupont, H. L., Wannemacher, R. W., Hornick, R. B., Bostian, K. A., and Beisel, W. R.**, Serum zinc, iron and copper concentrations during typhoid fever in man: effect of chloramphenicol therapy, *Clin. Chem.*, 21, 528, 1975.

1262. **Pekarek, R. S., Sandstead, H. H., Jacob, R. A., and Barcome D. F.**, Abnormal cellular immune responses during acquired zinc deficiency, *Am. J. Clin. Nutr.*, 32, 1466, 1979.

1263. **Pekarek, R. S., Wannemacher, R. W., and Beisel, W. R.**, The effect of leukocytic endogenous mediator (LEM) on the tissue distribution of zinc and iron, *Proc. Soc. Exp. Biol. Med.*, 140, 685, 1972.

1264. **Perez-Jimenez, F., Bockman, D. E., and Singh, M.**, Pancreatic acinar cell function and morphology in rats fed zinc deficient and marginal zinc deficient diets, *Gastroenterology*, 90, 946, 1986.

1265. **Petering, H. G.,** The effect of cadmium and lead on copper and zinc metabolism, in *Trace Element Metabolism in Animals,* Vol. 2, Hoekstra, W. G., Suttie, J. W., Ganther, H. E., and Mertz, W., Eds., University Park Press, Baltimore, 1974, 311.

1266. **Petering, H. G., Johnson, M. A., and Stemmer, K. L.,** Studies of zinc metabolism in the rat. I. Dose-response effects of cadmium, *Arch. Environ. Health,* 23, 93, 1971.

1267. **Petering, H. G., Murthy, L., and O'Flaherty, E.,** Influence of dietary copper and zinc on rat lipid metabolism, *J. Agric. Food Chem.,* 25, 1105, 1977.

1268. **Peters, A. J., Keen, C. L., Lonnerdal, B., and Hurley, L. S.,** Zinc-vitamin A interactions in pregnant and fetal rats: supplemental vitamin A does not prevent zinc deficiency-induced teratogenesis, *J. Nutr.,* 116, 1765, 1986.

1269. **Peters, H. A.,** Trace mineral metabolism in porphyria and other neuropsychiatric conditions — role of chelation therapy, in *Trace Element Metabolism in Animals,* Vol. 2, Hoekstra, W. G., Suttei, J. W., Ganther, H. E., and Mertz, W., Eds., University Park Press, Baltimore, 1974, 682.

1270. **Peters, H. A., Woods, S., Eichman, P. L., and Reese, H. H.,** Treatment of acute porphyria with chelating agents, *Ann. Intern. Med.,* 47, 889, 1957.

1271. **Peters, H. A., Eichman, P. L., and Reese, H. H.,** Therapy of acute, chronic and mixed hepatic porphyria patients with chelating agents, *Neurology,* 8, 621, 1958.

1272. **Peterson, D. A., Gerrard, J. M., Peller, J., Rao, G. H. R., and White, J. C.,** Interactions of zinc and arachidonic acid, *Prostagl. Med.,* 6, 91, 1981.

1273. **Pfeiffer, C. C. and Cott, A.,** A study of zinc and manganese dietary supplements in the copper-loaded schizophrenic, in *Clinical Applications of Zinc Metabolism,* Pories, W. J., Strain, W. H., Hsu, J. M., and Woolsey, R. L., Eds., Academic Press, New York, 1974, 260.

1274. **Pfeiffer, C. C. and Iliev, V.,** A study of zinc deficiency and copper excess in the schizophrenias, *Med. Clin. North Am.,* 60, 141, 1976.

1275. **Pfeiffer, C. C. and Jenney, E. H.,** Excess oral zinc in man lowers copper levels, *Fed. Proc. Fed. Am. Soc. Exp. Biol.,* 37, 324, 1978.

1276. **Pfeiffer, C. J., Builena, O., Espluges, J. V., Escolar, G., Navarro, C., and Espluges, J.,** Anti-ulcer and membrane stabilizing actions of zinc acexamate, *Arch. Int. Pharmacodyn. Ther.,* 285, 148, 1987.

1277. **Philip, B.,** Zinc and metabolism of lipids in normal and atheromatous rats, *Indian J. Exp. Biol.,* 16, 46, 1977.

1278. **Philip, B. and Kurup, P. A.,** Dietary zinc and levels of collagen, elastin and carbohydrate components of glycoproteins of aorta, skin and cartilage of rats, *Indian J. Exp. Biol.,* 16, 370, 1978.

1279. **Phillips, G. D. and Garnys, V. P.,** Trace element balance in adults receiving parenteral nutrition: preliminary data, *J. Parenteral Enteral Nutr.,* 5, 11, 1981.

1280. **Phillips, J. L.,** Uptake of transferrin-bound zinc by human lymphocytes, *Cell. Immunol.,* 35, 318, 1978.

1281. **Picciano, M. F. and Gutherie, H. A.,** Copper, iron and zinc contents of mature human milk, *Am. J. Clin. Nutr.,* 29, 242, 1976.

1282. **Pidduck, H. G., Wren, P. J. J., and Price-Evans, D. A.,** Hyperzincuria of diabetes mellitus and possible implications of this observation, *Diabetes,* 19, 240, 1970.

1283. **Piesse, J.,** Zinc and human male infertility, *Int. Clin. Nutr. Rev.,* 3, 4, 1983.

1284. **Piletz, J. E. and Ganschow, R. E.,** Is acrodermatitis enteropathica related to the absence of a zinc-binding ligand in bovine milk, *Am. J. Clin. Nutr.,* 32, 275, 1979.

1285. **Pilz, R. B., Willis, R. C., and Seegmiller, J. E.,** Regulation of human lymphblast plasma membrane 5′-nucleotidase by zinc, *J. Biol. Chem.,* 257, 13454, 1982.

1286. **Pippenger, C. E., Garlock, C., Fernandez, F., Slavin, W., and Iannarone, J.,** Effects of antiepileptic drugs on manganese, zinc and copper concentrations in whole blood, red blood cells and plasma of epileptics, in *Advances in Epileptology,* Vol. 11, Canger, R., Angeleri, F., and Penry, J. K., Eds., Raven Press, New York, 1980, 435.

1287. **Plishker, G. A.,** Effects of cadmium and zinc on calcium uptake in human red blood cells, *Am. J. Physiol.,* 247, C143, 1984.

1288. **Pohit, J., Saha, K. C., and Pal, B.,** A zinc tolerance test, *Clin. Chim. Acta,* 114, 279, 1981.

1289. **Pond, W. G., Chapman, P., and Walker, E.,** Influence of dietary zinc, corn oil and cadmium on certain blood components, weight gain and parakeratosis in young pigs, *J. Anim. Sci.,* 25, 122, 1966.

1290. **Ponteva, M., Elomaa, I., Backman, L., Hansson, L., and Kilpio, J.,** Blood cadmium and plasma zinc measurements in acute myocardial infarction, *Eur. J. Cardiol.,* 9, 379, 1979.

1291. **Pontremoli, S., Melloni, E., Salamino, F., Spartore, B., and Horecker, B. L.,** Interaction of zinc and magnesium with rabbit liver fructose 1,6-bisphosphate, *Arch. Biochem. Biophys.,* 188, 90, 1978.

1292. **Pories, W. J., Atawneh, A., Peer, R. M., Childers, R. C., Worland, R. L., Zaresky, S. A., and Strain, W. H.,** Mineral metabolism of the healing arterial wall, *Arch. Surg.,* 114, 254, 1979.

1293. **Pories, W. J., Dewys, W. D., Flynn, A., Mansour, E. G., and Strain, W. H.,** Implications of the inhibition of animal tumors by dietary zinc, *Adv. Exp. Med. Biol.,* 91, 243, 1977.

1294. **Pories, W. J., Mansour, E. G., Plecha, F. R., Flynn, A., and Strain, W. H.,** Metabolic factors affecting zinc metabolism in the surgical patient, in *Trace Elements in Human Health and Disease,* Vol. 1, Prasad, A. S. and Oberleas, D., Eds., Academic Press, New York, 1976, 115.

1295. **Porter, K. G., McMaster, D., Elmes, M. E., and Love, A. H. G.,** Anemia and low serum copper during zinc therapy, *Lancet,* ii, 774, 1977.

1296. **Portnoy, B. and Molokhia, M.,** Zinc and copper in psoriasis, *Br. J. Dermatol.,* 87, 291, 1972.

1297. **Pounds, J. G. and Morrison, D. R.,** Cellular metabolism of zinc. A kinetic analysis in cultured rat hepatocytes, in *Chemical Toxicology and Clinical Chemistry of Metals,* Brown, S. S. and Savory, J., Eds., Academic Press, New York, 1983, 251.

1298. **Powell-Beard, L., Lei, K. Y., and Shenker, L.,** Effect of long term oral contraceptive therapy before pregnancy on maternal and fetal zinc and copper status, *Obstet. Gynecol.,* 69, 26, 1987.

1299. **Prasad, A. S.,** Deficiency of zinc in man and its toxicity, in *Trace Elements in Human Health and Disease,* Vol. 1, Prasad, A. S. and Oberleas, D., Eds., Academic Press, New York, 1976, 1.

1300. **Prasad, A. S.,** Zinc in human nutrition, *CRC Crit. Rev. Clin. Lab. Sci.,* 8, 1, 1977.

1301. **Prasad, A. S.,** Nutritional deficiencies in man: zinc, in *CRC Handbook Series in Nutrition and Food,* Rechcigl, M., Ed., CRC Press, Boca Raton, Fla., 1978, 261.

1302. **Prasad, A. S.,** Clinical and biochemical spectrum of zinc deficiency in human subjects, in *Current Topics in Nutrition and Disease,* Vol. 6, Prasad, A. S., Ed., Alan R. Liss, New York, 1982, 3.

1303. **Prasad, A. S. and Bose, S. M.,** Effect of zinc deficiency on collagen cross-linking, *Indian J. Biochem. Biophys.,* 12, 249, 1975.

1304. **Prasad, A. S., Brewer, G. J., Schoomaker, E. B., and Rabbini, P.,** Hypocupremia induced by zinc therapy in adults, *JAMA,* 240, 2166, 1978.

1305. **Prasad, A. S. and Cossack, Z. T.,** Neutrophil zinc: an indicator of zinc status in man, *Am. J. Clin. Nutr.,* 35, 835, 1982.

1306. **Prasad, A. S. and Cossack, Z. T.,** Zinc supplementation and growth in sickle cell disease, *Ann. Intern. Med.,* 100, 367, 1984.

1307. **Prasad, A. S., Fernandez-Madrid, F., and Ryan, J. R.,** Deoxythymidine kinase of human implanted sponge connective tissue in zinc deficiency, *Am. J. Physiol.,* 236, E272, 1979.

1308. **Prasad, A. S., Halsted, J. A., and Nadimi, M.,** Syndrome of iron deficiency, anemia, hepatosplenomegaly, dwarfism, hypogonadism and geophagia, *Am. J. Med.,* 31, 532, 1961.

1309. **Prasad, A. S., Miale, A., Farid, Z., Sandstead, H. H., and Darby, W. J.,** Biochemical studies on dwarfism, hypogonadism and anemia, *Arch. Intern. Med.,* 111, 407, 1963.

1310. **Prasad, A. S. and Oberleas, D.,** Binding of zinc to amino acids and serum proteins in vitro, *J. Lab. Clin. Med.,* 76, 416, 1970.

1311. **Prasad, A. S. and Oberleas, D.,** Changes in activities of zinc dependent enzymes in zinc deficient tissues of rats, *J. Appl. Physiol.,* 31, 842, 1971.

1312. **Prasad, A. S. and Oberleas, D.,** Biochemical effects of zinc deficiency in experimental animals, in *Clinical Applications of Zinc Metabolism,* Pories, W. J., Strain, W. H., Hsu, J. M., and Woolsey, R. L., Eds., Academic Press, New York, 1974, 19.

1313. **Prasad, A. S., Oberleas, D., and Halsted, J. A.,** Determination of zinc in biological fluids by atomic absorption spectrophotometry in normal and cirrhotic subjects, *J. Lab. Clin. Med.,* 66, 508, 1965.

1314. **Prasad, A. S., Oberleas, D., Moghissi, K. S., and Stryker, J. C.,** Effect of oral contraceptive agents on nutrients. I. Minerals, *Am. J. Clin. Nutr.,* 28, 377, 1975.

1315. **Prasad, A. S., Oberleas, D., Wolf, P., and Horwitz, J. P.,** Studies on zinc deficiency: changes in trace elements and enzyme activities in tissues of zinc deficient rats, *J. Clin. Invest.,* 46, 549, 1967.

1316. **Prasad, A. S., Rabbini, P., Abbasii, A., Bowersox, E., and Spivey Fox, M. R.,** Experimental zinc deficiency in humans, *Ann. Intern. Med.,* 89, 483, 1978.

1317. **Prasad, A. S., Rabbini, P., Abbasii, A., Bowersox, E., and Spivey Fox, M. R.,** Experimental production of zinc deficiency in man, in *Trace Element Metabolism Man and Animals,* Vol. 3, Kirchgessner, M., Ed., Arbeitkreis fur Tierernahrungsfirschung, Weihenstephan, F. R. G., 1977, 280.

1318. **Prasad, A. S., Rabbini, P., and Warth, J. A.,** Effect of zinc on hyperammonemia in sickle cell anemia subjects, *Am. J. Hematol.,* 7, 323, 1980.

1319. **Prasad, A. S., Schoomaker, E. B., Ortega, J., Brewer, G. J., Oberleas, D., and Oelshlegel, F. J.,** The role of zinc in man and its deficiency in sickle cell disease, *Prog. Clin. Biol. Res.,* 1, 603, 1975.

1320. **Prasad, A. S., Schoomaker, E. B., Ortega, J., Brewer, G. J., Oberleas, D., and Oelshlegel, F. J.,** Zinc deficiency in sickle cell disease, *Clin. Chem.,* 21, 582, 1975.

1321. **Prasad, A. S., Schulert, A. R., Sandstead, H. H., Miale, A., and Farid, Z.,** Zinc, iron and nitrogen content of sweat in normal and deficient subjects, *J. Lab. Clin. Med.,* 62, 84, 1963.

1322. **Prasad, R., Lyall, V., and Nath, R.,** Effect of vitamin B6 and Vitamin B_1 deficiencies on intestinal uptake of calcium, zinc and cadmium, *Ann. Nutr. Metab.,* 26, 324, 1982.

1323. **Price, D. and Joshi, J. G.,** Ferritin. A zinc detoxicant and a zinc ion donor, *Proc. Natl. Acad. Sci. U.S.A.,* 79, 3116, 1982.

1324. **Principi, N., Guinta, A., and Gervasoni, A.,** The role of zinc in total parenteral nutrition, *Acta Pediatr. Scand.*, 68, 129, 1979.
1325. **Quarterman, J.,** The metabolic role of zinc with special reference to carbohydrate and lipid metabolism, *Rep. Rowett Inst.*, 24, 100, 1968.
1326. **Quarterman, J.,** The effect of zinc deficiency on the activity of the adrenal glands, *Proc. Nutr. Soc.*, 31, 74A, 1972.
1327. **Quarterman, J.,** The effects of zinc deficiency or excess on the adrenals and the thymus of the rat, in *Trace Element Metabolism in Animals*, Vol. 2, Hoekstra, W. G., Suttie, J. W., Ganther, H. E., and Mertz, W., Eds., University Park Press, Baltimore, 1974, 742.
1328. **Quarterman, J. and Florence, E.,** Observations of glucose tolerance and plasma levels of free fatty acids and insulin in the zinc deficient rat, *Br. J. Nutr.*, 28, 75, 1972.
1329. **Quarterman, J. and Humphries, W. R.,** The production of zinc deficiency in the guinea pig, *J. Comp. Pathol.*, 93, 261, 1983.
1330. **Quarterman, J., Mills, C. F., and Humphries, W. R.,** The reduced secretion of and sensitivity to insulin in zinc deficient rat, *Biochem. Biophys. Res. Commun.*, 25, 354, 1966.
1331. **Raab, W. P. and Gmeiner, B. M.,** Influence of ultra-violet light, various temperatures, and zinc ions on anthralin (dithranol), *Dermatologia*, 150, 267, 1975.
1332. **Rabbini, P. and Prasad, A. S.,** Plasma ammonia and liver ornithine transcarbamylase activity in zinc deficient rats, *Am. J. Physiol.*, 235, E203, 1978.
1333. **Rachlin, L.,** Aortic zinc in patients with peripheral vascular disease, *Angiology*, 23, 651, 1972.
1334. **Ramchandran, C. K. and Shah, S. N.,** Effect of feeding a zinc deficient diet to dams during lactation on brain development of the offspring: lipid composition of whole brain, myelin and synaptsomes, *Biochem. Arch.*, 1, 107, 1985.
1335. **Rana, S. V.,** Visual evidences on reversible dysenzymia by zinc and a new chelating agent in carbon tetrachloride poisoned liver of squirrels, *Mikroscopie*, 36, 233, 1980.
1336. **Rana, S. V.,** Influence of zinc, vitamin B12 and glutathione on the liver of rats exposed to carbon tetrachloride, *Ind. Health*, 19, 65, 1981.
1337. **Rana, S. V. S. and Tayal, M. K.,** Lipotrophic effects of zinc, vitamin B_{12} and glutathione on the fatty liver of the rat, A histochemical study, *Mikroscopie*, 38, 294, 1981.
1338. **Raulin, J.,** Etudes cliniques sur la vegetation, *Ann. Sci. Nat. Bot. Biol. Veg.*, 11, 93, 1869.
1339. **Reaven, E. P. and Cox, A. J.,** The histochemical localization of histidine in the human epidermis and its relation to zinc binding, *J. Histochem. Cytochem.*, 11, 782, 1963.
1340. **Rebello, T., Atherton, D. J., and Holden, C.,** The effect of zinc administration on sebum free fatty acids in acne vulgaris, *Arch. Dermatol. Venereol.*, 66, 305, 1986.
1341. **Record, I. R., Dreosti, I. E., and Tulsi, R. S.,** *In vitro* development of zinc deficient and replete rat embryos, *Aust. J. Exp. Biol. Med. Sci.*, 63, 65, 1985.
1342. **Record, I. R., Record, S. J., Dreosti, I. E., and Rohan, T. E.,** Dietary zinc intake of premenopausal women, *Hum. Nutr. Clin. Nutr.*, 39A, 363, 1985.
1343. **Record, I. R., Tulsi, R. S., Dreosti, I. E., and Fraser, F. J.,** Cellular necrosis in zinc deficient rat embryos, *Teratology*, 32, 397, 1985.
1344. **Reding, P., DuChateau, J., and Bataille, C.,** Oral zinc supplementation improves hepatic encephalopathy, *Lancet*, ii, 493, 1984.
1345. **Reeves, P. G., Frissell, S. G., and O'Dell, B. L.,** Response of serum corticosterone to ACTH and stress in the zinc deficient rat, *Proc. Soc. Exp. Biol. Med.*, 156, 500, 1977.
1346. **Reeves, P. G. and O'Dell, B. L.,** An experimental study of the effect of zinc on the activity of angiotensin-converting enzyme in serum, *Clin. Chem.*, 31, 581, 1985.
1347. **Reeves, P. G. and O'Dell, B. L.,** Effects of dietary zinc deprivation on the activity of angiotensin converting enzyme in serum of rats and guinea pigs, *J. Nutr.*, 116, 128, 1986.
1348. **Reimann, E. M., Sunde, M. L., and Hoekstra, W. G.,** Effect of chloroquine and certain amines, vitamins and arthritis-influencing agents on the zinc deficient chick, *Proc. Soc. Exp. Biol. Med.*, 137, 473, 1971.
1349. **Reinhold, E. W.,** Changes in zinc metabolism during the course of the nephrotic syndrome, *Am. J. Dis. Child*, 134, 46, 1980.
1350. **Reinhold, J. G., Faradji, B., Abadi, P., and Ismail-Beigi, F.,** Decreased absorption of calcium, magnesium, zinc and phosphorus by humans due to increased fibre and phosphorus consumption as wheat bread, *J. Nutr.*, 106, 493, 1976.
1351. **Reinhold, J. G. and Kfoury, G. A.,** Zinc dependent enzymes in zinc-depleted rats; intestinal alkaline phosphatase, *Am. J. Clin. Nutr.*, 22, 1250, 1969.
1352. **Reinstein, N. H., Lonnerdal, B., Keen, C. L., and Hurley, L. S.,** Zinc-copper interactions in the pregnant rat: fetal outcome and maternal and fetal zinc, copper and iron, *J. Nutr.*, 1266, 1984.
1353. **Reis, B. L. and Evans, G. W.,** Genetic influence on zinc metabolism in mice, *J. Nutr.*, 107, 1683, 1977.
1354. **Reiss, G., Przybyslawski, J., and Cheval, J.,** Twitch-reinforcing action, contractive effects and depressant effects of zinc ion on isolated rat diaphragm muscle fibres, *C. R. Soc. Biol., (Paris)*, 165, 465, 1971.

1355. **Reuss, J. D.,** *Reportorium Commentationum Scientica et Ars Medica et Chirurgica,* Vol. 11, Pharmacia, Franklin, New York, 1816, 286.

1356. **Reyes, A. S., Leary, W. P., Lockett, C. J., and Alcocer, L.,** Diuretics and zinc, *S. Afr. Med. J.*, 62, 373, 1982.

1357. **Richards, M. P. and Cousins, R. J.,** Influence of inhibitors of protein synthesis on zinc metabolism, *Proc. Soc. Exp. Biol. Med.*, 156, 505, 1977.

1358. **Rickli, E. E. and Edsall, J. T.,** Zinc-binding and the sulphydryl groups of human carbonic anhydrase, *J. Biol. Chem.*, 237, PC 258, 1961.

1359. **Rieder, H. P., Schoetti, G., and Seiler, H.,** Trace elements in whole blood of multiple sclerosis, *Eur. Neurol.*, 22, 85, 1983.

1360. **Rifkind, J. M. and Heim, J. M.,** Interaction of zinc with hemoglobin: binding of zinc and the oxygen affinity, *Biochemistry,* 16, 4438, 1977.

1361. **Rillema, J. A.,** Effect of zinc ions on the actions of prolactin on RNA and casein synthesis in mouse mammary gland explants, *Proc. Soc. Exp. Biol. Med.*, 162, 464, 1979.

1362. **Riordan, J. F. and Vallee, B. L.,** Structure and function of zinc metalloenzymes, *Med. Clin. North Am.*, 60, 227, 1976.

1363. **Robertson, A. F. and Putz, J.,** Serum and erythrocyte fatty acids in a case of acrodermatitis enteropathica, *J. Pediatr.*, 70, 279, 1967.

1364. **Robson, J. R. K., Self, K. S., Wadland, W., Hutson, A. C., and Deantonio, S.,** Relationship between zinc deficiency and Weber-Christian disease, *Am. J. Clin. Nutr.*, 33, 2221, 1980.

1365. **Rodger, R. S. C., Brook, A. C., Muirhead, N., and Kerr, D. N. S.,** Zinc metabolism does not influence sexual function in chronic renal insufficiency, *Contrib. Nephrol.*, 38, 112, 1984.

1366. **Rodriguez, A., Soto, G., Torres, S., Venegas, G., and Castillo-Duran, C.,** Zinc and copper hair and plasma levels in children with chronic diarrhea, *Acta Paediatr. Scand.*, 74, 770, 1985.

1367. **Roe, D. A. and Campbell, T. E., Eds.,** *Drugs and Nutrients: The Interactive Effects,* Marcel Dekker, New York, 1984.

1368. **Roman, W.,** Zinc in porphyria, *Am. J. Clin. Nutr.*, 22, 1290, 1969.

1369. **Roman, W., Oon, R., West, R. F., and Reid, D. P.,** Zinc sulphate in acute porphyria, *Lancet,* ii, 716, 1967.

1370. **Ronaghy, H. A., Reinhold, J. G., Mahloudji, M., Ghavami, P., Fox, M. R. S., and Halsted, J. A.,** Zinc supplementation of malnourished school boys in Iran, *Am. J. Clin. Nutr.*, 27, 112, 1974.

1371. **Ronquist, G., Frithz, G., Hedstrom, M., and Ericsson, P.,** Human red cell content of cyclic nucleotides and cations upon beta-adrenergic blockade, *Upsala J. Med. Sci.*, 83, 85, 1978.

1372. **Root, A. W., Duckett, G., Sweetland, M., and Reiter, E. D.,** Effects of zinc deficiency upon pituitary function in sexually mature and immature male rats, *J. Nutr.*, 109, 958, 1979.

1373. **Rose, G. and Willden, E. G.,** Whole blood, red cell and plasma total ultrafiltrable zinc levels in normal subjects and patients with chronic renal failure with and without hemodialysis, *Br. J. Urol.*, 44, 281, 1972.

1374. **Rosick, U., Rosick, E., Bratter, P., and Kynast, G.,** Determination of zinc in amniotic fluid in normal and high risk pregnancies, *J. Clin. Chem. Biochem.*, 21, 363, 1983.

1375. **Roth, H.-P. and Kirchgessner, M.,** Zum einfloss von Zinkmangel auf den Fettstoffwessel, *Int. Z. Vitaminforsch.*, 47, 277, 1977.

1376. **Roth, H.-P. and Kirchgessner, M.,** In vitro zinc-65 uptake by erythrocytes for the diagnosis of zinc deficiency, *Z. Tierphysiol. Tierernaehr. Futtermittelkd.*, 42, 101, 1979.

1377. **Rothbaum, R. J. and Maur, P. R.,** Serum alkaline phosphatase — a sensitive index of zinc undernutrition, *J. Pediatr.*, 98, 1023, 1981.

1378. **Rothman, R. J., Leure-duPree, A. E., and Fosmire, G. J.,** Zinc deficiency affects the composition of the rat adrenal gland, *Proc. Soc. Exp. Biol. Med.*, 182, 350, 1986.

1379. **Rubin, H.,** Inhibition of DNA synthesis in animal cells by EDTA and its reversal by zinc, *Proc. Natl. Acad. Sci. U.S.A.*, 69, 712, 1972.

1380. **Rumble, W. F., Aamodt, R. L., and Henkin, R. I.,** A rapid method for estimation of zinc absorption using zinc-69m, *Fed. Proc. Fed. Am. Soc. Exp. Biol.*, 36, 1138, 1977.

1381. **Russell, R. M., Cox, M. E., and Solomons, N. W.,** Zinc and the special senses, *Ann. Intern. Med.*, 99, 227, 1983.

1382. **Ruth, R. E. and Goldsmith, S. L.,** Interaction between zinc deprivation and acute ethanol intoxication during pregnancy in rats, *J. Nutr.*, 111, 2034, 1981.

1383. **Sabath, L. D. and Finland, M.,** Thiol-group binding of zinc to a beta-lactamase of *Bacillus cereus.* Differential effects on enzyme activity with penicillin and cephalosporins as substrates, *J. Bacteriol.*, 95, 1513, 1968.

1384. **Sadasivan, V.,** Studies on the biochemistry of zinc. I. Effect of feeding zinc on the liver and bones, *Biochem. J.*, 48, 527, 1951.

1385. **Sadasivan, V.,** Studies on the biochemistry of zinc. II. The effect of intake of zinc on the metabolism of rats maintained on a stock diet, *Biochem. J.*, 49, 186, 1951.

1386. **Sadasivan, V.,** Studies on the biochemistry of zinc. III. Further investigations on the influence of zinc on metabolism, *Biochem. J.*, 52, 452, 1952.

1387. **Safai-Kutti, S. and Kutti, J.,** Zinc and anorexia nervosa, *Ann. Intern. Med.*, 100, 317, 1984.

1388. **Sahenk, Z. and Mendell, J. R.,** Ultrastructural study of zinc pyridine thione-induced peripheral neuropathy, *J. Neuropathol. Exp. Neurol.*, 38, 532, 1979.

1389. **Saldeen, T.,** On the protective effect of zinc against experimental liver damage due to choline-free diet or carbon tetrachloride, *Z. Gesamte Exp. Med.*, 150, 251, 1969.

1390. **Salem, S. I., Coward, W. A., Lunn, P. G., Hemming, F., Louisot, P., and Richard, M.,** Response of the reproductive system of male rats to protein and zinc deficiency during puberty, *Ann. Nutr. Metab.*, 28, 44, 1984.

1391. **Salgo, L., Pal, A., Moholi, K., Gyurkovits, K., and Kovacs, L.,** Significance and the role of zinc in the antibacterial (group B streptococci) action of the amniotic fluid, in *Trace Element Analytical Chemistry in Medicine and Biology,* Bratter, P. and Schramel, P., Eds., Walter de Gruyter, New York, 1984, 677.

1392. **Salvioli, Z., Faldella, G., Alessandroni, R., Lanari, M., and Benfenati, L.,** Plasma zinc in iron supplemented low birth weight infants, *Arch. Dis. Child.*, 61, 346, 1986.

1393. **Samson, H. H. and Diaz, J.,** Altered development of brain by neonatal ethanol exposure: zinc levels during and after exposure, *Alcoholism Clin. Exp. Res.*, 5, 563, 1981.

1394. **Sandow, A. and Bien, S. M.,** Blockade of neuromuscular transmission by zinc, *Nature (London),* 193, 689, 1962.

1395. **Sandow, A. and Issacson, A.,** Effects of methylene blue, acridine orange and zinc on muscular contraction, *Biochem. Biophys. Res. Commun.*, 2, 455, 1960.

1396. **Sandow, A. and Issacson, A.,** Topochemical factors in potentiation of contraction by heavy metal cations, *J. Gen. Physiol.*, 49, 937, 1966.

1397. **Sandstead, H. H.,** Zinc nutrition in the United States, *Am. J. Clin. Nutr.*, 26, 1251, 1973.

1398. **Sandstead, H. H.,** Zinc interference with copper metabolism, *JAMA,* 240, 2188, 1978.

1399. **Sandstead, H. H.,** Availability of zinc and its requirement in human subjects, in *Clinical, Biochemical and Nutritional Aspects of Trace Elements,* Prasad, A. S., Ed., Alan R. Liss, New York, 1982, 83.

1400. **Sandstead, H. H.,** Requirement of zinc in human subjects, *J. Am. Coll. Nutr.*, 4, 73, 1983.

1401. **Sandstead, H. H., Al-Ubaidi, Y. Y., Halas, E., and Fosmire, G.,** Zinc deficiency during the critical period for growth, in *Trace Element Metabolism in Animals,* Vol. 2, Hoekstra, W. G., Suttie, J. W., Ganther, G. E., and Mertz, W., Eds., University Park Press, Baltimore, 1974, 745.

1402. **Sandstead, H. H., Gillespie, D. D., and Brady, R. N.,** Zinc deficiency: effect on brain of the suckling rat, *Pediatr. Res.*, 6, 119, 1972.

1403. **Sandstead, H. H., Henrilson, L. K., Greger, J. L., Prasad, A. S., and Good, R. A.,** Zinc nutriture in the elderly in relation to taste acuity, immune response and wound healing, *Am. J. Clin. Nutr.*, Suppl. 36, 1046, 1983.

1404. **Sandstead, H. H. and Howard, L.,** Zinc deficiency in Crohn's disease, *Nutr. Rev.*, 40, 109, 1982.

1405. **Sandstead, H. H., Prasad, A. S., Schulert, A. R., Farid, Z., Miale, A., Bassilly, S., and Darby, W. J.,** Human zinc deficiency: endocrine manifestations and response to treatment, *Am. J. Clin. Nutr.*, 20, 422, 1967.

1406. **Sandstead, H. H. and Rinaldi, R. A.,** Impairment of DNA synthesis by dietary zinc deficiency in the rat, *J. Cell. Physiol.*, 73, 81, 1969.

1407. **Sandstead, H. H., Vo-Khactu, K. P., and Solomons, N. W.,** Conditioned zinc deficiencies, in *Trace Elements in Human Health and Disease,* Vol. 1, Prasad, A. S. and Oberleas, D., Eds., Academic Press, New York, 1976, 33.

1408. **Sandstrom, B. M. and Cederblad, A.,** Zinc absorption from composite meals. II. Influence of the main protein source, *Am. J. Clin. Nutr.*, 33, 1778, 1980.

1409. **Sandstrom, B. M., Davidson, L., Cederblad, A., and Lonnerdal, B.,** Oral iron, dietary ligands and zinc absorption, *J. Nutr.*, 115, 411, 1985.

1410. **Sanecki, R. K., Corbin, J. E., and Forbes, R. M.,** Tissue changes in dogs fed a zinc deficient ration, *Am. J. Vet. Res.*, 43, 1642, 1982.

1411. **Sas, B. and Bremner, I.,** Effect of acute stress on the absorption and distribution of zinc and on zinc-metallothionein production in the liver of the chick, *J. Inorg. Biochem.*, 11, 67, 1979.

1412. **Sas, B. and Pethes, G.,** Relationship between zinc deficiency and malonaldehyde production in rats connected with stability of the membranes, *Acta Physiol. Acad. Sci. Hung.*, 53, 208, 1979.

1413. **Sato, M., Mehra, R. K., and Bremner, I.,** Measurement of plasma metallothionein in the assessment of the zinc status of zinc deficient and stressed rats, *J. Nutr.*, 114, 1683, 1984.

1414. **Savin, J. A.,** Skin disease: the link with zinc, *Br. Med. J.*, 289, 1476, 1984.

1415. **Saylor, W. W., Morrow, F. D., and Leach, R. M.,** Copper and zinc-binding proteins in sheep liver and intestine: effects of dietary levels of the metals, *J. Nutr.*, 110, 460, 1980.

1416. **Scharz, F. J.,** Changes in copper and zinc absorption and excretion after copper deficiency, *Z. Tierphysiol. Tierernaehr. Futtermittelkd.*, 41, 335, 1979.

1417. **Schechter, P. J., Giroux, E. L., Schlienger, J. L., Hoenig, V., and Sjoerdsma, A.,** Distribution of serum zinc between albumin and alpha$_2$-macroglobulin in patients with decompensated hepatic cirrhosis, *Eur. J. Clin. Invest.*, 6, 147, 1976.

1418. **Schechter, P. J., Giroux, E. L., and Sjoerdsma, A.,** Zinc distribution in human serum with data on alterations in pregnancy and hepatic cirrhosis, in *Trace Element Metabolism in Man and Animals*, Vol. 3, Kirchgessner, M., Ed., Arbeitskreis fur Tiererhnarunsforschung, Weihenstephan, F. R. G., 1978, 343.

1419. **Schechter, P. J. and Prakash, N. J.,** Failure of oral l-histidine to influence appetite or affect zinc metabolism in man: a double-blind study, *Am. J. Clin. Nutr.*, 32, 1011, 1979.

1420. **Schelling, J., Muller-Hess, S., and Thonney, F.,** Effect of food on zinc absorption, *Lancet*, ii, 968, 1973.

1421. **Schenker, J. G., Hellerstein, S., Jungreis, E., and Polishuk, W. Z.,** Serum copper and zinc levels in patients taking oral contraceptives, *Fertil. Steril.*, 22, 229, 1971.

1422. **Scheuhammer, A. M. and Cherian, M. G.,** The influence of manganese on the distribution of essential trace elements. I. Regional distribution of manganese, sodium, potassium, magnesium, zinc, iron and copper in rat brain after chronic manganese exposure, *Toxicol. Appl. Pharmacol.*, 61, 227, 1981.

1423. **Schmidt, K., Bayer, W., Geckler, K., and Schieferstein, G.,** Determination of trace element concentrations in psoriatic and non-psoriatic scales with special regard to zinc, in *Trace Element Analytical Chemistry in Medicine and Biology*, Vol. 1, Bratter, P. and Schramel, P., Eds., Walter de Gruyter, New York, 1980, 167.

1424. **Schneeman, B. O., Lacy, D., Nay, D., Lefevre, M. L., Keen, C. L., Lonnerdal, B., and Hurley, L. S.,** Similar effects of zinc deficiency and restricted feeding on plasma lipids and lipoproteins in rats, *J. Nutr.*, 116, 1889, 1986.

1425. **Schneider, U. A. and Kirchgessner, M.,** Changes in the retention of zinc during gravidity, *Nutr. Metab.*, 23, 241, 1979.

1426. **Schoelmerich, J., Becher, M. S., Hoppe-Seyler, P., Matern, S., Haeussinger, D., Loehle, E., Koettgen, E., and Gerok, W.,** Zinc and vitamin A deficiency in patients with Crohn's disease is correlated with activity but not with localization or extent of disease, *Hepatogastroenterology*, 32, 34, 1985.

1427. **Schoelmerich, J., Lohle, E., Kottgen, E., and Gerok, W.,** Zinc and vitamin A in liver cirrhosis, *Hepatogastroenterology*, 30, 119, 1983.

1428. **Schoenfeld, C., Amelar, R. D., Dubin, L., and Numeroff, M.,** Prolactin, fructose and zinc levels found in human seminal plasma, *Fertil. Steril.*, 32, 206, 1979.

1429. **Schoomaker, E. B., Brewer, G. J., and Oelshlegel, F. J.,** Zinc in the treatment of homozygous sickle cell anemia: studies in an animal model, *Am. J. Hematol.*, 1, 45, 1976.

1430. **Schott, G. D. and Delves, H. T.,** Plasma zinc levels with anticonvulsant therapy, *Br. J. Clin. Pharmacol.*, 5, 279, 1978.

1431. **Schroeder, H. A., Baker, J. T., Hansen, N. M., Size, J. G., and Wise, R. A.,** Vascular reactivity of rats altered by cadmium and a zinc chelate, *Arch. Environ. Health*, 21, 609, 1970.

1432. **Schroeder, H. A., Nason, A. P., Tipton, I. H., and Balassa, J. P.,** Essential trace elements in man: zinc relation to environmental cadmium, *J. Chronic. Dis.*, 20, 179, 1967.

1433. **Schwartz, A. E., Ledicotte, G. W., Fink, R. W., and Friedman, E. W.,** Trace elements in normal and malignant human breast tissue, *Surgery*, 76, 325, 1974.

1434. **Schwarz, F. J., Kirchgessner, M., and Roth, H.-P.,** Influence of picolinic acid and citric acid on intestinal absorption of zinc in vitro and in vivo, *Res. Exp. Med.*, 182, 39, 1983.

1435. **Schwarz, F. J., Kirchgessner, M., and Sherif, S. Y.,** Intestinal absorption of zinc during gravidity and lactation, *Res. Exp. Med.*, 179, 35, 1981.

1436. **Scott, B. J. and Bradwell, A. R.,** Zinc status and pregnancy outcome, *Lancet*, i, 894, 1981.

1437. **Scott, D. A.,** Crystalline insulin, *Biochem. J.*, 28, 1592, 1934.

1438. **Scott, D. B. M. and Sano, M. F.,** Disruption of the estrous cycle of hamsters on a zinc deficient diet, *Fed. Proc. Fed. Am. Soc. Exp. Biol.*, 34, 940, 1975.

1439. **Scribner, M. D.,** Zinc sulphate and axillary perspiration odor, *Arch. Dermatol.*, 113, 1302, 1977.

1440. **Schriener, G. E., Mahar, J. F., Freeman, R. B., and O'Connell, J. M. B.,** Problems of hemodialysis, *Proc. 3rd Int. Congr. Nephrol.*, 3, 316, 1967.

1441. **Seal, C. J. and Heaton, F. W.,** Chemical factors affecting the intestinal absorption of zinc in vitro and in vivo, *Br. J. Nutr.*, 50, 317, 1983.

1442. **Seal, C. J. and Heaton, F. W.,** Zinc transfer among proteins in rat duodenal mucosa, *Ann. Nutr. Metab.*, 31, 55, 1987.

1443. **Seelig, M. S.,** Auto-immune complications of D-penicillamine. A possible result of zinc and magnesium depletion and of pyridoxine inactivation, *J. Am. Coll. Nutr.*, 1, 207, 1982.

1444. **Segel, G. B., Simon, W., Lichtman, A. H., and Lichtman, M. A.,** The activation of lymphocyte plasma membrane (Na, K) ATPase by EGTA is explained better by zinc than by cadmium chelation, *J. Biol. Chem.*, 256, 6629, 1981.

1445. **Seifter, S., Takahashi, S., and Harper, E.,** Further demonstration that cystein reacts with the metal components of collagenase, *Biochim. Biophys. Acta,* 214, 559, 1970.

1446. **Sella, G. E., Cunnane, S. C., and McInnes, R. A.,** Zinc, copper, seminal volume, hormone correlations in a male infertility study, *Trace Subst. Environ. Health,* 14, 217, 1980.

1447. **Senapati, A. and Thompson, R. P. H.,** Zinc deficiency and the prolonged accumulation of zinc in wounds, *Br. J. Surg.,* 72, 583, 1985.

1448. **Serjeant, G. R., Galloway, R. E., and Gueri, M. C.,** Oral zinc sulphate in sickle cell ulcers, *Lancet,* ii, 891, 1970.

1449. **Seutton, E. and Sutorius, A. H. M.,** The quantitative analysis of some constituents of srude sweat. II. Zinc, copper, iron sialic acid content and oxidative activity, *Dermatologia,* 145, 203, 1972.

1450. **Sever, L. E. and Emanuel, I.,** Is ther a connection between maternal zinc deficiency and congenital malformations of the central nervous system in man?, *Teratology,* 7, 117, 1973.

1451. **Shah, B. G., Giroux, A., and Belonger, B.,** Bioavailability of zinc in infant cereals, *Nutr. Metab.,* 23, 286, 1979.

1452. **Shah, B. G., Giroux, A., Belonger, B., and Jones, J. D.,** Beneficial effect of zinc supplementation on reproduction in rats fed rapeseed protein concentrate, *Nutr. Metab.,* 23, 275, 1979.

1453. **Shapcott, D.,** Hair and plasma in the diagnosis of zinc deficiency, in *Clinical Applications of Recent Advances in Zinc Metabolism,* Prasad, A. S., Dreosti, I. E., and Hetzel, B. S., Eds., Alan R. Liss, New York, 1982, 121.

1454. **Shapcott, D., Giguere, R., and Lemeiux, B.,** Zinc and taurine in Freidreich's ataxia, *Can. J. Neurol. Sci.,* 11, 623, 1984.

1455. **Sharma, R., Ahuja, K. L., Prasad, S., and Kumar, A.,** Antiviral effect of zinc ions on aphthovirus in BHK-21 cell line, *Acta Virol.,* 29, 517, 1985.

1456. **Shaw, J. C. L.,** Trace elements in the fetus and young infant, *Am. J. Child. Dis.,* 133, 1260, 1979.

1457. **Shaw, N. A., Dickey, H. C., Bringham, H. H., Blamberg, D. L., and Witter, J. F.,** Zinc deficiency in female rabbits, *Lab. Anim.,* 8, 1, 1974.

1458. **Shears, M. A. and Fletcher, G. L.,** The binding of zinc to the soluble proteins of intestinal mucosa in winter flounder *(Pseudopleuronectes americanus), Comp. Biochem. Physiol.,* 64B, 297, 1979.

1459. **Sheldon, W. L., Aspillaga, M. O., Smith, P. A., and Lind, T.,** The effects of oral iron supplementation on zinc and magnesium levels during pregnancy, *Br. J. Obstet. Gynecol.,* 92, 892, 1985.

1460. **Sheline, G. E., Chaikoff, I. L., Jones, H. B., and Montgonery, M. L.,** Studies on the metabolism of zinc with the aid of its radioactive isotope. II. The distribution of administered radioactive zinc in the tissues of mice and dogs, *J. Biol. Chem.,* 149, 139, 1943.

1461. **Shingwehar, A. G., Mohanram, M., and Reddy, V.,** Effect of zinc supplementation on plasma levels of vitamin A and retinol-binding protein in malnourished children, *Clin. Chim. Acta,* 93, 97, 1979.

1462. **Shiraishi, N., Yamamoto, H., Kimoto, M., Shiragami, T., Togami, I., Niiya, H., and Aono, K.,** Distribution of protein-bound zinc in serum of analbuminemic rats, *Biochem. Biophys. Res. Commun.,* 125, 45, 1984.

1463. **Shyamala, G. and Yeh, Y.-F.,** Is the estrogen-binding protein of mammary glands a metalloprotein?, *Biochem. Biophys. Res. Commun.,* 64, 408, 1975.

1464. **Siegler, R. L., Eggert, J. V., and Udomkesmalee, E.,** Diagnostic indices of zinc deficiency in children with renal diseases, *Ann. Clin. Lab. Sci.,* 11, 428, 1981.

1465. **Silverman, B., Kwaitkowski, D., Pinto, J., and Rivlin, R.,** Disturbances in zinc binding to jejunal proteins induced by ethanol ingestion in rats, *Clin. Res.,* 27, 555A, 1979.

1466. **Simkin, P. A.,** Oral zinc sulphate in rheumatoid arthritis, *Lancet,* ii, 539, 1976.

1467. **Simkin, P. A.,** Zinc sulphate in rheumatoid arthritis, in *Zinc Metabolism: Current Aspects in Health and Disease,* Prasad, A. S. and Brewer, G. J., Eds., Alan R. Liss, New York, 1977, 343.

1468. **Simkin, P. A.,** Oral zinc and rheumatoid arthritis, *Arthritis Rheum.,* 24 865, 1981.

1469. **Simmer, K., Punchard, N. A., Murphy, G., and Thompson, R. P. H.,** Prostaglandin production and zinc depletion in human pregnancy, *Pediatr. Res.,* 19, 697, 1985.

1470. **Simmer, K. and Thompson, R. P. H.,** Zinc in the fetus and newborn, *Acta Paediatr. Scand.,* 319, 158, 1985.

1471. **Simmer, K. and Thompson, R. P. H.,** Maternal zinc and intrauterine growth retardation, *Clin. Sci.,* 68, 395, 1985.

1472. **Simpson, R. I. D. and Bryce-Smith, D.,** Cutaneous manifestations of zinc deficiency during treatment with anticonvulsants, *Br. Med. J.,* i, 1215, 1985.

1473. **Singal, P. K., Kapur, N., Dhillon, K. S., Beamish, P. E., and Dhalla, N. S.,** Role of free radicals in catecholamine-induced cardiomyopathy, *Can. J. Physiol. Pharmacol.,* 60, 1390, 1982.

1474. **Sinquin, G., Morfin, K., Charles, J.-F., and Floch, H. H.,** Testosterone metabolism by homogenates of human prostates with benign hyperplasia, *J. Steroid Biochem.,* 17, 395, 1982.

1475. **Sinquin, G., Morfin, R. F., Charles, J.-F., and Floch, H. H.,** Testosterone metabolism by homogenates of human prostate with benign hyperplasia: effects of zinc, cadmium and other bivalent cations, *J. Steroid Biochem.*, 20, 773, 1984.

1476. **Sinthusek, G. and Magee, A. C.,** Relationships of dietary zinc/copper ratios to plasma cholesterol and liver trace mineral deposition in young rats fed saturated and unsaturated fats, *Nutr. Res.*, 4, 841, 1984.

1477. **Skandhan, K. P., Skandhan, S., and Mehta, Y. B.,** Semen electrolytes in normal and infertile subjects. II. Zinc, *Experientia*, 34, 1476, 1978.

1478. **Slaby, I., Lind, B., and Holmgren, A.,** T7 DNA polymerase is not a zinc metalloenzyme and the polymerase and exonuclease activities are inhibited by zinc ions, *Biochem. Biophys. Res. Commun.*, 122, 1410, 1984.

1479. **Slavik, M., Danilson, D., Keiser, H. R., and Henkin, R. I.,** Alteration in metabolism of copper and zinc after administration of 6-azauridine triacetate, *Biochem. Pharmacol.*, 22, 2349, 1973.

1480. **Smit, A. J., Hoorntje, S. J., and Donker, A. J. M.,** Zinc deficiency during captopril treatment, *Nephron*, 34, 196, 1983.

1481. **Smit, P. and Gibson, R. S.,** Relationship of growth to biochemical and dietary zinc status in some preschool children, *Proc. Can. Fed. Biol. Soc.*, 28, PA-23, 1985.

1482. **Smith, D. K.,** Effect of topical zinc on delayed hypersensitivity responsiveness (DHR), *J. Am. Coll. Nutr.*, 3, 292, 1984.

1483. **Smith, J. C., Jr.,** Heritable hyperzincemia in humans, in *Zinc Metabolism: Current Aspects in Health and Disease*, Prasad, A. S. and Oberlease, D., Eds., Alan R. Liss, New York, 1977, 181.

1484. **Smith, J. C., Jr.,** The vitamin A-zinc connection: a review, *Ann. N.Y. Acad. Sci.*, 355, 62, 1980.

1485. **Smith, J. C., Jr.,** Interrelationships of zinc and vitamin A metabolism: a review, in *Clinical, Biochemical and Nutritional Aspects of Trace Elements*, Prasad, A. S., Ed., Alan R. Liss, New York, 1982, 239.

1486. **Smith, J. C., Jr., Brown, E. D., and Cassidy, W. A.,** Zinc and vitamin A: interrelationships, in *Zinc Metabolism: Current Aspects in Health and Disease*, Prasad, A. S., Ed., Alan R. Liss, New York, 1977, 29.

1487. **Smith, J. C. Jr., Brown, E. D., McDaniel, E. G., and Chan, W.,** Alterations in vitamin A metabolism during zinc deficiency and food and growth restriction, *J. Nutr.*, 106, 569, 1976.

1488. **Smith, J. C., Jr., McDaniel, E. G., Fann, F. F., and Halsted, J. A.,** Zinc: a trace metal essential in vitamin A metabolism, *Science*, 181, 954, 1973.

1489. **Smith, J. C., Jr., McDaniel, E. G., McBean, L. D., Doft, F. S., and Halsted, J. A.,** Effect of microorganisms upon zinc metabolism using germ-free and conventional rats, *J. Nutr.*, 102, 711, 1972.

1490. **Smith, J. C., Jr., Zeller, J. A., Brown, E. D., and Ong, S. C.,** Elevated plasma zinc: a heritable anomaly, *Science*, 193, 996, 1976.

1491. **Smith, J. E., Brown, E. D., and Smith, J. C., Jr.,** The effect of zinc deficiency on the metabolism of retinol-binding protein in the rat, *J. Lab. Clin. Med.*, 84, 692, 1974.

1492. **Smith, K. T., Cousin, R. J., Silbon, B. L., and Failla, M. L.,** Zinc absorption and metabolism by isolated vascularly prefused rat intestine, *J. Nutr.*, 108, 1849, 1978.

1493. **Smith, R. M., King, R. A., Spargo, R. M., Cheek, D. M., Field, J. B., and Veitch, L. G.,** Growth-retarded aboriginal children with low plasma zinc levels do not show a growth response to supplementary zinc, *Lancet*, i, 923, 1985.

1494. **Smith, S. E. and Larson, E. J.,** Zinc toxicity in rats. Antagonistic effects of copper and silver, *J. Biol. Chem.* 163, 29, 1946.

1495. **Snaith, S. M., and Lewy, G. A.,** Purification and properties of alpha-D-mannosidase from Jack-bean meal, *Biochem. J.*, 110, 663, 1968.

1496. **Snyder, D. R., Gralla, E. J., and Coleman, G. L.,** Preliminary neurological evaluation of generalized weakness in zinc-pyrithione treated rats, *Food Cosmet. Toxicol.*, 15, 43, 1977.

1497. **Sobocinski, P. Z.,** Induction of hypozincemia and hepatic metallothionein synthesis in hypersensitivity reactions, *Proc. Soc. Exp. Biol. Med.*, 160, 175, 1979.

1498. **Sobocinski, P. Z., Knutsen, G. L., Canterbury, W. J., and Hauer, E. C.,** Altered zinc homeostasis and hepatic accumulation of metallothionein in indomethacin-induced enteropathy, *Toxicol. Appl. Pharmacol.*, 50, 557, 1979.

1499. **Solomons, N. W.,** On the assessment of zinc and copper nutriture in man, *Am. J. Clin. Nutr.*, 32, 856, 1979.

1500. **Solomons, N. W.,** Zinc and copper in human nutrition, in *Zinc and Copper in Medicine*, Karcioglu, Z. A. and Sarper, R. M., Eds. Charles C Thomas, Springfield, Ill., 1980, 224.

1501. **Solomons, N. W.,** Zinc and copper in hepatobiliary and pancreatic disorders, in *Zinc and Copper in Medicine*, Karcioglu, Z. A. and Sarper, R. M., Eds., Charles C Thomas, Springfield, Ill., 1980, 317.

1502. **Solomons, N. W.,** Biological availability of zinc in humans, *Am. J. Clin. Nutr.*, 35, 1046, 1982.

1503. **Solomons, N. W. and Jacob, R. A.,** Studies on the bioavailability of zinc in man. IV. Effect of heme and non-heme iron on the absorption of zinc, *Am. J. Clin. Nutr.*, 34, 475, 1981.

1504. **Solomons, N. W., Helitzer-Allen, D. L., and Villar, J.,** Zinc needs in pregnancy, *Clin. Nutr.*, 5, 63, 1986.
1505. **Solomons, N. W., Jacob, R. A., Pineda, O., and Viteri, F. E.,** Studies on the bioavailability of zinc in man. I. Effects of the Guatemalan rural diet and of the iron-fortifying agent NaFeEDTA, *J. Nutr.*, 109, 1519, 1979.
1506. **Solomons, N. W., Jacob, R. A., Pineda, O., and Viteri, F. E.,** Studies on the bioavailability of zinc in man. II. Absorption of zinc from organic and inorganic sources, *J. Lab. Clin. Med.*, 94, 335, 1979.
1507. **Solomons, N. W., Jacob, R. A., Pineda, O., and Viteri, F. E.,** Studies on the bioavailability of zinc in man. III. Effects of ascorbic acid on zinc absorption, *Am. J. Clin. Nutr.*, 32, 2495, 1979.
1508. **Solomons, N. W., Khactu, K. V., and Sandstead, H. H.,** Zinc nutrition in regional enteritis, *Clin. Res.*, 22, 582A, 1974.
1509. **Solomons, N. W., Reiger, C. H. L., Jacob, R. A., Rothberg, R., and Sandstead, H. H.,** Zinc nutriture and taste acuity in patients with cystic fibrosis, *Nutr. Res.*, 1, 13, 1981.
1510. **Solomons, N. W., Rosenberg, I. H., and Sandstead, H. H.,** Zinc nutrition in celiac sprue, *Am. J. Clin. Nutr.*, 29, 371, 1976.
1511. **Solomons, N. W., Rosenberg, I. H., Sandstead, H. H., and Vo-Khactu, K. P.,** Zinc deficiency in Crohn's disease, *Digestion*, 16, 87, 1977.
1512. **Solomons, N. W., Rosenfield, R. L., Jacob, R. A., and Sandstead, H. H.,** Growth retardation and zinc nutrition, *Pediatr. Res.*, 10, 923, 1976.
1513. **Solomons, N. W., Rosenfield, R. L., Jacob, R. A., and Sandstead, H. H.,** A reexamination of the effect of human growth hormone (HGH) on trace mineral metabolism, *Clin. Res.*, 27, 377A, 1979.
1514. **Solomons, N. W. and Russell, R. M.,** The interaction of vitamin A and zinc: implications for human nutrition, *Am. J. Clin. Nutr.*, 33, 2030, 1980.
1515. **Somers, M. and Underwood, E. J.,** Ribonuclease activity and nucleic acid and protein metabolism in the testes of zinc deficient rats, *Aust. J. Biol. Sci.*, 22, 1277, 1969.
1516. **Son, S. M. and Magee, A. C.,** Zinc and vitamin B_6 interrelationships on growth and trace mineral deposition of young rats fed adequate and marginal protein, *Nutr. Rep. Int.*, 35, 191, 1986.
1517. **Sondheimer, J. H. and Mahajan, S. K.,** Relationship of plasma zinc to serum lipids in hemodialysis patients, *Clin. Res.*, 32, 740A, 1984.
1518. **Sondheimer, J. H. and Mahajan, S. K.,** Inverse relationship of plasma zinc to serum lipids in hemodialysis patients, *Am. J. Coll. Nutr.*, 3, 283, 1984.
1519. **Sonoki, S. and Ikezana, H.,** Studies of phospholipase C from *Pseudomonas aureofaciens*. II. Further studies on the properties of the enzyme, *J. Biochem. (Tokyo)*, 80, 361, 1976.
1520. **Song, M. K. and Adham, N. F.,** A possible role for a prostaglandin-like substance in zinc absorption, *Fed. Proc. Fed. Am. Soc. Exp. Biol.*, 35, 1667, 1976.
1521. **Song, M. K. and Adham, N. F.,** Role of prostaglandin E_2 in zinc absorption in the rat, *Am. J. Physiol.*, 234, E99, 1978.
1522. **Song, M. K. and Adham, N. F.,** Evidence for an important role of prostaglandins E_2 and $F_{2\alpha}$ in the regulation of zinc transport in the rat, *J. Nutr.*, 109, 2152, 1979.
1523. **Song, M. K. and Adham, N. F.,** Influence of zinc on prostaglandin E_2 and F_{2alpha} metabolism in plasma and small intestine of rats, *Fed. Proc. Fed. Am. Soc. Exp. Biol.*, 43, 478, 1984.
1524. **Song, M. K. and Adham, N. F.,** Relationship between zinc and prostaglandin metabolism in plasma and small intestine of rats, *Am. J. Clin. Nutr.*, 41, 1201, 1985.
1525. **Song, M. K., Adham, N. F., and Ament, M. E.,** Metabolism of zinc binding ligands in rat small intestine, *Biol. Trace Elem. Res.*, 6, 181, 1984.
1526. **Song, M. K., Littner, M. R., Adham, N. F., Kazmi, G. M., and Lott, F. D.,** Effect of oral administration of arachidonic acid on prostaglandin and zinc metabolism in plasma and small intestine of the rat, *Prostagl. Leukotr Med.*, 17, 159, 1985.
1527. **Soskel, N. T., Watanabe, S., Hammond, E., Sandberg, L. B., Renzetti, A. D., and Crapo, J. D.,** A copper deficient, zinc supplemented diet produces emphysema in pigs, *Am. Rev. Respir. Dis.*, 126, 316, 1982.
1528. **Southon, S., Gee, J. M., Bayliss, C. E., Wyatt, G. M., Horn, N., and Johnson, I. T.,** Intestinal microflora, morphology and enzyme activity in zinc deficient and zinc-supplemented rats, *Br. J. Nutr.*, 55, 603, 1986.
1529. **Southon, S., Gee, J. M., and Johnson, I. T.,** Intestinal uptake of galactose in rats recovering from experimental zinc deficiency, *Proc. Nutr. Soc.*, 42, 90A, 1983.
1530. **Southon, S., Gee, J. M., and Johnson, I. T.,** Hexose absorption from jejunal loops *in situ* in zinc deficient and zinc-supplemented rats, *Br.J. Nutr.*, 55, 193, 1986.
1531. **Southon, S., Gee, J. M., and Johnson, I. T.,** Hexose transport and mucosal morphology in the small intestine of the zinc deficient rat, *Br. J. Nutr.*, 52, 371, 1984.
1532. **Southon, S., Johnson, I. T., and Gee, J. M.,** Anorexia, depression and zinc deficiency, *Lancet*, ii, 1162, 1984.

1533. **Southon, S., Johnson, I. T., Gee, J. M., and Gee, M. G.,** Effect of zinc deficiency on intestinal uptake of galactose in the rat, *Proc. Nutr. Soc.,* 41, 134A, 1984.

1534. **Southon, S., Livesey, G., Gee, J. M., and Johnson, I. T.,** Intestinal cellular proliferation and protein synthesis in zinc deficient rats, *Br. J. Nutr.,* 53, 595, 1985.

1535. **Spears, J. W., Hatfield, E. E., and Forbes, M. R.,** Interrelationship between nickel and zinc in the rat, *J. Nutr.,* 108, 307, 1978.

1536. **Spencer, H., Kramer, L., Norris, C., and Osis, D.,** Effect of calcium and phosphorus on zinc metabolism in man, *Am. J. Clin. Nutr.,* 40, 1213, 1984.

1537. **Spencer, H., Kramer, L., and Osis, D.,** Zinc balance in humans, in *Clinical, Biochemical and Nutritional Aspects of Trace Elements,* Prasad, A. S., Ed., Alan R. Liss, New York, 1982, 103.

1538. **Spencer, H., Rasmussen, C. R., Holtzman, R. B., and Kramer, L.,** Metabolic balances of cadmium, copper, manganese and zinc in man, *Am. J. Clin. Nutr.,* 32, 1867, 1979.

1539. **Spencer, H., Rosoff, B., Lewin, I., and Samachson, J.,** Studies of zinc-65 metabolism in man, in *Zinc Metabolism,* Prasad, A. S., Ed., Charles C Thomas, Springfield, Ill., 1966, 339.

1540. **Spencer, H., Vankinscott, V., Lewin, I., and Samachson, J.,** Zinc-65 metabolism during low and high calcium intake in man, *J. Nutr.,* 86, 169, 1965.

1541. **Spencer, J. C.,** Direct relationship between the body's copper/zinc ratio, ventricular premature beats and sudden coronary death, *Am. J. Clin. Nutr.,* 32, 1184, 1979.

1542. **Spray, C. M. and Widdowson, E. M.,** The effect of growth and development on the composition of mammals, *Br. J. Nutr.,* 4, 332, 1951.

1543. **Sprenger, K. B. G., Bundschu, D., Lewis, K., Spohn, B., Schmitz, J., and Franz, H.-E.,** Improvement of uremic neuropathy and hypogeusia by dialysate zinc supplementation: a double-blind study, *Kidney Int.,* Suppl. 16, 5315, 1983.

1544. **Srinivasan, S. and Balwani, J. H.,** Effects of zinc sulphate on carbon tetrachloride hepatotoxicity, *Acta Pharmacol. Toxicol.,* 27, 424, 1969.

1545. **Srivastava, A. and Setty, B. S.,** The distribution of zinc in the subcellular fractions of the rhesus monkey testes, *Biol. Trace Elem. Res.,* 7, 83, 1985.

1546. **Stacey, N. H. and Klassen, C. D.,** Zinc uptake by isolated rat hepatocytes, *Biochim. Biophys. Acta,* 640, 693, 1981.

1546a. **Stankovic, H. and Mikac-Devic, D.,** Zinc and copper in human semen, *Clin. Chim. Acta,* 70, 123, 1976.

1547. **Startcher, B. C., Hill, C. H., and Madaras, J. G.,** Effect of zinc deficiency on bone collagenase and collagen metabolism, *J. Nutr.,* 110, 2095, 1980.

1548. **Statter, M. and Krieger, I.,** Zinc transport in human fibroblasts, *Pediatr. Res.,* 17, 239, 1983.

1549. **Steele, T. H.,** Flow-related characteristics of zinc excretion in man, *J. Lab. Clin. Med.,* 78, 1019, 1971.

1550. **Steger, J. W.,** Acute zinc depletion syndrome during parenteral hyperalimentation, *Int. J. Dermatol.,* 18, 472, 1979.

151. **Steinhardt, H. J. and Adibi, S. A.,** Interaction between transport of zinc and other solutes in human intestine, *Am. J. Physiol.,* 247, G176, 1984.

1552. **Steinhauer, H. B., Batsford, S., Schollemeyer, P., and Kluthe, R.,** Studies on thromboxane B_2 and prostaglandin E_2 production in the course of murine autoimmune disease; Inhibition by oral histidine and zinc supplementation, *Clin. Nephrol.,* 24, 63, 1985.

1553. **Stengaard-Pedersen, K.,** Inhibition of enkephalin binding to opiate receptors by zinc ions: possible physiological importance for the brain, *Acta Pharmacol. Toxicol.,* 50, 213, 1982.

1554. **Stengaard-Pedersen, K., Fredens, K., and Larsson, L.-I.,** Enkephalin and zinc in the hippocampal mossy fibre system, *Brain Res.,* 212, 230, 1981.

1555. **Stengaard-Pedersen, K., Fredens, K., and Larsson, L.-I.,** Inhibition of opiate receptor binding by zinc ions: possible physiological importance in the hippocampus, *Peptides,* Suppl. 2, 27, 1981.

1556. **Stengaard-Pedersen, K., Larsson, L.-I., Fredens, K., and Rehfeld, J. F.,** Modulation of cholecystokinin concentrations in the rat hippocampus by chelation of heavy metals, *Proc. Natl. Acad. Sci. U.S.A.,* 81, 5876, 1984.

1557. **Stephan, J. K. and Hsu, J. M.,** Effect of zinc deficiency and wounding on DNA synthesis in rat skin, *J. Nutr.,* 103, 548, 1973.

1558. **Stephenson, R. A., Luft, B. A., Pedrotti, P. W., and Remington, J. S.,** Inhibition of mouse natural killer cell activity by zinc, *J. Natl. Cancer Inst.,* 74, 1067, 1980.

1559. **Stevens, M. D., MacKenzie, W. F., and Anand, V. D.,** A simplified method for determination of zinc in whole blood, plasma and erythrocytes by atomic absorption spectrophotometry, *Biochem. Med.,* 18, 158, 1977.

1560. **Stirn, F. E., Elvehjem, C. A., and Hart, E. B.,** The indispensibility of zinc in the nutrition of the rat, *J. Biol. Chem.,* 109, 347, 1935.

1561. **Stocks, P. and Davies, R. I.,** Epidemiological evidence from chemical and spectrographic analyses that soil is concerned in the causation of cancer, *Br. J. Cancer,* 14, 8, 1960.

1562. **Stowe, H. D.,** Biliary excretion of cadmium by rats: effects of zinc, cadmium and selenium pre-treatments, *J. Toxicol. Environ. Health,* 2, 45, 1976.

1563. **Strain, W. H., Hirsh, F. S., and Michel, B.,** Increased copper/zinc ratios in acrodermatitis enteropathica, *Lancet,* i, 1196, 1975.

1564. **Strain, W. H., Huegin, F., Lankau, C. A., Berliner, W. P., McCovey, R. K., and Pories, W. J.,** Zinc-65 retention by aortic tissue of rats, *Int. J. Appl. Radiat.,* 15, 231, 1964.

1565. **Strain, W. H., Macon, W. L., Pories, W. J., Perim, C., Adams, F. D., and Hill, O. A.,** Excretion of trace elements in bile, in *Trace Element Metabolism in Aniamsl,* Vol. 2, Hoekstra, W. H., Suttie, J. W., Ganther, H. E., and Mertz, W., Eds., University Park Press, Baltimore, 1974, 644.

1566. **Strain, W. H. and Pories, W. J.,** Zinc levels of hair as tools in zinc metabolism, in *Zinc Metabolism,* Prasad, A. S., Ed., Charles C Thomas, Springfield, Ill., 1966, 363.

1567. **Stromberg, H. E. and Agren, M. S.,** Topical Zinc oxide treatment improves arterial and venous leg ulcers, *Br. J. Dermatol.,* 111, 461, 1984.

1568. **Sturniolo, G. C., Martin, A., Gurrieri, G., and Naccarato, R.,** The effects of prostaglandin synthetase inhibition on the oral zinc tolerance test in man, *Gastroenterol. Clin. Biol.,* 7, 933, 1983.

1569. **Sturniolo, G. C., Molokhia, M. M., Sheilds, R., and Turnberg, L. A.,** Zinc absorption in Crohn's disease, *Gut,* 21, 387, 1980.

1570. **Sturtevant, F. M.,** Zinc deficiency, acrodermatitis, optic atrophy, subacute myelo-optic neuropathy and 5,7-dihalo-8-quinolinols, *Pediatrics,* 65, 610, 1980.

1571. **Suh, S. M. and Firek, A. F.,** Magnesium and zinc deficiency and growth retardation in offspring of alcoholic rats, *J. Am. Coll. Nutr.,* 1, 193, 1983.

1572. **Suita, S., Ikeda, K., Hayashida, Y., Naito, K., Handa, N., and Doki, T.,** Zinc and copper requirements during parenteral nutrition in the newborn, *J. Pediatr. Surg.,* 19, 126, 1984.

1573. **Sullivan, J. F.,** Effect of alcohol on urinary zinc excretion, *Q. J. Stud. Alcohol,* 23, 216, 1962.

1574. **Sullivan, J. F., Blotcky, A. J., Jetton, M. M., Hahn, H. K. J., and Burch, R. E.,** Serum levels of selenium, calcium, copper, magnesium and zinc in various human diseases, *J. Nutr.,* 109, 1432, 1979.

1575. **Sullivan, J. F. and Burch, R. E.,** Potential role of zinc in liver disease, in *Trace Elements in Human Health and Disease,* Vol. 1, Prasad, A. S. and Oberleas, D., Eds., Academic Press, New York, 1976, 67.

1576. **Sullivan, J. F., Burch, R. E., Qigley, H. J., and Magee, D. F.,** Zinc deficiency and decreased pancreatic secretory response, *Am. J. Physiol.,* 227, 105, 1974.

1577. **Sullivan, J. F. and Heaney, R. P.,** Zinc metabolism in alcoholic liver disease, *Am. J. Clin. Nutr.,* 23, 170, 1970.

1578. **Sullivan, J. F., Jetton, M. M., and Burch, R. E.,** A zinc tolerance test, *J. Lab. Clin. Med.,* 93, 485, 1979.

1579. **Sullivan, J. F., Jetton, M. M, Hahn, H. K. J., and Burch, R. E.,** Enhanced lipid peroxidation in liver microsomes of zinc deficient rats, *Am. J. Clin. Nutr.,* 33, 51, 1980.

1580. **Sullivan, J. F. and Lankford, H. G.,** Zinc metabolism and chronic alcoholism, *Am. J. Clin. Nutr.,* 17, 57, 1965.

1581. **Sullivan, J. F., O'Grady, J., and Lankford, H. G.,** The zinc content of pancreatic secretions, *Gastroenterology,* 48, 438, 1965.

1582. **Sullivan, J. F., Williams, R. V., and Burch, R. E.,** Metabolism of zinc and selenium in cirrhotic patients during 6 weeks of zinc ingestion, *Alcoholism,* 3, 235, 1979.

1583. **Sun, I. L. and Crane, F. L.,** Evidence for zinc function in the magnesium/calcium-stimulated ATPase of *E. coli* membranes, *Biochem. Biophys. Res. Commun.,* 65, 1334, 1975.

1584. **Sunamoto, J., Shironita, M., and Kawauchi, N.,** Liposomal membranes. V. Interaction of zinc (II) ion with egg phosphatidylcholine liposomes, *Bull. Chem. Soc. Jpn.,* 53, 2778, 1980.

1585. **Suso, F. A. and Edwards, H. M.,** Binding of EDTA, histidine and acetylsalicylic acid in zinc-protein complexes in intestinal content, intestinal mucosa and blood plasma, *Nature (London),* 236, 230, 1972.

1586. **Sutton, W. R. and Nelson, V. E.,** Studies of zinc, *Proc. Soc. Exp. Biol. Med.,* 36, 211, 1937.

1587. **Suzuki, H., Igarashi, Y., Konno, T., and Arai, N.,** Inclusion bodies in the Paneth cells in zinc deficiency, *Lancet,* i, 734, 1979.

1588. **Svenson, K. L. G., Hallgren, R., Johansson, E., and Lindh, U.,** Reduced zinc in peripheral blood cells from patients with inflammatory connective tissue disease, *Inflammation,* 9, 189, 1985.

1589. **Swaminathan, R., Chapman, C., Segall, N. H., and Morgan, D. B.,** Red blood cell composition in thyroid disease, *Lancet,* ii, 1382, 1976.

1590. **Swann, J. C., Reynolds, J. J., and Galloway, W. A.,** Zinc metalloenzyme properties of active and latent collagenase from rabbit bone, *Biochem. J.,* 195, 41, 1981.

1591. **Swanson, C. A. and King, J. C.,** Zinc utilization in pregnant and non-pregnant women fed controlled diets providing the zinc RDA, *J. Nutr.,* 112, 697, 1982.

1592. **Swanson, C. A., Turnlund, J. R., and King, J. C.,** Effect of dietary zinc sources and pregnancy on zinc utilization in adult women fed controlled diets, *J. Nutr.,* 113, 2557, 1983.

1593. **Swenerton, H. and Hurley, L. S.,** Severe zinc deficiency in male and female rats, *J. Nutr.,* 95, 8, 1968.

1594. **Swenerton, H. and Hurley, L. S.**, Teratogenic effects of a chelating agent and their prevention by zinc, *Science,* 173, 62, 1971.

1595. **Swenerton, H., Shrader, R., and Hurley, L. S.**, Zinc deficient embryos: reduced thymidine incorporation, *Science,* 166, 1014, 1969.

1596. **Tamura, T., Shane, B., Baer, M. T., and King, J. C.**, Absorption of mono- and polyglutamyl folates in zinc-depleted men, *Am. J. Clin. Nutr.*, 31, 1984, 1978.

1597. **Tanaka, H., Inomata, K., and Arima, M.**, Zinc supplementation in ethanol-treated pregnant rats increases the metabolic activity in the fetal hippocampus, *Brain Dev.*, 5, 549, 1983.

1598. **Tanaka, H., Nakazawa, K., Suzuki, N., and Arima, M.**, Prevention possibility for brain dysfunction in the rat with the fetal alcohol syndrome — low zinc status and hypoglycemia, *Brain Dev.*, 4, 429, 1982.

1599. **Tapazoglou, E., Prasad, A. S., Hill, G., Brewer, G. J., and Kaplan, J.**, Decreased natural killer cell activity in patients with zinc deficiency with sickle cell disease, *J. Lab. Clin. Med.*, 105, 19, 1985.

1600. **Taper, L. J., Minners, M. L., and Ritchey, S. J.**, Effects of zinc intake on copper balance in adult females, *Am. J. Clin. Nutr.*, 33, 1077, 1980.

1601. **Tasic, V., Gordova, A., Delidzhakova, M., and Kozhinkova, N.**, Zinc toxicity, *Pediatrics,* 70, 660, 1982.

1602. **Tasman-Jones, C.**, Zinc and copper deficiency with particular reference to parenteral nutrition, *Surg. Ann.*, 10, 23, 1978.

1603. **Tasman-Jones, C. and Kay, R. G.**, Zinc deficiency and skin lesions, *N. Engl. J. Med.*, 293, 830, 1975.

1604. **Taylor, C. J., Moore, G., and Davidson, D. C.**, The effect of treatment on zinc, copper, and cadmium status in children with phenylketonuria, *J. Inherit. Metab. Dis.*, 7, 160, 1984.

1605. **Taylor, M. L., Butler, L. C., McCurdy, P. R., and Mahmood, L.**, Zinc and copper metabolism in sickle cell anemia, *Clin. Res.*, 25, 542A, 1977.

1606. **Terry, C. W., Terry, B. E., and Davies, J.**, Transfer of zinc across the placenta and fetal membranes of the rabbit, *Am. J. Physiol.*, 198, 303, 1960.

1607. **Theuer, R. C. and Hoekstra, W. G.**, Oxidation of carbon-14 labelled carbohydrate, fat and amino acid substrates by zinc deficient rats, *J. Nutr.*, 89, 448, 1966.

1607a. **Thiers, R. E. and Vallee, B. L.**, Distribution of metals in subcellular fractions of rat liver, *J. Biol. Chem.*, 226, 911, 1957.

1608. **Thind, G. S. and Fischer, G. M.**, Relationship of plasma zinc to human hypertension, *Clin. Sci. Mol. Med.*, 46, 137, 1974.

1609. **Thind, G. S. and Fischer, G. M.**, Plasma cadmium and zinc in human hypertension, *Clin. Sci. Mol. Med.*, 51, 483, 1976.

1610. **Thomas, J. P., Bachowski, G. J., and Girotti, A. W.**, Inhibition of cell membrane lipid peroxidation by cadmium and zinc metallothioneins, *Biochim. Biophys. Acta,* 884, 448, 1986.

1611. **Thompson, D. M., Balenovich, W., Hornich, L. H. M., and Richardson, M. F.**, Reactions of metals with vitamins. IV. The crystal structure of a zinc complex of pyridoxamine, *Inorg. Chim. Acta,* 46, 199, 1980.

1612. **Thompson, R. W., Gilbreath, R. L., and Bielk, F.**, Alterations of porcine skin acid mucopolysaccharides in zinc deficiency, *J. Nutr.*, 105, 154, 1975.

1613. **Thurnham, D. I., Rathakette, P., Hambidge, K. M., Munoz, N., and Crespi, M.**, Riboflavin vitamin A and zinc status in Chinese subjects in a high risk area for esophageal cancer, *Hum. Nutr. Clin. Nutr.*, 36, 337, 1982.

1614. **Todd, W. R., Elvehjem, C. A., and Hart, E. B.**, Zinc in the nutrition of the rat, *Am. J. Physiol.*, 107, 146, 1934.

1615. **Topping, D. L., Clark, D. G., and Dreosti, I. E.**, Impaired thermoregulation in cold-exposed zinc deficient rats — effects of nicotine, *Nutr. Rep. Int.*, 24, 643, 1981.

1616. **Toskes, P., Dawson, W., Duncan, D., Storms, L., and Fitzgerald, C.**, Treatment of non-diabetic retinopathy in patients with chronic pancreatitis, *Am. J. Clin. Nutr.*, 31, 719, 1978.

1617. **Toskes, P. P., Dawson, W., Curlington, C., and Levy, N. S.**, Non-diabetic retinal abnormalities in chronic pancreatitis, *N. Engl. J. Med.*, 300, 942, 1979.

1618. **Toskes, P., Storms, L., and Duncan, D.**, Zinc deficiency in chronic pancreatitis, *Clin. Res.*, 26, 762A, 1978.

1619. **Tsai, S. L., Craig-Schmidt, M. C., Weete, J. D., and Keth, R. E.**, Effects of zinc deficiency on delta-6 desaturase activity in rat liver, *Fed. Proc. Fed. Am. Soc. Exp. Biol.*, 42, 823, 1983.

1620. **Tsai, R. C. Y. and Lei, K. Y.**, Dietary cellulose, zinc and copper: effects on tissue levels of trace minerals in the rat, *J. Nutr.*, 109, 1117, 1979.

1621. **Tsambaos, D. and Orfanos, C. E.**, Zinc distribution disorder in psoriasis, *Arch. Dermatol. Res.*, 259, 97, 1977.

1622. **Tsukamoto, I., Yoshinaga, T., and Sano, S.**, Zinc and cysteine residues in the active site of bovine liver delta-amino levulenic dehydratase, *Int. J. Biochem.*, 12, 751, 1980.

1623. **Tucker, H. F. and Salmon, W. D.,** Parakeratosis or zinc deficiency disease in the pig, *Proc. Soc. Exp. Biol. Med.*, 88, 613, 1955.

1624. **Tucker, S. B., Schroeter, A. L., Brown, P. W., and McCall, J. T.,** Acquired zinc deficiency, *JAMA*, 235, 2399, 1976.

1625. **Tupper, R., Watts, R. W. E., and Wormall, A.,** Some observations on zinc in carbonic anhydrase, *Biochem. J.*, 50, 429, 1952.

1626. **Turner, S. R., Turner, R. A., Smith, D. M., and Johnson, J. A.,** Effects of heavy metal ions on phospholipid metabolism in human neutrophils: relationship to ionophore-mediated cytotoxicity, *Prostaglandins*, 32, 919, 1986.

1627. **Turnlund, J. R., King, J. C., Keyes, W. R., Gong, B., and Michel, M. C.,** A stable isotope study of zinc absorption in young men: effects of phytate and alpha-cellulose, *Am. J. Clin. Nutr.*, 40, 1071, 1984.

1628. **Turnlund, J. and Margen, S.,** Effect of glucocorticoids and zinc deficiency on femur and liver zinc in rats, *J. Nutr.*, 109, 467, 1979.

1629. **Twomey, S. L. and Baxter, C. F.,** Some aspects of pyridoxal phosphokinase in chick brain, *J. Neurochem.*, 21, 1253, 1973.

1630. **Tyrala, E. E.,** Zinc and copper balances in preterm infants, *Pediatrics*, 77, 513, 1986.

1631. **Urban, E. and Campbell, M. E.,** In vivo zinc transport by rat small intestine after extensive small bowel resection, *Am. J. Physiol.*, 247, G88, 1984.

1632. **Valberg, L. S., Flanagan, P. R., Brennan, J., and Chamberlain, M. T.,** Does the oral zinc tolerance test measure zinc absorption?, *Am. J. Clin. Nutr.*, 41, 37, 1985.

1633. **Valberg, L. S., Flanagan, P. R., Ghent, C. N., and Chamberlain, M. J.,** Zinc absorption and leucocyte zinc in alcoholic and non-alcoholic cirrhosis, *Dig. Dis. Sci.*, 30, 329, 1985.

1634. **Vallee, B. L.,** Biochemistry, physiology and pathology of zinc, *Physiol. Rev.*, 39, 443, 1959.

1635. **Vallee, B. L.,** Zinc, in *Mineral Metabolism An Advanced Treatise*, Comar, C. L. and Bronner, F., Eds., Academic Press, New York, 1962, 443.

1636. **Vallee, B. L. and Altschule, M. D.,** Zinc in the mammalian organism with particular reference to carbonic anhydrase, *Physiol. Rev.*, 29, 370, 1949.

1637. **Vallee, B. L. and Gibson, J. G.,** The zinc content of whole blood, plasma, leucocyte and erythrocytes in the anemias, *Blood*, 4, 455, 1949.

1638. **Vallee, B. L. and Wacker, W. A. C.,** Zinc, a component of rabbit muscle lactic dehydrogenase, *J. Am. Chem. Soc.*, 78, 1771, 1956.

1639. **Vallee, B. L., Wacker, W. A. C., Bartholomy, A. F., and Robin, E. D.,** Zinc metabolism in hepatic dysfunction. I. Serum zinc concentrations in Laennac's cirrhosis and their evaluation by sequential analysis, *N. Engl. J. Med.*, 255, 403, 1956.

1640. **Vallee, B. L., Wacker, W. A. C., Bartholomy, A. F., and Hoch, F. L.,** Zinc metabolism in hepatic dysfunction. II. Correlation of metabolic patterns with biochemical findings, *N. Engl. J. Med.*, 257, 1055, 1957.

1641. **Valquist, A., Michelsson, G., and Juhlin, L.,** Acne treatment with oral zinc and vitamin A: effect on the serum levels of zinc and retinol-binding protein (RBP), *Arch. Dermatol. Venerol.*, 58, 437, 1978.

1642. **Van Caille-Bertrand, M., Degenhart, H. J., Visser, H. K., Sinaasappel, M., and Bouquet, J.,** Oral zinc sulphate for Wilson's disease, *Arch. Dis. Child.*, 60, 656, 1985.

1643. **Van Campen, D. R. and House, W. A.,** Effect of a low protein diet on retention of an oral dose of zinc-65 and on tissue concentrations of zinc, iron and copper in rats, *J. Nutr.*, 104, 84, 1974.

1644. **Van Campen, D. R. and Scaife, P. U.,** Zinc interference with copper absorption in rats, *J. Nutr.*, 91, 473, 1967.

1645. **Vander, A. J., Vistery, W., Germain, C., and Holloway, D.,** Insulin is a physiological inhibitor of urinary zinc excretion in anesthetized dogs, *Am. J. Physiol.*, 244, E536, 1983.

1646. **Vanderhoof, J. A., Park, J. H. Y., and Grandjean, C. J.,** Effect of zinc on mucosal hyperplasia following 70% bowel resection, *Am. J. Clin. Nutr.*, 44, 670, 1986.

1647. **Van Reen, R.,** Zinc toxicity in man and experimental species, in *Zinc Metabolism*, Prasad, A. S., Ed., Charles C Thomas, Springfield, Ill., 1966, 411.

1648. **Van Rij, A. M.,** Zinc supplements in surgery, in *Zinc and Copper in Medicine*, Karcioglu, Z. A. and Sarper, R. M., Eds., Charles C Thomas, Springfield, Ill., 1982, 259.

1649. **Van Rij, A. M. and Pories, W. J.,** Zinc and copper in surgery, in *Zinc and Copper in Medicine*, Karcioglu, Z. A. and Sarper, R. M., Eds., Charles C Thomas, Springfield, Ill., 1980, 535.

1650. **Varagaftig, B. B., Tranier, Y., and Chignard, M.,** Blockade by metal complexing agents and by catalase of the effects of arachidonic acid on platelets: relevance to the study of anti-inflammatory mechanisms, *Eur. J. Pharmacol.*, 33, 19, 1975.

1651. **Varas Lorenzo, M. J.,** Zinc acexamate and ranitidine in short and mid-term management of gastrointestinal ulcers, *Curr. Ther. Res.*, 39, 19, 1986.

1652. **Verma, K. C., Saini, A. S., and Dhamija, S. K.,** Oral zinc sulphate therapy in acne vulgaris: a double-blind trial, *Acta Dermatol. Venereol.*, 60, 337, 1980.

1653. **Versieck, J. and Cornelis, R.,** Normal levels of trace elements in human blood or serum, *Anal. Chim. Acta,* 116, 217, 1980.

1654. **Vesieck, J., Hoste, J., and Barbier, F.,** Determination of manganese, copper and zinc in serum in normal controls and patients with liver metastases, *Acta Gastro Enterol. Belg.*, 39, 340, 1976.

1655. **Vertongen, F., Neve, J., Cauchie, P., and Molle, L.,** Zinc, copper, selenium and glutathione peroxidase in plasma and erythrocytes of Fown's syndrome (Trisomy 21) patients. Interpretation of some variations, in *Trace Element Analytical Chemistry in Medicine and Biology,* Vol. 3, Bratter, P. and Schramel, P., Eds., Walter de Gruyter, New York, 1984, 175.

1656. **Villa-Elizaga, I. and Da Cuhna Ferriera, R. M. C.,** Zinc, pregnancy and parturition, *Acta Paediatr. Scand.*, Suppl. 319, 150, 1985.

1657. **Vikbladh, I.,** Studies on zinc in blood, *Scand. J. Clin. Lab. Invest.*, 3(Suppl. 2), 1, 1951.

1658. **Vir, S. C. and Love, A. H. G.,** Zinc and copper status of the elderly, *Am. J. Clin.Nutr.*, 32, 1472, 1979.

1659. **Vojnik, C. and Hurley, L. S.,** Abnormal prenatal lung development resulting from maternal zinc deficiency in rats, *J. Nutr.*, 107, 862, 1977.

1660. **Von Glos, K. I. and Boursnell, J. C.,** Formation of a double salt of phosphatidylcholine and zinc chloride, *Biochem. J.*, 193, 1017, 1981.

1661. **Vormann, J., Hollriegel, V., Merker, H.-J., and Gunther, T.,** Effect of valproate on zinc metabolism in fetal and maternal rats fed normal and zinc deficient diets, *Biol. Trace Elem. Res.*, 10, 25, 1986.

1662. **Vreman, H. J., Venter, C., Leegwater, J., Oliver, C., and Weiner, M. W.,** Taste, smell and zinc metabolism in patients with chronic renal failure, *Nephron,* 26, 163, 1980.

1663. **Wachtel, L. W., Hove, E., Elvehjem, C. A., and Hart, E. B.,** Blood uric acid and liver uricase of zinc deficient rats on various diets, *J. Biol. Chem.*, 138, 361, 1941.

1664. **Wacker, W. A. C.,** Role of zinc in wound healing: a critical review, in *Trace Elements in Human Health and Disease,* Vol. 1, Prasad, A. S. and Oberleas, D. Eds., Academic Press, New York, 1976, 107.

1665. **Wacker, W. A. C., Ulmer, D. D., and Vallee, B. L.,** Metalloenzymes and myocardial infarction. II. Malic and lactic dehydrogenase activities and zinc in serum, *N. Engl. J. Med.*, 255, 449, 1956.

1666. **Wada, L., Turnlund, J. R., and King, J. C.,** Zinc utilization in young men fed adequate and low zinc intakes, *J. Nutr.*, 115, 1345, 1985.

1667. **Wade, J. V., Agrawal, P. R., and Poisner, A. M.,** Induction of metallothionein in a human trophoblast cell line by cadmium and zinc, *Life Sci.*, 39, 1361, 1986.

1668. **Walker, B. E., Dawson, J. B., Kelleher, J., and Losowsky, M. S.,** Plasma and urinary zinc in patients with malabsorption syndromes or hepatic cirrhosis, *Gut,* 14, 943, 1973.

1669. **Walldius, G., Michaelsson, G., Hardell, L.-I., and Aberg, H.,** The effects of diet and zinc treatment on the fatty acid composition of serum lipids, and adipose tissue and on serum liporproteins in two adolescent patients with acrodermatitis enteropathica, *Am. J. Clin. Nutr.*, 38, 512, 1983.

1670. **Wallwork, J. C., Botnen, J. H., and Sandstead, H. H.,** Effect of dietary zinc on rat brain catecholamines, *J. Nutr.*, 112, 514, 1982.

1671. **Wallwork, J. C. and Duerre, J. A.,** Effect of zinc deficiency on methionine metabolism, methylation reactions and protein synthesis in isolated perfuced rat liver, *J. Nutr.*, 115, 252, 1985.

1672. **Wallwork, J. C., Milne, D. B., Sims, R. L., and Sandstead, H. H.,** Severe zinc deficiency: effects on the distribution of 9 elements (potassium, magnesium, calcium, iron, zinc, copper, and manganese) in regions of the rat brain, *J. Nutr.*, 113, 1895, 1983.

1673. **Walravens, P. A.,** Zinc metabolism and its implications in clinical medicine, *West. J. Med.*, 130, 133, 1979.

1674. **Walravens, P. A.,** Acrodermatitis enteropathica: pathogenesis and implications for treatment, in *Metabolism of Trace Elements in Man,* Vol. 2, Rennert, O. M. and Chan, W.-Y., Eds., CRC Press, Boca Raton, Fla., 1984, 71.

1675. **Walravens, P. A. and Hambidge, K. M.,** Nutritional zinc deficiency in infants and children, in *Zinc Metabolism: Current Aspects in Health and Disease,* Prasad, A. S., Ed., Alan R. Liss, New York, 1977, 61.

1676. **Walshe, J. M.,** Treatment of Wilson's disease with zinc sulphate, *Br. Med. J.*, 289, 558, 1984.

1677. **Walton, K. E., Fitzgerald, P. C., Herrmann, M. S., and Behnke, W. D.,** A fully active DNA polymerase I from *E. coli* lacking stochiometric zinc, *Biochem. Biophys. Res. Commun.*, 108, 1353, 1982.

1678. **Wannemacher, J. R., Pekarek, R. S., Klainer, A., Bartelloni, P., Dupont, H., Hornick, R., and Beisel, W.,** Detection of a leucocyte endogenous mediator-like mediator of serum amino acid and zinc depression during various infectious illnesses, *Infect. Immun.*, 11, 873, 1975.

1679. **Wapnir, R. A., Khani, D. E., Bayne, M. A., and Lipshitz, F.,** Absorption of zinc by the rat ileum: effects of histidine and other low molecular weight ligands, *J. Nutr.*, 113, 1346, 1983.

1680. **Wapnir, R. A. and Steil, L.,** Zinc intestinal absorption in rats: specificity of amino acids as ligands, *J. Nutr.*, 116, 2171, 1986.

1681. **Wastney, M. E., Aamodt, R. L., Rumble, W. F., and Henkin, R. I.,** Kinetic analysis of zinc metabolism and its regulation in normal humans, *Am. J. Physiol.*, 251, R398, 1986.

1682. **Watkins, D. W., Antoniou, L. D., and Shaloub, R. J.,** Urinary zinc in relation to other cations and urine flow during volume expansion and intravenous chlorthiazide, *Can. J. Physiol. Pharmacol.*, 59, 562, 1981.

1683. **Watkinson, M., Aggett, P. J., and Cole, T. J.,** Zinc and acute tropical ulcers in Gambian children and adolescents, *Am. J. Clin. Nutr.*, 41, 43, 1985.

1684. **Watson, C. J. and Schwartz, S.,** The excretion of zinc uroporphyrin in idiopathic porphyria, *J. Clin. Invest.*, 20, 440, 1941.

1685. **Wazewska-Czyewska, M., Wesierska-Gadek, J., and Legutko, L.,** Immunostimulatory effect of zinc in patients with actue lymphocytic leukemia, *Folia Haematol.*, 105, 727, 1978.

1686. **Webb, M.,** Protection by zinc against cadmium toxicity, *Biochem. Pharmacol.*, 21, 2767, 1972.

1687. **Webb, M., Plastow, S. R., and Magos, L.,** Copper-zinc-thionein in pig liver, *Life Sci.*, 24, 1901, 1979.

1688. **Wegger, I. and Palludan, B.,** Zinc metabolism in swine with special emphasis on reproduction, in *Trace Element Metabolism in Man and Animals*, Vol. 3, Kirchgessner, M., Ed., Arbeitskreis fur Tierernahrungs-forschung, Weihenstephan, F.R.G., 1978, 428.

1689. **Weigand, E.,** Homeostatic adjustments in zinc digestion to widely varying dietary zinc intake, *Nutr. Metab.*, 22, 101, 1978.

1690. **Weigand, E. and Kirchgessner, M.,** Total positive efficiency of zinc utilization: determination and homeostatic dependence upon the zinc supply status in young pigs, *J. Nutr.*, 110, 469, 1980.

1691. **Weiner, A. L. and Cousins, R. J.,** Differential regulation of copper and zinc metabolism in rat liver parenchymal cells in primary culture, *Proc. Soc. Exp. Biol. Med.*, 173, 486, 1983.

1692. **Weismann, K.,** Lines of Beau: possible markers of zinc deficiency, *Acta Dermatol. Venereol.*, 57, 88, 1977.

1693. **Weismann, K.,** Dystrophic epidermolysis bullosa treated unsuccessfully with oral zinc, *Arch. Dermatol.*, 277, 404, 1985.

1694. **Weismann, K., Asboe-Hansen, G., Secher, L., Pedersen, E., and Hansen, H. J.,** Plasma zinc levels in multiple sclerosis, *Metab. Pediatr. Syst. Ophthalmol.*, 6, 137, 1982.

1695. **Weismann, K., Christensen, E., and Dreyer, V.,** Zinc supplementation in alcoholic cirrhosis, *Acta Med. Scand.*, 205, 361, 1979.

1696. **Weismann, K. and Hoyer, H.,** Serum alkaline phosphatase activity in acrodermatitis enteropathica. An index of the serum zinc level, *Acta Dermatol. Venereol.*, 59, 89, 1979.

1697. **Weismann, K. and Hoyer, H.,** Serum alkaline phosphatase and serum zinc levels in the diagnosis and exclusion of zinc deficiency in man, *Am. J. Clin. Nutr.*, 41, 1214, 1985.

1698. **Weismann, K. and Hoyer, H.,** Serum zinc levels during oral glucocorticoid therapy, *J. Invest. Dermatol.*, 86, 715, 1986.

1699. **Weismann, K. and Knudsen, L.,** Effects of penicillamine and hydroxyguinoline on absorption of orally ingested zinc-65 in the rat, *J. Invest. Dermatol.*, 71, 242, 1978.

1700. **Weismann, K., Knudsen, L., and Hoyer, H.,** Phenytoin increases zinc-65 absorption in the rat, *J. Invest. Dermatol.*, 71, 396, 1978.

1701. **Weismann, K. and Mikkelsen, H. I.,** Osmotic lysis of erythrocytes in relation to the zinc concentration of the medium, *Arch. Dermatol. Res.*, 269, 105, 1980.

1702. **Weismann, K., Wanscher, B., and Krakauer, R.,** Oral zinc therapy in geriatric patients with selected skin manifestations and a low plasma zinc, *Acta Dermatol. Venereol.*, 58, 157, 1978.

1703. **Weitzel, G., Buddecke, E., Fretzdoff, A.-M., Strecker, F. J., and Roester, U.,** Strucker der im Tapetum lucidum von Hund und Fuchs enthalenen Zinkferbindung, *Hoppe-Seyler's Z. Physiol. Chem.*, 299, 193, 1955.

1704. **Weizman, Z.,** Zinc deficiency: cause of hypoproteinemia or its result?, *Pediatrics*, 75, 128, 1985.

1705. **Wells, M. A.,** Spectral perturbations of *Crotalus adamanteus* phospholipase A2 induced by divalent cation binding, *Biochemistry*, 12, 1080, 1973.

1706. **Wenk, G. L. and Stemmer, K. L.,** Suboptimal dietary zinc intake increases aluminum accumulation into the rat brain, *Brain Res.*, 288, 393, 1984.

1707. **Weser, U., Seeber, S., and Warnecke, P.,** Reactivity of zinc on nuclear DNA and RNA biosynthesis of regenerating rat liver, *Biochim. Biophys. Acta*, 179, 422, 1969.

1708. **West, K. R., Dreosti, I. E., Gargett, C. E., and Record, I.,** Aggregation by platelets from pregnant zinc deficient rats, *Nutr. Rep. Int.*, 22, 1, 1980.

1709. **Westmorland, N.,** Connective tissue alterations in zinc deficiency, *Fed. Proc. Fed. Am. Soc. Exp. Biol.*, 30, 1001, 1971.

1710. **Westmorland, N. and Hoekstra, W. G.,** Pathological defects in the epiphyseal cartilage of zinc deficient chicks, *J. Nutr.*, 98, 76, 1969.

1711. **Weston, W. L., Huff, J. C., Humbery, J. R., Hambidge, K. M., Neldner, K. H., and Walravens, P. A.,** Zinc correction of defective chemotasis in acrodermatitis enteropathica, *Arch. Dermatol.*, 113, 422, 1977.

1712. **Wester, P. O.,** Trace elements in human myocardial infarction determined by neutron activation analysis, *Acta Med. Scand.*, Suppl. 439, 1, 1965.

1713. **Wester, P. O.,** Zinc during diuretic treatment, *Lancet,* i, 578, 1975.

1714. **Wester, P. O.,** Urinary zinc excretion during treatment with different diuretics, *Acta Med. Scand.*, 208, 209, 1980.

1715. **Wester, P. O.,** Zinc balance before and during treatment with bendroflumethazide, *Acta Med. Scand.*, 209, 265, 1980.

1716. **Wester, P. O.,** Tissue zinc at autopsy. Relation to medication with diuretics, *Acta Med. Scand.*, 208, 269, 1980.

1717. **Whanger, P. D. and Weswig, P. H.,** Effects of supplementary zinc on the intracellular distribution of hepatic copper in rats, *J. Nutr.*, 101, 1093, 1971.

1718. **White, C. L.,** Increased glutathione peroxidase activity in zinc deficient sheep, *Proc. Nutr. Soc. Aust.*, 5, 182, 1980.

1719. **White, H. B. and Montalvo, J. M.,** Serum fatty acids before and after recovery from acrodermatitis enteropathica: comparison of an infant with her family, *J. Pediatr.*, 83, 999, 1973.

1720. **Whitehouse, M. W., Hanley, W. S., and Field, L.,** A potential hazard: toxicity of zinc with penicillamine, *Arthritis Rheum.*, 20, 1035, 1977.

1721. **Whitehouse, R. C., Prasad, A. S., Rabbini, P., and Cossack, Z. T.,** Zinc in plasma, neutrophils, lymphocytes and erythrocytes as determined by flameless atomic absorption spectrophotometry, *Clin. Chem.*, 28, 475, 1982.

1722. **Whiting, F. and Bezeau, L. M.,** Calcium, phosphorus and zinc balance in pigs as influenced by the weight of pig and the level of calcium, zinc and vitamin D in the ration, *Can. J. Anim. Sci.*, 38, 109, 1958.

1723. Trace Elements in Human Nutrition, WHO Tech. Rep. Ser. No. 532, World Health Organization, 1973.

1724. **Wibell, L., Gebre-Medhin, M., and Lindmark, G.,** Magnesium and zinc in diabetic pregnancy, *Acta Paediatr. Scand.*, Suppl. 320, 100, 1985.

1725. **Widdowson, E. M., Dauncey, J., and Shaw, J. C. L.,** Trace elements in foetal and early neonatal development, *Proc. Nutr. Soc.*, 33, 275, 1974.

1726. **Williams, R. B. and Chesters, J. K.,** Effects of zinc deficiency on nucleic acid synthesis in the rat, in *Trace Element Metabolism in Animals,* Vol. 1, Mills, C. F., Ed., Churchill Livingstone, Edinburgh, 1970, 164.

1727. **Williams, R. B. and Chesters, J. K.,** The effects of early zinc deficiency on DNA and protein synthesis in the rat, *Br. J. Nutr.*, 24, 1053, 1970.

1728. **Williams, R. B., Demertzis, P., and Mills, C. F.,** The effects of dietary zinc concentrations on reproduction in the rat, *Proc. Nutr. Sco.*, 32, 3A, 1973.

1729. **Williams, R. B., Mills, C. F., and Dawson, R. J. L.,** Relationships between zinc deficiency and folic acid status in the rat, *Proc. Nutr. Soc.*, 32, 2A, 1973.

1730. **Williams, R. B., Russell, R. M., Dutta, S. K., and Giovetti, A. C.,** Alcoholic pancreatitis patients at high risk of acute zinc deficiency, *Am. J. Med.*, 66, 889, 1979.

1731. **Williams, K. J., Meltzer, R., Brown, P. A., Tanaka, Y., and Kay, C. J.,** The effect of topically-applied zinc on the healing of open wounds, *J. Surg. Res.*, 27, 62, 1979.

1732. **Willson, R. L.,** Metroindazole and tissue zinc/iron ratio in cancer therapy, *Lancet,* i, 1407, 1976.

1733. **Wilson, E. L., Burger, P. E., and Dowdle, E. B.,** Beef liver 5-amino levulinic acid dehydratase. Purification and properties, *Eur. J. Biochem.*, 29, 563, 1972.

1734. **Wilson, M. C., Fischer, T. J., and Riordan, M. M.,** Isolated IgG hypogammaglobulinemia in acrodermatitis enteropathica — correction with zinc therapy, *Ann. Allergy*, 48, 288, 1982.

1735. **Wingender, E., Dilloo, D., and Seifert, K. H.,** Zinc ions are differentially required for the transcription of ribosomal 5S RNA and tRNA in a HeLa cell extract, *Nucleic Acids Res.*, 12, 8971, 1984.

1736. **Wolfe, J. A., Margolis, S., Bujdoso-Wolfe, K., Matusick, E., and MacLean, W. C.,** Plasma and red blood cell fatty acid composition in children with protein-calorie malnutrition, *Pediatr. Res.*, 18, 162, 1984.

1737. **Wolman, S. L., Anderson, G. H., Marliss, E. B., and Jeejeebhoy, K. N.,** Zinc in total parenteral nutrition: requirements and metabolic effects, *Gastroenterology*, 76, 458, 1979.

1738. **Wong, E. K., Enomoto, H., and Leopold, I. H.,** Plasma zinc levels in multiple sclerosis, *Metab. Pediatr. Ophthalmol.*, 4, 3, 1980.

1739. **Wong, E. K. and Leopold, I. H.,** Zinc deficiency and visual dysfunction, *Metab. Pediatr. Ophthalmol.*, 3, 1, 1979.

1740. **Woo, W., Gibbs, D. L., Hooper, P. L., and Garry, P. J.,** Zinc and lipid metabolism, *Am. J. Clin. Nutr.*, 34, 120, 1981.

1741. **Woo, W., Gibbs, D. L., Hooper, P. L., and Garry, P. J.,** The effect of dietary zinc on high density lipoprotein synthesis, *Nutr. Rep. Int.*, 27, 499, 1983.

1742. **Woodward, W. D., Filteau, S. M., and Allen, O. B.,** Decline in serum zinc level throughout adult life in the laboratory mouse, *J. Gerontol.*, 39, 521, 1984.

1743. **Wootten, A. C.,** *Chronicles of Pharmacy,* Vols. 1 and 2, Macmillan, New York, 1910.

1744. **Wright, C. E., Gaull, G. E., and Pasentes-Morales, H.,** Protective effects of taurine, zinc and vitamin E on human cell membranes: possible relevance to retina, *J. Am. Coll. Nutr.*, 3, 248, 1984.

1745. **Wright, E. B. and Dormandy, T. L.,** Liver zinc in carcinoma, *Nature (London)*, 237, 166, 1972.

1746. **Wu, C.-T., Lee, J.-N., Shen, W. W., and Lee, S.-L.,** Serum zinc, copper and ceruloplasmin levels in male alcoholics, *Biol. Psychiatr.*, 19, 1333, 1984.

1747. **Wysochi, K., Owczarek, L., Fenrych, W., Gorski, S., and Majewski, C.,** The metabolism of radioactive zinc in the liver of rats damaged by single administration of carbon tetrachloride, *Acta Med. Pol.*, 7, 97, 1966.

1748. **Chen, X.-C., Yin, T.-A., He, J.-S., Ma, Q.-Y., Han, Z.-M., and Li, L.-X.,** Low levels of zinc in hair and blood, pica, anorexia and poor growth in Chinese pre-school children, *Am. J. Clin. Nutr.*, 42, 694, 1985.

1749. **Yadav, H. S., Nagpal, K. K., Sharma, B. N., and Chaundhuri, B. N.,** Influence of thyroxine and temperature on zinc metabolism, *Indian J. Exp. Biol.*, 18, 993, 1980.

1750. **Yalouris, A. G.,** Zinc deficiency and haem synthesis: an additional problem in uremia, *Nephron*, 43, 72, 1986.

1751. **Yamaguchi, M., Katayama, K., and Okada, S.,** Hypocalcemic effect of zinc and its mechanism in rats, *J. Pharamcobio-Dyn.*, 4, 656, 1981.

1752. **Yamaguchi, M. and Sakashita, T.,** Enhancement of vitamin D_3 effect on bone metabolism in weanling rats orally administered zinc sulphate, *Acta Endocrinol.*, 111, 285, 1986.

1753. **Yamaguchi, M., Takahashi, K., and Okada, S.,** Zinc-induced hypocalcemia and bone resorption in rats, *Toxicol. Appl. Pharmacol.*, 67, 224, 1983.

1754. **Yip, R., Reeves, J. D., Lonnerdal, B., Keen, C. L., and Dallman, P. R.,** Does iron supplementation compromise zinc nutrition in healthy infants, *Am. J. Clin. Nutr.*, 42, 683, 1985.

1755. **Yoshino, M., Murakami, K., and Tusushima, K.,** Inhibition of AMP deaminase by zinc ions, *Biochem. Pharmacol.*, 27, 2651, 1978.

1756. **Youinou, P., Leguse, D., Garre, M., Menez, J. F., and Miossec, P.,** The respective roles of zinc and high-density lipoprotein-cholesterol in the formation of human autologous-rosettes during protein-calorie malnutrition, *IRCS Med. Sci.-Biochem.*, 10, 273, 1982.

1757. **Younoszai, H. D.,** Clinical zinc deficiency in total parenteral nutrition: zinc supplementation, *J. Parenter. Enter. Nutr.*, 7, 72, 1983.

1758. **Yunice, A. A., Czerwinski, A. W., and Lindeman, R. D.,** Influence of synthetic corticosteroids on plasma zinc and copper levels in humans, *Am. J. Med. Sci.*, 282, 68, 1981.

1759. **Yunice, A. A. and Lindeman, R. D.,** Effect of ascorbic acid and zinc sulphate on ethanol toxicity and metabolism, *Proc. Soc. Exp. Biol. Med.*, 154, 146, 1977.

1760. **Zahradka, P. and Ebisuzaki, K.,** Poly(ADP-ribose)polymerase is a zinc metalloenzyme, *Eur. J. Biochem.*, 142, 503, 1984.

1761. **Zarling, E. J., Mobarhan, S., Makino, D., Friedman, H., and Kunigk, A.,** Does severe zinc deficiency affect intestinal protein content or disaccharidase activity, *J. Am. Coll. Nutr.*, 4, 360, 1985.

1762. **Zelkowitz, M., Verghese, J. P., and Anterl, J.,** Copper and zinc in the nervous system, in *Zinc and Copper in Medicine*, Karcioglu, Z. A. and Sarper, R. M., Eds., Charles C Thomas, Springfield, Ill., 1980, 418.

1763. **Zhukov, N. A. and Bakhina, T. S.,** Pathways and significance of redistribution of zinc in patients with chronic pancreatitis, *Ter. Arkh.*, 44, 64, 1972.

1764. **Zimmerman, A. W.,** Hyperzincemia in anencephaly and spina bifida: a clue to the pathogenesis of neural tube defects?, *Neurology*, 34, 443, 1984.

1765. **Zimmerman, A. W., Dunham, B. S., Nochimson, D. J., Kaplan, B. M., Clive, J. M., and Kunkel, S. L.,** Zinc transport in pregnancy, *Am. J. Obstet. Gynecol.*, 149, 523, 1984.

1766. Subcommittee on Zinc, National Research Council, *Zinc*, University Park Press, Baltimore, 1979.

1767. **Zipper, A., Medel, M., Pastene, L., Torres, L., Osorio, A., Rivera, A., and Toscanini, C.,** Studies on the physiological activity of intrauterine devices containing copper, *Contraception*, 12, 1, 1976.

1768. **Zlotkin, S. H. and Buchanan, B. E.,** Meeting zinc and copper intake requirements in parenterally-fed preterm and fullterm infants, *J. Pediatr.*, 103, 441, 1983.

1769. **Zumkley, H., Bertram, H. P., Lison, A., Knoll, O., and Losse, H.,** Aluminum, zinc and copper concentrations in plasma in chronic renal insufficiency, *Clin. Nephrol.*, 12, 18, 1979.

1770. **Zumkley, H., Vetter, H., Bertram, H. P., Tank, B., and Wirth, W.,** Plasma zinc and magnesium alterations in acute myocardial infarction, *Klin. Wochenschr.*, 58, 1143, 1980.

1771. **Hammermueller, J. D., Bray, T. M., and Bettger, W. J.,** *J. Nutr.*, 117, 894, 1987.

1772. **Prasad, A. S.,** unpublished data.

GENERAL READING

Journal Articles/Chapters/Books

Aggett, P. J. and Davies, N. T., Some nutritional aspects of trace metals, *J. Inherit. Metab. Dis.*, 6 (Suppl. 1), 22, 1984.

Aggett, P. J. and Harries, J. T., Current status of zinc in health and disease states, *Arch. Dis. Child.*, 54, 909, 1979.

Davies, S., Zinc, nutrition and health, in *Yearbook of Nutritional Medicine*, 1st ed., Bland, J., Ed., Keats Publishing, New Canaan, Conn., 1984, 113.

Forbes, R. M., Use of laboratory animals to define physiological function and bioavailability of zinc, *Fed. Proc. Fed. Am. Soc. Exp. Biol.*, 43, 2835, 1984.

Golden, M. H. N., Trace elements in human nutrition, *Human Nutr. Clin. Nutr.*, 36, 185, 1982.

Gordon, E. F., Gordon, R. C., and Passal, D. B., Zinc metabolism: basic clinical and behavioural aspects, *J. Pediatr.*, 99, 341, 1981.

Halsted, J. A., Smith, J. C., Jr., and Irwin, M. I., A conspectus of research on zinc requirements of man, *J. Nutr.*, 104, 345, 1974.

McClain, C. J., Kasarskis, E. J., and Allen, J. J., Functional consequences of zinc deficiency, *Prog. Food Nutr. Sci.*, 9, 185, 1985.

Prasad, A. S., Zinc in human nutrition, *Crit. Rev. Clin. Lab. Sci.*, 8, 1, 1977.

Prasad, A. S., Trace elements: biochemical and clinical effects of zinc and copper, *Am. J. Hematol.*, 6, 77, 1979.

Prasad, A. S., Clinical manifestations of zinc deficiency, *Annu. Rev. Nutr.*, 5, 341, 1985.

Riordan, J. F., Biochemistry of zinc, *Med. Clin. North Am.*, 60, 661, 1976.

Solomons, N. W. and Cousins, R. J., Zinc, in *Absorption and Malabsorption of Mineral Nutrients*, Solomons, N. W. and Rosenberg, I. H., Eds., Alan R. Liss, New York, 1984, 125.

Books

Clinical Applications of Recent Advances in Zinc Metabolism, Prasad, A. S., Dreosti, I. E., and Hetzel, B., Eds., Alan R. Liss, New York, 1982.

Clinical Aspects of Zinc Metabolism, Pories, W. J., Strain, W. H., Hsu, J. M., and Woolsey; R. L., Eds., Academic Press, New York, 1974.

Clinical, Biochemical and Nutritional Aspects of Trace Elements, Prasad, A. S., Ed., Alan R. Liss, New York, 1982.

Trace Element Metabolism in Animals, Vol. 1, Mills, C. F., Ed., Churchill Livingstone, Edinburgh, 1969.

Trace Element Metabolism in Animals, Vol. 2, Hoekstra, W. G., Suttie, J. W., Ganther, H. E., and Mertz, W., Eds., University Park Press, Baltimore, 1974.

Trace Element Metabolism in Man and Animals, Vol. 3, Kirchgessner, M., Ed., Arbeitskreis fur Tiernahrungsforschung, Weihenstephan, F.R.G., 1978.

Trace Element Metabolism in Man and Animals, Vol. 4, Howell, J. McC., Gawthorne, J. M., and White, C. L., Eds., Australian Academy of Sciences, Canberra, 1981.

Trace Element Metabolism in Man and Animals, Vol. 5, Mills, C. F., Bremner, I., and Chesters, J. K., Eds., Commonwealth Bureaux of Nutrition, Slough, U.K., 1985.

Trace Elements in Human and Animal Nutrition, Vol. 4, Underwood, E. J., Ed., Academic Press, New York, 1977.

Trace Elements in Human Health and Disease, Vol. 1, Prasad, A. S., Ed., Academic Press, New York, 1976.

National Research Council, Subcommittee on Zinc, *Zinc*, University Park Press, Baltimore, 1979.

Zinc and Copper in Medicine, Karcioglu, Z. A. and Sarper, R. M., Eds., Charles C Thomas, Springfield, Ill., 1980.

Zinc Deficiency in Human Subjects, Prasad, A. S., Cavdar, A. O., Brewer, G. J., and Aggett, P. J., Eds., Alan R. Liss, New York, 1983.

Zinc Metabolism: Current Aspects in Health and Disease, Prasad, A. S. and Brewer, G. J., Eds., Alan R. Liss, New York, 1977.

Index

INDEX

A

B

C

D

E

I

K

L

M

N

O

P

R

U

V

W

X

Z